MEMORY

MEMORY

The enchanted loom property in search of self

ALAIN L FYMAT

Memory
Copyright © 2023 by Alain L Fymat

The information in this book has been compiled by way of general guidance concerning the specific subjects addressed. It is not a substitute, and should not be relied on, for medical, healthcare, pharmaceutical or other professional advice on specific circumstances, and in specific locations. Please consult your General Practitioner or Physician Specialist before starting, changing, or stopping any medical treatment. So far as the author is aware, the information given is correct and current as of November 2023. Practice, laws, and regulations all change and the reader should obtain up-to-date professional advice on any such issue. As far as the laws allow, the author disclaims any liability arising directly or indirectly from the use or misuse of the information contained in this book.

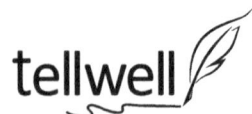

tellwell

Tellwell Talent
www.tellwell.ca

ISBN
9781-7-7941-528-8 (Hardcover)
978-1-77941-527-1 (Paperback)

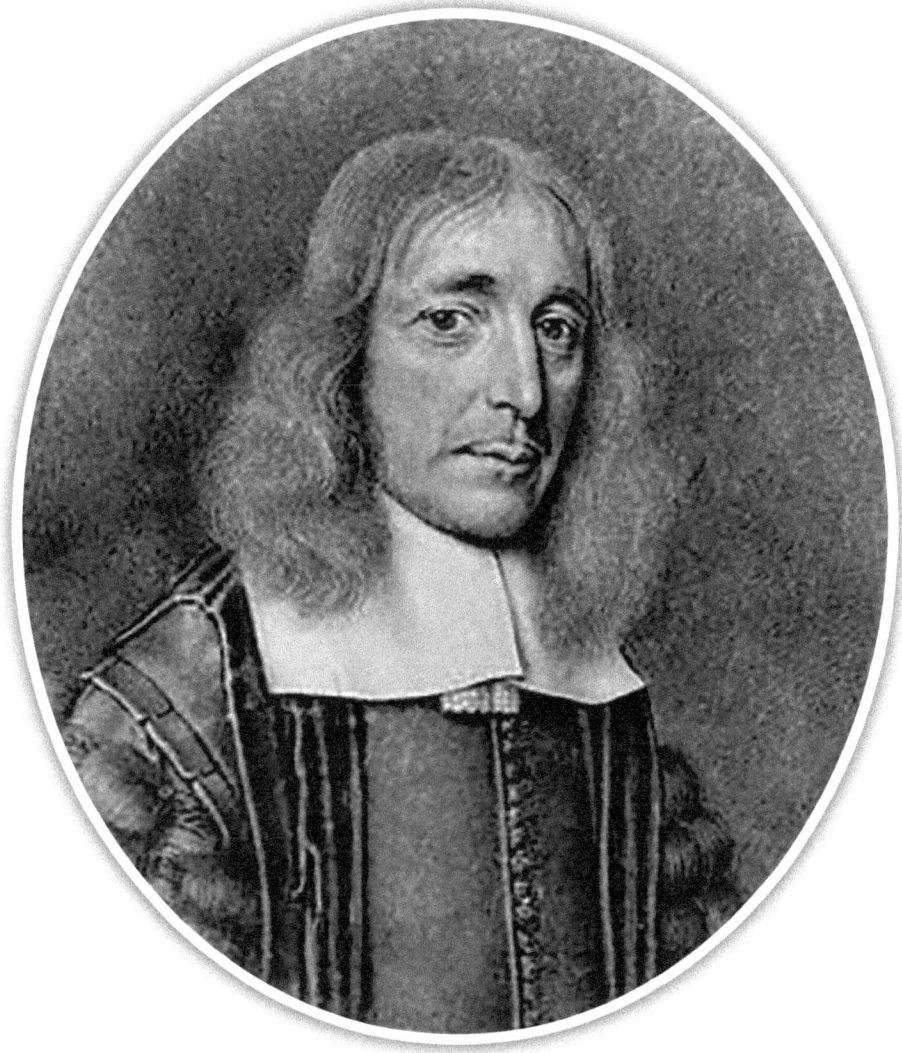

Table of Contents

Part F: Memory

Part G: Memory treatment portfolio

Part H: Hope for the future

Preface

"The ability of neurons to grow in an adult and their power to create new connections can explain learning".
(Statement by Santiago Ramón y Cajal to the
Royal Society of London, 1894)

The history of the brain (its anatomy, neurology, pathology, and physiology) and the fulcrum of memory can be dated back to humanity's early history in the 17th century BCE in ancient Egypt. Through the intervening centuries to modern days, that history continues unabated as we still do not truly comprehend the detailed subtleties of the brain's functioning in health and disease.

Memory, that wonderful but critical property of the brain, refers to the psychological processes of acquiring, retaining, storing, and later retrieving information. How memories are formed has been a perplexing puzzle for over a century, and there are still many questions that remain about the underpinning biological mechanisms. Memories are created through the connections (synapses) that exist between neurons so that strengthening them helps commit information to memory. Here, a select amount of perceived information is converted into a more permanent form, a subset of which will be secured in long-term storage, accessible for future use. It is a continually unfolding process, reflecting real-world experience with varying levels of fidelity and accuracy. The malleability of memories over time means internal and external factors can introduce errors and certain stimuli can sometimes act as powerful triggers that draw memories into conscious awareness. When memory becomes dysfunctional, problematic changes in our behavior and emotions devolve and potentially contribute to a variety of mental health disorders. The causes for memory issues and aging are still unclear. Six tentative theories have so far been advanced to explain memory loss and age-related memory loss has been associated with several possible mechanisms.

Numerous memory constructs (more than 20! of them) have been identified so far, including: Autobiographical; declarative; emotional; episodic; explicit; implicit; intrusive; kinesthetic; long term; motor; non-declarative; objective; procedural; prospective; semantic; sensory (verbal, visual-spatial or iconic, auditory or echoic, olfactory, haptic); short-term; spatial; subjective; and working memory. Nonetheless, there is not always consensus on the definition of many of them. For example, in 2010, a specialized workshop (the first in a planned series of the same) was organized by the (U.S.) National Institutes of Health merely on working memory. One of the main goals of that workshop was to arrive at an agreed-upon definition that incorporated how the field viewed it, and how it is distinguished from other similar constructs in cognition.

In addition, it also behooves us to clearly differentiate within the brain age spectrum (young to aging brain) and also within the brain health spectrum (healthy to diseased brain). Normal aging is associated with a decline in various memory abilities in many cognitive tasks. Age-related memory loss, sometimes described as "normal aging", is qualitatively different from memory loss associated with brain diseases that involve different brain mechanisms such as any one or a mixture of several dementia types (including Alzheimer's, vascular, Lewy bodies, frontotemporal, syphilitic, senilitic, etc.).

Because of the gap in understanding the biological mechanisms of memory, the lack of consensus on the multiple memory definitions and constructs advanced, and the requirements to discriminate within the brain age and health spectra, the root cause(s) of memory problems have not been identified. And, as is unfortunately the case for many medical problems, we have been content to treat symptoms. In consequence, there are no pharmacological interventions that can be taken to improve memory. No drug treatment can effectively cure memory loss. Indeed, the (U.S.) National Institute on Aging has stated that "*people should avoid any treatment that promises to restore brain function and improve memory"*. It further noted that these medications are typically unsafe and can cause negative drug interactions with other medications. However, certain medications can and do help individuals ease the symptoms and manage the condition's progression. Health experts recommend that those with memory loss follow doctor-approved prescriptions only.

In rare cases where patients may not improve using customary approaches, surgery can be an option when offered by specialized centers with experience in such procedures. Surgeries include electroconvulsive therapy, transcranial electrotherapy stimulation, continuous theta burst stimulation, repetitive transcranial magnetic stimulation, vagus nerve stimulation, magnetic seizure therapy, and deep brain stimulation. Brain stimulation is a means to potentially remediate symptoms in a range of neurological and psychiatric diseases, however, precise targeting of stimulation is necessary to ensure efficacy. Nonetheless, hope looms in the horizon, as research is making many strides along these different paths and numerous resources and support organizations exist for assisting and providing help.

Having deeply immersed myself in the subject of memory in health, aging, and disease, I hope this book will also be of interest to those other individuals and organizations who could do their part, however small, in helping get rid of this scourge that will continue to terribly afflict humanity. Otherwise, it would be a tragic dereliction of our collective duties and responsibilities to humanity as a whole. It is also hoped that patients (and other interested readers) will be empowered to get hold of, and contribute to, the better understanding of their disease and the associated treatment options available to them.

Introduction

This book is divided into seven sequentially arranged parts (Parts A through G). **Part A,** titled "**Once upon a time**", one of the three briefest of them all, spans only two chapters. **Chapter 1** is a brief chronicle of the brain from early history through the Renaissance to the modern period. The history of the brain's anatomy, neurology, pathology, and physiology, and the fulcrum of memory can be dated back to humanity's early history in the 17th century BCE in ancient Egypt. Through the intervening centuries to modern days, that history continues unabated as we still do not truly comprehend the detailed subtleties of the brain's functioning and diseases. This is chronicled in this introductory chapter that will serve for laying bare the current state of the brain's understanding and research, and particularly of memory in the aging and diseased brains. **Chapter 2** narrates the life, time, and works of Santiago Ramón y Cajal, the founder of 20th century Neuroscience.

Part B, titled "**Wonders of the healthy brain**" comprises three chapters (Chapters 3-5). **Chapter 3** discusses the wonders of the human brain beginning from the developing brain, continuing by a description of its protective barriers, and its gross anatomy including the cerebral hemispheres and the cerebral cortex (cerebrum, prefrontal cortex, cortex, brainstem, cerebellum, meninges, basal ganglia, and the limbic system). It will evidence those brain structures and corresponding control(s) or function(s) of importance in controlling or regulating memory and cognition. It will show that there is not any single brain structure that is totally responsible for these functions. It is equally important to also note that the brain does not respond linearly to any stimulus and that we still do not understand the particularities of this non-linear system, hampering us from truly fathoming the workings of the brain. From that vantage point, **Chapter 4** explores the microanatomy of the brain, including the various cell types (neurons, glial cells, mast cells), and the cerebrospinal fluid and its associated glymphatic system (the cerebral veins that drain deoxygenated blood from the brain). The brain has two main networks of veins (exterior and interior), the blood drainage consisting of two communicating surface networks and the blood-brain barrier. This barrier is lined with cells joined by tight junctions so fluids do not seep-in or leak-out to the same degree as they do in other capillaries while remaining permeable to water, carbon dioxide, oxygen, and most fat-soluble substances (including anesthetics and alcohol). A similar blood–cerebrospinal fluid barrier serves the same purpose, but facilitates the transport of different substances into the brain due to the distinct structural characteristics between the two barrier systems. **Chapter 5** devotes special attention to the several control functions exerted by the various brain structures. It encompasses the healthy brain, its autonomic functions, and its physiology. Among its several other functions, the brain is responsible for **cognition**, which functions through numerous processes and executive functions. It also plays a critical role in the body's perception of stress and its response to it. Thus, higher-order executive functions require the simultaneous use of multiple basic executive functions. Also, **working memory** manipulation involves the dorsolateral prefrontal cortex, the inferior frontal gyrus, and areas of the parietal cortex.

Part C titled "**Disorders of the neurodegenerated brain**" includes four chapters (Chapters 6-9). **Chapter 6** gives a synoptic overview of most (if not all) the brain diseases so as to position those diseases of interest to this book within their proper context. That view is multiply charted so as to present the constellation of brain diseases due to inflammation, or encephalopathy (degenerative, demyelinating, episodic/paroxysmal, cerebrospinal fluid, and other causes), or else spinal cord/myelopathy and/or degenerative encephalopathy and spinal cord/myelopathy. Such a view greatly helped to evidence the multiple possible contributors to memory impairments, which would theoretically need to be considered, as appropriate, for a correct diagnosis and treatment. The sidebar to this chapter examines the kindling observations of a growing list of pathogens (bacteria, viruses, fungi, and other microbes) found in the brains of patients with neurodegenerative diseases. For such diseases not previously thought to be infectious, finding pathogens in the brain is both surprising and concerning. **Chapters 7-9** are brief primers on Alzheimer's, dementias, and other neurodegenerative diseases. For more elaborate treatments of these diseases, I refer the reader to my books on these subjects. According to current knowledge, Alzheimer's disease (**Chapter 7**) is an age-related (not age-caused), progressive, irreversible neurological disorder in which brain cells die slowly, destroying **memory** and thinking skills, eventually even the ability to carry out the simplest tasks. In most people with this disease, symptoms first appear after age 60. The **memory loss** and the associated cognitive decline had developed over a period of years or decades. The four major hallmarks (*not* causes) of the disease are analyzed. Whereas these hallmarks are still considered the main features, many other complex brain changes are thought to play a role in Alzheimer's. Based on identified risk factors, no less that 19 theories (rather hypotheses) have been propounded for its cause(s), spanning genetics, the environment, and lifestyle. Such a wide array of hypotheses is by itself indicative of our lack of true understanding and knowledge of the disease and a sad testimonial to this shortcoming. It is my contention that Alzheimer's disease is but a runaway autoimmune disease. The chapter also discusses the diagnostic tests utilized (including the individualized gold standard), the staging scales, and the treatments to change the disease progression of cognitive symptoms (**memory** and thinking), and of non-cognitive symptoms (behavioral and psychological). **Chapter 8** is dedicated to dementia, which describes symptoms of a major neurocognitive disorder that interferes with the patient's ability to perform everyday functions and activities. The main contributors to dementia include: Alzheimer's, vascular, Lewy body, Parkinson's, frontotemporal, mixed, progressive supranuclear palsy, corticobasal degeneration, Creutzfeldt-Jakob disease, encephalopathy, immunologically-mediated, inherited, and other conditions. Other minor contributors include senilitic dementia or senility, normal pressure hydrocephalus, and syphilis. Most of these forms are covered. There is currently no cure for the disease and medical interventions remain therefore palliative with aim to alleviate pain and suffering. While much is known about dementia and the underlying and contributing factors, and much has been published on the subject, we still do not understand the deep biology of the disease. Lacking this understanding, we have so far failed to find a cure and continue to be limited to symptomatic treatments that have limited or no effect. **Chapter 9** covers other neurodegenerative diseases, which are caused by the progressive loss of structure or function of neurons, in the process known as neurodegeneration. Such neuronal damage may ultimately involve cell death. There are approximately 400 known neurological disorders, some of which having been classified as mental disorders.They include Alzheimer's disease, amyotrophic lateral sclerosis, Huntington's disease, multiple sclerosis, multiple system atrophy, Parkinson's disease, and prion diseases. Neurodegeneration can be found in the brain at many different levels of neuronal circuitry, ranging from molecular to systemic. Because there is no known way to reverse the progressive degeneration of neurons, these diseases are considered to be incurable; however, research has shown that the two major contributing factors to neurodegeneration are oxidative stress and inflammation. Biomedical research has also revealed many similarities between these diseases at the subcellular level, including atypical protein assemblies (like proteinopathy) and induced cell death. These similarities suggest that therapeutic advances against one neurodegenerative disease might ameliorate other diseases as well.

Part D titled "The aging brain" comprises only two chapters (Chapter 10 and 11). **Chapter 10** looks into the aging brain, that process of transformation of the brain in older age. It encompasses changes experienced by all healthy individuals as well as those changes caused by illnesses (including unrecognized illnesses). The aging process is associated with several structural, chemical, and functional changes in the brain as well as a host of neurocognitive changes. In addition, there are distinct changes in the expression of genes at the single neuron level. Aging entails many physical, biological, chemical, and psychological changes. The brain is no exception to this phenomenon. These various changes are briefly explored, especially in relation to **memory** and **cognition** functions. In particular, neuropsychological changes include changes in orientation, attention, **memory**, language, and behavioral flexibility. Nonetheless, while much research has focused on diseases of aging, there are few informative studies on the molecular biology of the aging brain in the absence of neurodegenerative disease and likewise for the neuropsychological profile of healthy older adults. The current state of biomedical technology does not allow to stop and reverse aging. However, one may potentially delay the effects and severity of the symptoms of aging. While there is no consensus of efficacy, several factors have been reported as delaying cognitive decline. **Chapter 11** focuses on superagers, those octogenarians and older with the memory function of people decades younger than them. They are resistant to age-related memory loss, may possibly do more physically demanding activities, exhibit no significant difference in biomarkers or genetic risk factors for neurodegenerative diseases, and exhibit similar concentrations of dementia blood biomarkers. They are cognitively healthier and resistant to age-related memory decline because they have better brain and physical health and are aging at a different rate than the rest of the population. Their greater performance relative to typical older adults might not only be a result of better memory function but could also reflect differences in motivation, executive function, and persistence in the face of difficulty, which suggests that they have a higher level of tenacity than typical older adults.

Part E titled "Memory" spans three chapters (Chapters 12 to 14). **Chapter 12** studies memory and its particulars. Memory refers to the psychological processes of acquiring, retaining, storing, and later retrieving information. There are four major processes involved: encoding, preservation, storage, and retrieval. However, this is not a flawless process. When memory becomes dysfunctional, problematic changes in our behavior and our emotions devolve and potentially contribute to a variety of mental health disorders. Memories are created through the connections (synapses) that exist between neurons. Strengthening them helps commit information to memory. This creation is a transformation process in which a select amount of perceived information is converted into a more permanent form, a subset of which will be secured in long-term storage, accessible for future use. It is a continually unfolding process, reflecting real-world experience with varying levels of fidelity and accuracy. The malleability of memories over time means internal and external factors can introduce errors. Certain stimuli can sometimes act as powerful triggers that draw memories into conscious awareness. Nonetheless, human memory remains a complex process that researchers are still trying to better understand. Memory in the aging brain is explored in **Chapter 13**. Brains do change over time, and it is helpful to be able to distinguish normal changes from those that require medical and psychological attention.

The brain remains capable of regrowth and of learning and retaining new facts and skills throughout life. Some types of memory improve or stay the same; other types decline somewhat over time. Age-related memory loss, sometimes described as "normal aging" is qualitatively different from memory loss associated with types of dementia such as Alzheimer's disease, and has a different brain mechanism. Normal aging is associated with a decline in various memory abilities in many cognitive tasks. There is a positive correlation between early life education and memory gains in older age. The causes for memory issues and aging are still unclear. Six tentative theories have so far been advanced to explain memory loss and age-related memory loss has been associated with several possible mechanisms, two of which will be reviewed. **Chapter 14** looks into memory and the diseased brain, and particularly in the cases of Alzheimer's and Lyme. With increasing lifespan in the developed world, dementia has emerged as an increasing public health concern. But dementia is not an emerging disease! To this day, the causal etiology of many types of dementia, including Alzheimer's disease, still remains unclear. Many different diseases can cause dementia, including Alzheimer's, vascular disease, Lewy bodies, frontotemporal disorders, syphilis, senility, and even stroke. However, not being a specific disease, the above potential contributors do not reach to the primary cause of the disease and there lies our greatest shortcoming. Several years ago (in 2017), I posited that the *root cause* (not a risk factor) of Alzheimer's and other neurodegenerative diseases is but a runaway autoimmune disease – an explanation that has so far remained unchallenged. While we continue to unravel the complex brain changes involved in the onset and progression of the disease, it seems likely that damage to the brain started a decade or more before **memory and other cognitive problems** appeared. These problems are abundantly illustrated here using different neuroradiological images. In addition, Lyme neuroborreliosis, a disorder of the central nervous system, also affects **memory.**

Part F titled "Memory treatment portfolio" encompasses six chapters (Chapters 15 to 20). **Chapter 15** deals with memory degradation, its prediction and prevention. Forgetfulness is common and happens to most people, including memory champions. Most episodes of forgetfulness are simply temporary and not a harbinger of Alzheimer's or other memory disorder. Such episodes are frequently linked to situational factors and normal age-related changes. It is important to distinguish between normal age-related memory changes and signs of a memory disorder. It may be noted that the vast potential of the human brain is especially clear in the domain of memory. For example, hyperthymesic people are able to remember an abnormally large number of their life experiences in vivid detail in the absence of extensive training. Likewise, people endowed with highly superior autobiographical memory are able to remember far more about one's own life than is typical. A memory champion can accomplish impressive feats of memory not because of a radical difference in cognitive functioning relative to other people, but through training and the use of techniques for enhancing memory. In **Chapter 16**, nutrition and supplementation are considered for brain health. In particular, creatine supplementation appears to moderately improve memory function in healthy adults and moderately improves mental health conditions and mild traumatic brain injury. However, the optimal dosing schedule of creatinine or/ and vitamin B12 supplementation for brain benefits remains unclear. Also, digital puzzle strategic gaming seems to improve working memory more for older adults than for younger adults who play action games. Unfortunately, there are presently no disease-modifying medications for memory loss. Cholinesterase inhibitors and N-Methyl-D-aspartic Acid (NMDA) glutamate regulators can only stop memory loss symptoms for a short time. They can help manage a person's memory loss symptoms and modify the progression of their condition. However, they cannot stop or reverse that progression. **Chapter 17** reviews the available pharmacotherapy for brain diseases, outlining the various medications for memory loss, their indications, and potential side effects as well as their management. Medications can help manage a person's memory loss symptoms and eventually modify the progression of their condition. However, they cannot stop or reverse the progression of the condition. Without medication, symptoms of memory loss can become severe. For the treatment of Alzheimer's disease, five drugs are currently FDA-approved: Donepezil, Galantamine, Rivastigmine, Tacrine and, as of July 2023, Leqembi. Nonetheless, while helping ease symptoms and manage the condition's progression, medications are typically unsafe and can cause negative drug interactions with other medications. Additionally, the safety profile and efficacy of many medications in people with dementia are undetermined due to their active exclusion from 85% of published clinical trials. Medication management is complicated for people with dementia so that careful consideration should be given to the initiation and continuation of all medications. It is a complex task as it is unclear what constitutes optimal medication management for them due to the shifting focus of health priorities and the balance between the benefits and harms of medications. In rare cases where patients may not improve using standard approaches, surgery can be an option. These other approaches are reviewed in **Chapter 18,** including electroconvulsive therapy, transcranial electrotherapy stimulation, continuous theta burst stimulation, repetitive transcranial magnetic stimulation, vagus nerve stimulation, magnetic seizure therapy, and deep brain stimulation. The chapter discusses the principles and applications of these several procedures, which still need to be further investigated and used only at centers with expertise in them. Brain stimulation therapies treat serious mental illnesses and can play an important role in treating mental disorders. Of the above therapies, the authorized ones include: Electroconvulsive therapy, repetitive transcranial magnetic stimulation, and vagus nerve stimulation whereas the experimental therapies include: magnetic seizure therapy and deep brain stimulation. Other brain stimulation therapies may also hold promise for treating mental disorders, including: Transcranial alternating current stimulation, transcranial direct current stimulation, transcranial random noise stimulation, and transcranial ultrasound stimulation. Surgical procedures need to be further investigated and used only at expert centers. **Chapter 19** is a detailed presentation of clinical trials. These are prospective biomedical or biobehavioral research studies on human participants designed to answer specific questions about biomedical or biobehavioral interventions, including new treatments (such as novel vaccines, drugs, dietary choices, dietary supplements, and medical devices) and known interventions that warrant further study and comparison. Their overriding goal is to determine if a new test or treatment works and is safe. People with memory problems and others may be able to take part in them. The particulars of the several trial categories are provided, including: Memory functions and physiological processes; memory processes; memory lapse /consolidation /reactivation; memory delays, deficits, impairments, and disorders; memory and mental health; various types of memory (autobiographical, declarative, emotional, episodic, intrusive, motor, prospective, spatial, subjective, verbal and visual, working); memory aids and tools; and the virtual reality helmet. **Chapter**

20 takes a cursory look at complementary and alternative treatments, including manipulating memories to discover novel methods to treat post-traumatic stress disorder, depression, and Alzheimer's; increasing working memory by playing strategic digital games; resorting to alternative therapies (aromatherapy and massage, cannabinoids, omega-3 fatty acid supplements, and dental hygiene); various sleep medications; and lifestyle changes (cognitive behavioral therapy, herbal remedies, relaxation techniques, engaging in healthy sleep habits, and increased exercise).

Lastly, **Part G** titled "Hope for the future" comprises four chapters (Chapters 21 through 24). **Chapter 21** answers most of the frequently asked questions which, for convenience, have been grouped under the following categories concerning: Mild forgetfulness, serious memory problems, emotional problems, mild cognitive impairment, dementia, Alzheimer's disease, vascular dementia, Lewy body dementia, mixed dementia, sleep-related myths, medication approval, clinical trials and research studies, and help from family members. **Chapter 22** lists the available federal resources along with their particulars, including several (U.S.) institutions and private organizations. It also provides information concerning agnosia, palliative care, and caregiving. **Chapter 23** covers the results of current research and latest developments from the (U.S.) National Institutes of Health (NIH), National Institute of Mental Health (NIMH), National Institute on Aging (NIA), National Library of Medicine (NLM), and the Alzheimer's Association (AA). The concluding **Chapter 24** sets forth my conclusions including the presentation of a roadmap for tackling, diagnosing, and treating the memory issues presented by a patient. The medical professional would begin by understanding the memory issues presented, identifying the memory types involved, conducting a differential diagnosis to eliminate as many confounding diseases as possible, determining the applicable causal theory(ies), and prescribing the appropriate medication(s), as applicable. It also provide a brief incursion into the domain of artificial intelligence (AI) and how the rain's memory replay mechanism could, in turn, enhance AI capabilities.

-o-o-o-

For the reader's convenience, each Chapter ends with a take-away points section to summarize what we have learned from it. Additionally, one or more Sidebars are provided at the end of Chapters 1, 3, 4, 6, 10, 12, 13, 16, 17, 18, and 19 for those readers interested in the more specialized aspects they discuss.

PART A
ONCE UPON A TIME

1

A brief chronicle of the brain

Contents

1

A brief chronicle of the brain

The history of the brain's anatomy, neurology, pathology, and physiology, and the fulcrum of memory can be dated back to humanity's early history in the 17th century BCE in ancient Egypt. It begun with the discovery of the Edwin Smith papyrus, the oldest known treatise on surgery and trauma. Through the intervening centuries to modern days, that history continues unabated as we still do not truly comprehend the detailed subtleties of the brain's functioning and diseases, as epitomized by the continued lack of cures for neurodegenerative and other brain diseases. This is chronicled in this introductory chapter that will serve for laying bare the current state of the brain's understanding and research, and particularly of memory in the aging and diseased brains.

Early history

In the 17th century BCE: The **Edwin Smith Papyrus,** named after Edwin Smith who bought it in 1862, is an ancient Egyptian medical treatise, which was written in the 17th century BCE. It is the oldest known treatise on surgery and trauma. It may have been known to ancient surgeons as the *Secret Book of the Physician*. It may also have been a manual of military surgery, describing 48 cases of injuries, fractures, wounds, dislocations, and tumors. It dates to Dynasties 16–17 of the Second Intermediate Period in ancient Egypt (circa 1600 BCE). The papyrus is unique among the four principal medical papyri in existence that survive today. While other papyri, such as the Ebers Papyrus and the London Medical Papyrus are medical texts based in magic, the Edwin Smith Papyrus presents a rational and scientific approach to medicine in ancient Egypt in which medicine and magic do not conflict. It contains the earliest recorded reference to the brain. The hieroglyph for brain occurs no less than eight times in this papyrus, describing the symptoms, diagnosis, and prognosis of two traumatic injuries to the head. It also mentions the external surface of the brain, the effects of injury (including seizures and aphasia), the meninges, and the cerebrospinal fluid (CSF). (Figure 1.1.) The recto columns 6 (right) and 7 (left) of the papyrus, pictured in Figure 1.2, discuss facial trauma (Cases 12-20). Sidebar 1.1 will present other hieroglyphs and various ancient scripts.

In the 5ᵗʰ century BCE: Alcmaeon of Croton, an early Greek medical writer and philosopher- scientist whose work in biology has been praised as remarkable and of pioneering originality. He has been described as one of the most eminent natural philosophers and medical theorists of Antiquity and also been referred to as "*a thinker of considerable originality and one of the greatest philosophers, naturalists, and neuroscientists of all time*". He first considered the brain to be the seat of the mind. Also in Athens, the unknown author of the medical treatise *On the Sacred Disease*, a part of the *Hippocratic Corpus* traditionally attributed to Hippocrates, also believed the brain to be the seat of intelligence.

Figure 1.1 – Egyptian hieroglyph for the word 'brain' (circa 1700 BCE)

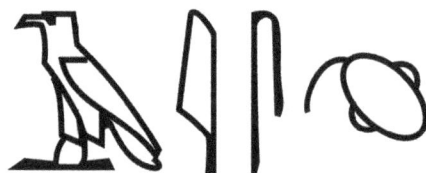

Source: Riccardo Metere

In the 5ᵗʰ to 4ᵗʰ century BCE: Hippocrates of Kos (also known as **Hippocrates II**) was a Greek physician of the classical period who is considered one of the most outstanding figures in the history of medicine.

He is traditionally referred to as the "Father of Medicine" in recognition of his lasting contributions to the field, such as the use of prognosis and clinical observation, the systematic categorization of diseases, and the formulation of humoral theory. The Hippocratic school of medicine revolutionized ancient Greek medicine, establishing it as a discipline distinct from other fields with which it had traditionally been associated (theurgy and philosophy), thus establishing medicine as a profession. However, the achievements of the writers of the *Hippocratic Corpus*, the practitioners of Hippocratic medicine, and the actions of Hippocrates himself were often conflated so that very little is known about what Hippocrates actually thought, wrote, and did. Hippocrates is commonly portrayed as the paragon of the ancient physician and credited with coining the *Hippocratic Oath*, which is still relevant and in use today. He is also credited with greatly advancing the systematic study of clinical medicine, summing up the medical knowledge of previous schools, and prescribing practices for physicians through the Hippocratic Corpus and other works.

Figure 1.2 - Plates vi & vii of the Edwin Smith Papyrus

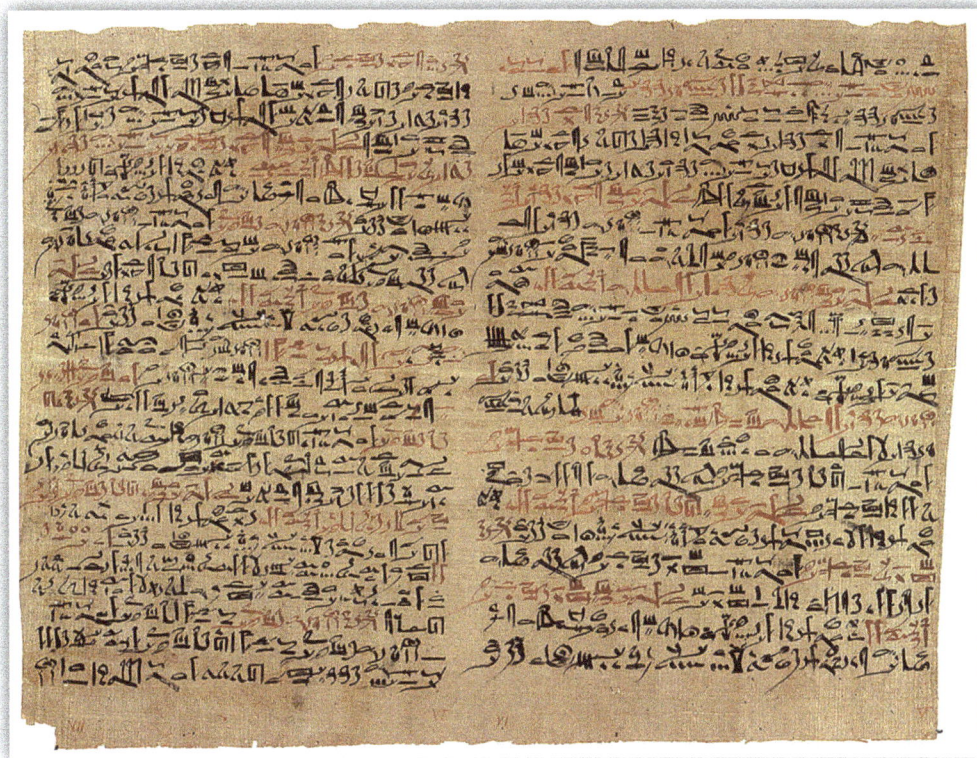

Reference: Rare Book Room, New York Academy of Medicine

In the 4ᵗʰ century BCE: Aristotle, the Ancient Greek philosopher and polymath, covered in his writings a broad range of subjects spanning the natural sciences, philosophy, linguistics, economics, politics, psychology, and the arts. He set the ground work for the development of modern science. In his biology, he initially believed the heart to be the seat of intelligence, seeing the brain as a cooling mechanism for the blood. He reasoned that humans are more rational than the beasts because, among other reasons, they have a larger brain to cool their hot-bloodedness. Aristotle did also describe the meninges and distinguished between the cerebrum and cerebellum.

In the 4ᵗʰ to 3ʳᵈ century BCE: Herophilus of Chalcedon (335-280 BCE) was a Greek physician and anatomist who performed human dissections at the world-renowned Museum of Alexandria. He gained fame as a physician and medical instructor and, because of his careful human dissections, he has been called the "Father of Anatomy." Frequently quoted by the medical colossus **Galen,** his careful and detailed works on the brain, eyes, nerves, liver, and arteries greatly advanced the understanding of both human anatomy and physiology. He distinguished the cerebrum and the cerebellum, and provided the first clear description of the ventricles. With **Erasistratus of Ceos**, he also experimented on living brains. Their works are now mostly lost, and we know about their achievements mostly from secondary sources. Some of their discoveries had to be re-discovered a millennium after their deaths.

In the 3ʳᵈ to 2ⁿᵈ century BCE: The Greek-controlled city of Alexandria, Egypt, was fast becoming a growing center of scholarly activities when **Herophilus** established himself there at the invitation of King Ptolemy (323-285 BCE), and he became the leading physician and anatomist at the Museum of Alexandria. He is believed to have produced at least nine written works that are known to have influenced his contemporaries and future generations of physicians, including the most influential of all physicians, **Galen**, whose writings dominated human medicine for centuries after his death. Unfortunately, none of the works of Herophilus survived directly, and we are left with only the frequent quotes of his writings made by others, especially Galen, **Dioscorides** (c.40-90 AD), **Pliny** (AD 23-79), and **Plutarch** (c. AD 46-after 119). Herophilus worked in Alexandria during a single brief period that saw the ruling Greeks relax their long-held prohibition on human dissections. This allowed Herophilus to study human internal anatomy in considerable detail, and he was able to advance overall knowledge of human anatomical design and function tremendously. Herophilus was a follower of the Hippocratic doctrine of medicine, which saw health and disease as a balance or imbalance of the four humors of the body. He believed that proper diet and exercise were the necessary ingredients to good health. Herophilus sought to advance understanding of the system of arteries and veins that had been described by **Praxagoraswas** (fl. 4th century BCE). He concentrated on the structures and functions of the three important organs that were subject to generations of great debate: the liver, the heart, and the brain.

In the 2nd century AD: Aelius Galenus (or **Claudius Galenus,** often Anglicized as **Galen** or **Galen of Pergamon (216 – 129 BCE)** was a Roman-Greek physician, surgeon, and philosopher during the time of the Roman Empire. Considered to be one of the most accomplished of all medical researchers of Antiquity, he influenced the development of various scientific disciplines, including anatomy, physiology, pathology, pharmacology, and neurology, as well as philosophy and logic. Galen's understanding of anatomy and medicine was principally influenced by the then-current theory of the four humors: black bile, yellow bile, blood, and phlegm, as first advanced by the author of *On the Nature of Man* in the *Hippocratic corpus*. His views dominated and influenced Western medical science for more than 1,300 years. His anatomical reports were based mainly on the dissection of Barbary apes. However, when he discovered that their facial expressions were too much like those of humans, he switched to other animals, such as sheep, dogs, and pigs. His anatomical reports remained uncontested until 1543, when printed descriptions and illustrations of human dissections were published in the seminal work *De humani corporis fabrica* by **Andreas Vesalius**, where Galen's physiological theory was accommodated to these new observations. Galen's theory of the physiology of the circulatory system remained unchallenged until c. 1242. He further theorized that the brain functioned by movement of animal spirits through the ventricles.

In 1316: Mondino de Luzzi (or **de Liuzzi** or **de Lucci,** also known as **Mundinus) (c. 1270 – 1326),** was an Italian physician, anatomist, and professor of surgery who lived and worked in Bologna. He is often credited as the restorer of anatomy because he made seminal contributions to the field by reintroducing the practice of public dissection of human cadavers and writing the first modern anatomical text. His *Anathomia* began the modern study of brain anatomy.

In 1536: Niccolò Massa (1485–1569) was an Italian anatomist. He was the author of several works beginning with a 1524 book *Liber morbo gallico* (the French disease), which is commonly equated to modern-day syphilis. This was followed by a book on anatomy, *Anatomiae Libri Introductorius*, a book on fevers, the *Liber de febre pestilentiali*, the work *La loica divisa in sette libri,* and a collection of his letters, *Epistolae medicinales.* He wrote two more books, *Raggionamento... sopra le infermitia che vengono dall'aere pestilentiale del presente anno MDL* and *Diligens examen de venaesectione in febribus ex humorum putredine ortis.* Massa was a regular dissector of bodies and performed dissections both to study anatomy and understand the causes of diseases like syphilis. He described the cerebrospinal fluid and discovered that the ventricles were filled with fluid.

In the early-to-mid 16th century: Matteo Realdo Colombo (or **Realdus Columbus**) was an italian apothecary, anatomist, and surgeon. He put an emphasis on vivisection (the practice of experimentation or scientific research on live animals) in order to learn about the different bodily functions of the human body. According to his book *De Re Anatomica Libri XV,* he put energy into dissecting, in particular the cadavers of men. He anatomized the live, active body whereas his contemporaries had anatomized the dead body. His concentration on vivisection revived the practice of ancient Alexandrian anatomists using live instead of dead animals, which led him to adopting this new way of conceptualizing the body. The vivisection method enabled Colombo to study the operation of the voice, the motions of the lungs, the heart, and the arteries; the dilation and contraction of the brain; and variations of the pulse and other functions. With the centrality of vivisection, the three 'rivers' was also emphasized in Colombo's book, specifically Book XI. "*There are three fountain-heads, the liver, heart, and brain, from which are distributed throughout the body the three rivers of the natural blood, the vital blood, and the animal spirits, respectively*". The view of the three rivers does not come from any known ancient source. Although there were many important organs like the liver in the abdomen area and the heart, for Columbo, the supreme organ was the brain.

Colombo described the organs in the form of hierarchy and because the brain was said to be the most noble of organs, it was the 'King of the principal members' of the body. The supremacy of the brain was directly related to his view of the three rivers. "*What is generated in the brain and distributed through the nerves, is what differentiates the live body from the dead one*". Among other reasons, the most important one for the brain being King of all organs, is the fact that the brain is the source of sense and motion.

Figure 1.3 - Drawing of the base of the brain

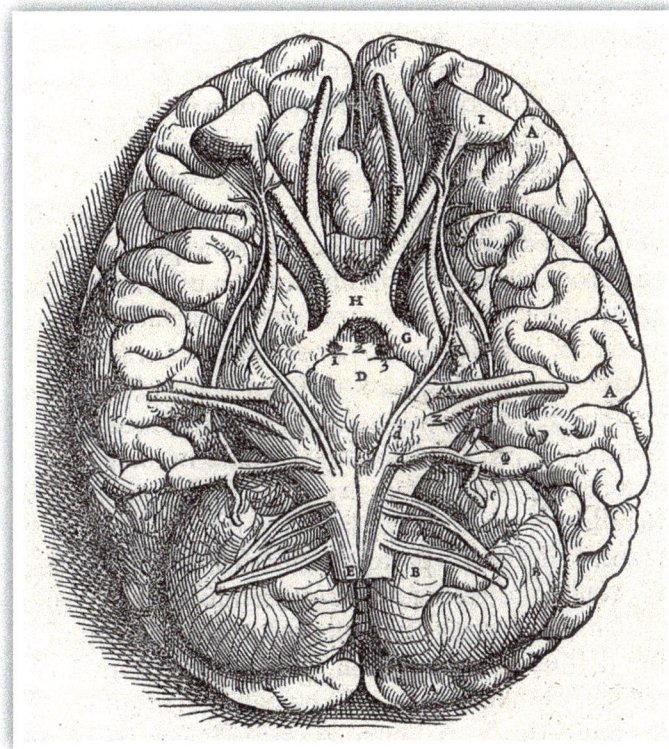

Reference: Andreas Vesalius's 1543 work *De humani corporis fabrica*

In 1543: Andries van Wezel (latinized as **Andreas Vesalius**) **(1514 – 1564)**, a Belgian/Dutch anatomist and physician, was often referred to as the founder of modern human anatomy. He wrote *De Humani Corporis Fabrica Libri Septem* (On the fabric of the human body) in seven books, which were considered to be the most influential books on human anatomy and a major advance over the long-dominant work of Galen. The seventh book, in particular, covered the brain and the eyes, with detailed images of the ventricles, cranial nerves, pituitary gland, meninges, structures of the eye, the vascular supply to the brain and spinal cord, and an image of the peripheral nerves. He rejected the common belief that the ventricles were responsible for brain function, arguing that many animals have a similar ventricular system to humans, but no true intelligence (Figure 1.3, 4).

Figure 1.4 – One of Leonardo da Vinci's (1452 – 1519) sketches of the human skull

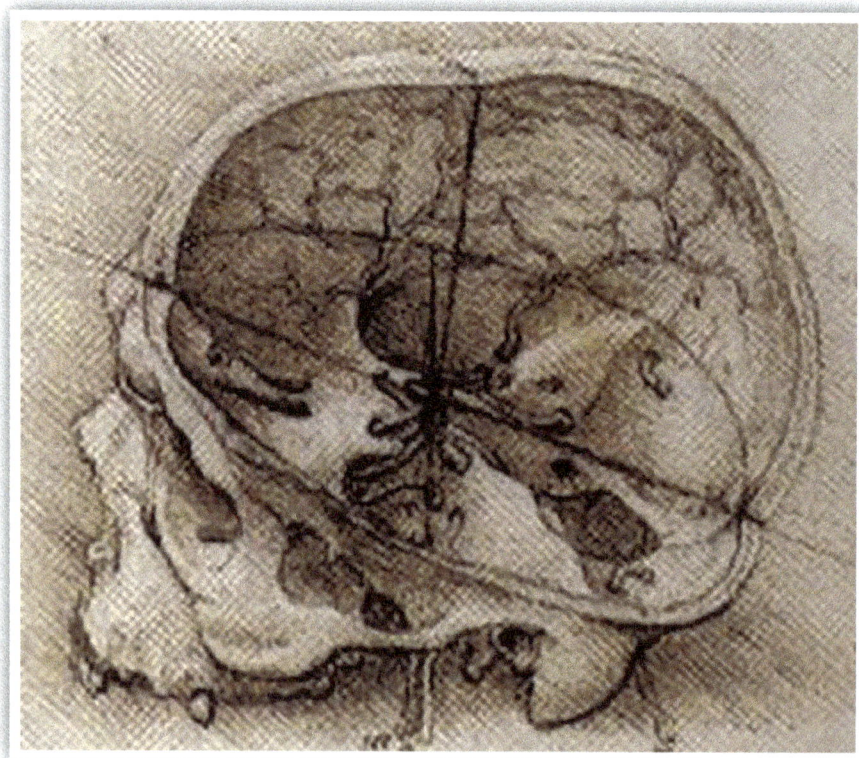

In the early-to-mid 16th century: Jacques Dubois (Latinized as **Jacobus Sylvius**) **(1478 - 1555)** was a French anatomist who first described venous valves, although their function was later discovered by **William Harvey**. He made a valuable service by giving a name to the muscles, which, until then, had simply been referred to by numbers. These numbers were arbitrarily assigned by different authors. He was the first anatomist to publish descriptions of satisfactory pterygoid process, the sphenoid bone, and the clinoid bone tear. He gave a good description of the sphenoid sinus in an adult, but denied its existence in children. He also wrote about the vertebrae, but described incorrectly the sternum. Although the cerebral aqueduct (Aqueduct of Sylvius) and Sylvian (lateral) sulcus of the brain have been said to be his contributions to anatomy, the aqueduct was described by Galen nearly 1300 years before, *albeit* the name aqueduct in this context was first mentioned by another Sylvius (**Franciscus Sylvius**, 1614–1672), who apparently also described the sulcus which bears his name.

In 1553: Miguel de Villanueva (or **Michael Servetus**, or **Miguel Servet**, or **Miguel Revés**, or else **Michel de Villeneuve**) **(1509 or 1511 - 1553)** was a Spanish theologian, physician, cartographer, and Renaissance humanist. He was the first European to correctly describe the function of pulmonary circulation, as discussed in *Christianismi Restitutio (1553)*. He was also a polymath versed in many sciences: mathematics, astronomy and meteorology, geography, human anatomy, medicine and pharmacology, as well as jurisprudence, translation, poetry, and the scholarly study of the Bible in its original languages. He is renowned in the history of several of these fields, particularly medicine. His work on the circulation of blood and his observations on pulmonary circulation were particularly important.

In 1556: Archangelo Piccolomini (or Arcangelo Piccolomini) (1525–1586) was an Italian anatomist and personal physician to a number of popes. He compiled a broad commentary on the treatise of Galen *De Humoribus* in 1556. He became the personal physician to several succeeding popes, Paul IV, Pius IV, and Gregory XIII. In 1586 he published the anatomical treatise *Anatomicae praelectiones explicantes mirificam corporis humani fabricam.* He was the first to describe and differentiate the white matter of the cerebrum from the grey matter of the cortex. His observations led to the anatomical study of the cortex by **Marcello Malphigi** and **Antonie van Leeuwenhoek.**

In the early-to-mid 17th century: William Harvey (1578 – 1657), an English physician, made influential contributions in anatomy and physiology. He was the first known physician to describe completely, and in detail, the systemic circulation and properties of blood being pumped to the brain and the rest of the body by the heart, though earlier writers, such as Realdo Colombo, Michael Servetus, and Jacques Dubois, had provided precursors of the theory.

In 1658: Jan (or **Johannes**) **Swammerdam (1637 - 1680)** was a Dutch biologist and microscopist whose work on insects demonstrated that the various phases during the life of an insect—egg, larva, pupa, and adult—are different forms of the same animal. As part of his anatomical research, he carried out experiments on muscle contraction. In 1658, he was the first to observe and describe red blood cells under a microscope. He was also one of the first people to use the microscope in dissections, and his techniques remained useful for hundreds of years.

In 1664: René Descartes (latinized **Renatus Cartesius**) **(1596 – 1650)** was a French philosopher, scientist, and mathematician, widely considered a seminal figure in the emergence of modern philosophy and science. Many elements of his philosophy have precedents in late Aristotelianism, the revived Stoicism of the 16th century, or in earlier philosophers like **Augustine**. In his natural philosophy explaining natural phenomena, he differed from the schools on two major points, rejecting the splitting of corporeal substance into matter and form and also rejecting any appeal to final ends, divine or natural. He wrote *Passions of the Soul*, an early modern treatise on emotions. Descartes has often been called the father of modern philosophy, and is largely seen as responsible for the increased attention given to epistemology in the 17th century. He proposed the theory of dualism to tackle the issue of the brain's relation to the mind. He suggested that the pineal gland was where the mind interacted with the body, serving as the seat of the soul and as the connection through which animal spirits passed from the blood into the brain. This dualism likely provided impetus for later anatomists to further explore the relationship between the anatomical and functional aspects of brain anatomy.

1664-7: Considered a second pioneer in the study of neurology and brain science, the Englishman **Thomas Willis** wrote *Cerebri Anatome* (Latin: Anatomy of the brain) in 1664, followed by *Pathologicae cerebri* (Cerebral pathology) in 1667, itself followed by *Nervosi generis specimen* (Generic nervous specimen). In these, he described the structure of the cerebellum, the ventricles, the cerebral hemispheres, the brainstem, and the cranial nerves. He proposed functions associated with different areas of the brain. The 'circle of Willis 'was named after his investigations into the blood supply of the brain. He was the first to use the word "neurology". Willis removed the brain from the body when examining it, and rejected the commonly held view that the cortex only consisted of blood vessels, and the view of the last millennium that the cortex was only incidentally important.

In 1666: Marcello Malpighi (1628 – 1694), an Italian biologist and physician, was referred to as the "Founder of microscopical anatomy and histology" and "Father of physiology and embryology". His name is borne by several physiological features related to the biological excretory system, such as the 'Malpighian corpuscles', the 'Malpighian pyramids' of the kidneys and the 'Malpighian tubule system' of insects. The splenic lymphoid nodules are often called the 'Malpighian bodies of the spleen' or 'Malpighian corpuscles'.The botanical family *Malpighiaceae* is also named after him. He was the first person to see capillaries in animals. Further, he discovered the link between arteries and veins that had eluded William Harvey. Malpighi was one of the earliest people to observe red blood cells under a microscope, after **Jan Swammerdam**. His treatise *De polypo cordis* (1666) was important for understanding blood composition, as well as how blood clots form. In it, he described how the form of a blood clot differed in the right against the left sides of the heart. Malpighi also studied the anatomy of the brain and concluded this organ is a gland. In terms of modern endocrinology, a correct deduction because the hypothalamus of the brain has long been recognized for its hormone- secreting capacity.

In the 1670's: Antonie Philips van Leeuwenhoek (1632 – 1723), a Dutch pioneer of microscopy and microbiology, helped establish microbiology as a scientific discipline. As one of the first microscopists and microbiologists, he is commonly known as "the Father of Microbiology". In the 1670s, he started to explore microbial life with his microscope. Using single-lensed microscopes of his own design and make, van Leeuwenhoek was the first to observe and experiment with microbes, which he originally referred to as dierkens, diertgens or diertjes.

(Dutch for "small animals" [translated into English as 'animalcules', from Latin *animalculum* "tiny animal"]). He was the first to relatively determine their size. Most of the "animalcules" are now referred to as unicellular organisms, although he observed multicellular organisms in pond water. He was also the first to document microscopic observations of muscle fibers, bacteria, spermatozoa, red blood cells, and crystals in gouty tophi. In addition, van Leeuwenhoek was among the first to see blood flow in capillaries.

In the early 19th century: Johannes Peter Müller (1801 – 1858), a German physiologist, comparative anatomist, ichthyologist, and herpetologist, was known not only for his discoveries but also for his ability to synthesize knowledge. The paramesonephric duct ('Müllerian duct') was named in his honor. His view that the nerve impulse was a vital function that could not be measured was later discarded when his students **Emil Heinrich du Bois-Reymond** and **Hermann von Helmholtz** demonstrated the contrary (see below).

In the 1820s: Marie Jean-Pierre Flourens (1794 – 1867), a French physiologist, was the founder of experimental brain science and a pioneer in anesthesia. He pioneered the experimental method of damaging specific parts of animal brains describing the effects on movement and behavior.

In the mid-19th century: Emil Heinrich du Bois-Reymond (1818 – 1896), a German physiologist, co-discovered with Hermann von Helmholtz the nerve action potential and developed experimental electrophysiology.

In the 1860s: Pierre Paul Broca (1824 – 1880) was a French physician, anatomist, and anthropologist. He is best known for his research on regions of the brain associated with specific functions, in particular language, following work on brain-damaged patients. 'Broca's area' is a region of the frontal lobe that is named after him. It is involved with language. His work revealed that the brains of patients with aphasia contained lesions in a particular part of the cortex, in the left frontal region. This was the first anatomical proof of localization of brain function. Broca's work also contributed to the development of physical anthropology, advancing the science of anthropometry and craniometry, in particular, the now-discredited practice of determining intelligence.

In the mid-19ᵗʰ century: John Hughlings Jackson (1835 – 1911), an English neurologist bestknown for his research on epilepsy, described the function of the motor cortex by watching the progression of epileptic seizures through the body. Together with his friends **Sir David Ferrier** and **Sir James Crichton-Browne**, two eminent neuropsychiatrists of his time, Jackson was one of the founders of the important journal *Brain* (still being published today), which was dedicated to the interaction between experimental and clinical neurology. Its inaugural issue was published in 1878. In 1892, Jackson was one of the founding members of the National Society for the Employment of Epileptics (now the National Society for Epilepsy), along with **Sir William Gowers** and **Sir David Ferrier**.

In 1875: Richard Caton (1842 – 1926) was a British physician and physiologist who was crucial in discovering the electrical nature of the brain by demonstrating electrical impulses in the cerebral hemispheres of rabbits and monkeys. He laid the groundwork for **Hans Berger** to discover alpha-wave activity in the human brain.

In 1880: Sir David Ferrier (1843 - 1928) was a pioneering Scottish neurologist and psychologist. He conducted experiments on the brains of animals such as monkeys. In 1881, he became the first scientist to be prosecuted under the 1876 Cruelty to Animals Act, which had been enacted following a major public debate over vivisection.

In 1886: Sir William Richard Gowers (1845 – 1915), a British neurologist, was described by **Macdonald Critchley** in 1949 as "probably the greatest clinical neurologist of all time". He published extensively, but is probably best remembered for his two-volume *Manual of Diseases of the Nervous System* (1886, 1888), affectionately referred to at Queen Square as the Bible of Neurology.

In the mid- to late 19th century: Hermann Ludwig Ferdinand von Helmholtz (1821 - 1894), a German physician, physicist, and philosopher made significant contributions in several scientific fields, particularly hydrodynamic stability. In the fields of physiology and psychology, he is known for his mathematics concerning the eye, theories of vision, ideas on the visual perception of space, color vision research, the sensation of tone, perceptions of sound, and empiricism in the physiology of perception. In physics, he is known for his theories on the conservation of energy and on the electrical double layer, work in electrodynamics, chemical thermodynamics, and on a mechanical foundation of thermodynamics. As a philosopher, he is known for his philosophy of science, ideas on the relation between the laws of perception and the laws of nature, the science of esthetics, and ideas on the civilizing power of science. He used a galvanometer to show that electrical impulses passed at measurable speeds along nerves, refuting the view of his teacher **Johannes Peter Müller** that the nerve impulse was a vital function that could not be measured.

In 1873: Camillo Golgi (1843 - 1926) was an Italian biologist and pathologist known for his works on the central nervous system. His discovery of a staining technique called *black reaction* (sometimes called 'Golgi's method' or 'Golgi's staining' in his honor) in 1873 was a major breakthrough in neuroscience. Several structures and phenomena in anatomy and physiology are named for him, including the 'Golgi apparatus', the 'Golgi tendon organ' and the 'Golgi tendon reflex'. He and the Spanish biologist **Santiago Ramón y Cajal** were jointly given the 1906 Nobel Prize in Physiology or Medicine "in recognition of their work on the structure of the nervous system".

In the 1880s: Studies of the brain became more sophisticated with the use of the microscope and the development of the silver staining method of Camillo Golgi. This research showed the intricate structures of single neurons. This was used by Santiago Ramón y Cajal, leading to the formation of the "neuron doctrine", the then revolutionary hypothesis that the neuron is the functional unit of the brain. Cajal used microscopy to uncover many cell types, and proposed functions for the cells he saw. For this, Golgi and Cajal are considered the founders of twentieth century neuroscience.

Modern period

In the late 19ᵗʰ century – beginning 20ᵗʰ century: Carl (or **Karl**) **Wernicke (1848 – 1905),** a German physician, anatomist, psychiatrist and neuropathologist, is known for his influential research into the pathological effects of specific forms of encephalopathy and also the study of receptive aphasia. Both of these conditions are commonly associated with Wernicke's name and referred to as 'Wernicke encephalopathy' and 'Wernicke's aphasia', respectively. He described a region associated with language comprehension, and production. His research, along with that of Paul Broca, led to groundbreaking realizations of the localization of brain function, specifically in speech. As such, Wernicke's area (a.k.a. 'Wernicke's speech area') has been named after him.

In the late 19ᵗʰ to the beginning of the 20ᵗʰ century: Korbinian Brodmann (1868 - 1918) was a German neuropsychiatrist known for mapping the cerebral cortex and defining 52 distinct cortical regions grouped into 11 histological areas. Based on their cytoarchitectonic (histological) characteristics, they are known as 'Brodmann's areas'. His work to characterize the brain cytoarchitecture was strongly influenced by **Oskar Vogt**, who postulated over 200 distinct areas in the brain. He used a variety of criteria to map the human brain, including attention to both gross anatomical features and cortical micro-structures. He postulated that areas with different structures performed different functions and some were later associated to nervous functions, such as the following:

- Areas 41 and 42 in the temporal lobe, related to hearing;
- Areas 45 and 44 overlap with the Broca's area for language in humans;
- Areas 1, 2, and 3 in the post-central gyrus of the parietal lobe (the somatosensory region);

- Area 4 in the pre-central gyrus of the frontal lobe (the primary motor area); and
- Areas 17 and 18 in the occipital lobe (the primary visual areas).

In modern science, the regions that were identified by Brodmann are frequently referred to by their function, rather than by the number Brodmann assigned to them. However, in some situations, the use of Brodmann numbers persists.

In 1906: Sir Charles Scott Sherrington (1857 – 1952) was an eminent English neurophysiologist. His experimental research established many aspects of contemporary neuroscience, including the concept of the spinal reflex as a system involving connected neurons (the "neuron doctrine"), and the ways in which signal transmission between neurons can be potentiated or depotentiated. Sherrington himself coined the word "synapse" to define the connection between two neurons. He also examined the function of reflexes, the evolutionary development of the nervous system, the functional specialization of the brain, and the layout and cellular function of the central nervous system. He published his influential *The Integrative Action of the Nervous System,* a synthesis of this work, in recognition of which he was awarded the 1932 Nobel Prize in Physiology or Medicine (along with **Edgar Adrian**). In addition to his work in physiology, Sherrington did research in histology, bacteriology, and pathology.

In the early 20th century: Harvey Cushing (1869–1939) is recognized as the first proficient brain surgeon in the world.

In the early-to-mid 20th century: Santiago Ramón y Cajal (1852 – 1934) was a Spanish neuroscientist, pathologist, and histologist specializing in neuroanatomy and the central nervous system. He and Camillo Golgi jointly received the 1906 Nobel Prize in Physiology or Medicine. His original investigations of the microscopic structure of the brain made him a pioneer of modern neuroscience. Since the mid-20th century, hundreds of his drawings illustrating the arborizations ("tree growing") of brain cells are still in use for educational and training purposes.

In the 1930s: John Farquhar Fulton (1899 - 1960) was an American neurophysiologist and historian of science. His main contributions were in primate neurophysiology and the history of science. He created the first primate research laboratory in the United States. Through the 1930s, he and other scientists did comparative studies on functional localization in the cerebral cortex. They found that lesioning the prefrontal cortex created calming effects in the monkeys. Fulton proposed, but did not implement, the idea of using this technique on humans to relieve mental diseases. His team's findings influenced Portuguese neurologist **Egas Moniz,** who developed the medical practice of the frontal lobotomy in humans, which won him the 1949 Nobel Prize for his work. In 1928, he founded the *Journal of Neurophysiology* and published the first comprehensive textbook on the physiology of the nervous system.

In 1936: Margaret Alice Kennard (1899 – 1975) was a neurologist who principally studied the effects of neurological damage on primates during the 1930-40s. The capacity of the brain to re- organize and change with age, and a recognized critical development period, were attributed to neuroplasticity, which she pioneered. She worked closely with **John Fulton** in her famous infant brain studies. Her work led to the creation of the 'Kennard Principle', which posits a negative linear relationship between age of a brain lesion and the outcome expectancy. In other words, the earlier in life a brain lesion occurs, the more likely it is for some compensation mechanism to reverse at least some of the lesion's bad effects; in other words, how well a brain can reorganize itself after damage is a function of the developmental stage. This research led to one of the earliest experimental evidence for age effects on neuroplasticity.

In 1937: James Wenceslas Papez (1883–1958) was an American neuroanatomist, most famous for his 1937 description of the 'Papez circuit', a neural pathway in the brain thought to be involved in the cortical control of emotion. Specifically, he hypothesized that the hippocampus, the cingulate gyrus ('Broca's callosal lobe'), the hypothalamus, the anterior thalamic nuclei, and the interconnections among these structures constituted a harmonious mechanism that elaborate the functions of emotions. He never mentioned 'Broca's limbic lobe' but others noted that his circuit was very similar to Broca's great limbic lobe.

In the mid-20th century: António Caetano de Abreu Freire Egas Moniz (also known as **Egas Moniz**) **(1874 – 1955)** was a Portuguese neurologist and the developer of cerebral angiography. He is regarded as one of the founders of modern psychosurgery, having developed the surgical procedure leucotomy—better known today as lobotomy—for which he became the first Portuguese national to receive the 1949 Nobel Prize (shared with **Walter Rudolf Hess**).

In 1942: Sherrington coined the term 'enchanted loom' as a metaphor for the brain.

In the early to mid-1940s: Walter Edward Dandy (1886 – 1946), an American neurosurgeon and scientist, is considered one of the founding fathers of neurosurgery, along with **Victor Horsley (1857–1916)** and Harvey Cushing (1869–1939). In 1937, he began the practice of vascular neurosurgery by performing the first surgical clipping of an intracranial aneurysm. He is credited with numerous neurosurgical discoveries and innovations, including the description of the circulation of the cerebrospinal fluid in the brain, the surgical treatment of the hydrocephalus, the invention of air ventriculography and pneumoencephalography, the description of brain endoscopy, the establishment of the first intensive care unit, and the first clipping of an intracranial aneurysm, which marked the birth of cerebrovascular neurosurgery. The importance of his numerous contributions to neurosurgery, in particular, and to medicine, in general, has increased as the field of neurosurgery has evolved.

By 1950: Sherrington, Papez, and **MacLean** had identified many of the brainstem and limbic system functions.

In the 1950s: David McKenzie Rioch, Francis O. Schmitt, and **Stephen Kuffler** played critical roles in establishing Neuroscience as a distinct unified academic discipline. Rioch originated the integration of basic anatomical and physiological research with clinical psychiatry at the Walter Reed Army Institute of Research. During the same period, Schmitt established the Neuroscience Research Program, an inter-university and international organization bringing together biology, medicine, and psychological and behavioral sciences. The word neuroscience itself arose from this program.

In the mid-to-late 20ᵗʰ century: David McKenzie Rioch (1900 - 1985) was a psychiatric research scientist and neuroanatomist, known as a pioneer in brain research and for leading the interdisciplinary neuropsychiatry division at the (U.S.) Walter Reed Army Institute of Research (1951–1970), a program that contributed to the formation of the then-nascent field of neuroscience.

In the mid-to-late 20ᵗʰ century: Stephen William Kuffler (1913 - 1980) was a Hungarian- American neurophysiologist. He is often referred to as the "Father of Modern Neuroscience". He made numerous seminal contributions to our understanding of vision, neural coding, and the neural implementation of behavior. He is known for his research on neuromuscular junctions in frogs, presynaptic inhibition, and the neurotransmitter Gamma-AminoButyric Acid (GABA).

-o-o-o-

July 23, 2023 is World Brain Day!

Sidebar 1.1 – Hieroglyphs and various ancient scripts

A hieroglyph (Greek for "sacred carvings") was a character of the ancient Egyptian writing system. The word *hieroglyphics* actually refers to a hieroglyphic script. We distinguish the several scripts below:

➢ **Egyptian:** The Egyptians invented the pictorial script. The appearance of these distinctive figures in 3000 BCE marked the beginning of ancient Egyptian civilization. Though based on images, Egyptian script was more than a sophisticated form of picture-writing. Each picture (or glyph) served three functions: (1) to represent the image of a thing or action, (2) to stand for the sound of a syllable, and (3) to clarify the precise meaning of adjoining glyphs. Writing hieroglyphs required some artistic skill, limiting the number of people chosen to learn it. Only those privileged with an extensive education (i.e. the Pharaohs, nobles, and priests) were able to read and write hieroglyphs; others used simpler 'joined-up' called demotic and hieratic script.

> **Logographic:** These are pictographic in form in a way reminiscent of ancient Egyptian; they are sometimes called "logographs". In Neoplatonism, especially during the Renaissance, a "logograph" was an artistic representation of an esoteric idea, which Neoplatonists believed actual Egyptian hieroglyphs were.

> **Chinese:** These logograms have been adapted to write a number of Asian languages. They constitute the oldest continuously used system of writing throughout the Sinosphere and in the world. They number in the tens of thousands, though most of them are minor graphic variants encountered only in historical texts. Unlike an alphabet, a character-based writing system associates each logogram with an entire sound and thus may be compared in some aspects to a syllabary. They remain a key component of the Japanese writing system where they are known as *kanji*.

> **Anatolian:** This indigenous logographic script native to central Anatolia consists of some 500 signs. They were once commonly known as Hittite hieroglyphs, but the language they encode proved to be Luvian, not Hittite. There is no demonstrable connection to the Hittite cuneiform script.

> **Luwian:** They are typologically similar to Egyptian hieroglyphs, but do not derive graphically from that script. Also, they are not known to have played the sacred role of hieroglyphs in Egypt.

> **Minoan:** Undeciphered Linear A (1800 to 1450 BCE) has been used to write the hypothesized Minoan language. During the second millennium BC, there were four major branches: Linear A, Linear B, Cypro-Minoan, and Cretan hieroglyphic. In the 1950s, Linear B was deciphered as Mycenaean Greek. It shares many symbols with Linear A, and both

scripts may notate similar syllabic values. But neither those nor any other proposed readings lead to a language that scholars can read.

> **Olmec:** A possible system of writing or proto-writing was developed by the Olmec. This is the earliest known major Mesoamerican civilization, flourishing during the formative period (1500 BCE to 400 BCE) in the tropical lowlands of the modern-day Mexican states of Veracruz and Tabasco. The successor Epi-Olmec culture (300 BCE to 250 BCE) featured a full-fledged writing system, the Isthmian (or Epi-Olmec) script.

> **Nahuatl** (or **Aztec**): A pre-Columbian writing system that combines ideographic writing with specific phonetic logograms and syllabic signs. It was adopted from writing systems also used in Central Mexico such as Zapotec writing and Mixtec writing which descends from it.

> **Mi'kmaq:** A writing system and memory aid used by the Mi'kmaq, a First Nations people of the east coast of Canada. They were derived from a pictograph and petroglyph tradition. In Mi'kmaq the glyphs are called *komqwejwi'kasikl,* or "sucker-fish writings", which refers to the tracks the sucker fish leaves on the muddy river bottom.

> **Ojibwe:** Similar to Mi'kmaq, found as petroglyphs, on story-hides and on Midewiwin wiigwaasabakoon.

> **Muisca:** Numerals written with hieroglyphs that appear as rock art and on textiles. The frog is the most important; it is represented in the numbers from one (*ata*) to twenty (*gueta*) five times because the Muisca did not have hieroglyphs for the numbers 11 to 19.

> **Hebrew (עִבְרִית):** A Northwest Semitic language of the Israelites, Judeans, and their ancestors, it dates back to the 10th century BCE. It belongs to the Northwest Semitic branch of the Afroasiatic language family. It ceased to be an everyday spoken language somewhere between 200 and 400 CE but survived into the medieval period and was revived as a spoken and literary language. It is the only Canaanite language still spoken and the only truly successful example of a revived dead language.

> ➢ **Arabic (اللَّعَرَبِيّة):** A Semitic language that first emerged in the 1st to 4th centuries CE, it has influenced many other languages around the globe throughout its history, but has also borrowed from these other languages. It is written with the Arabic alphabet, which is an abjad script written from right to left, although the spoken varieties are sometimes written in ASCII Latin from left to right with no standardized orthography.

-o-o-o-

And so, after this brief historical detour, It is now time to explore the mysteries of the brain.

2

Santiago Ramón y Cajal, ...the founder of 20th century Neuroscience

Contents

2

Santiago Ramón y Cajal, ... the founder of 20th century Neuroscience

Our story begins with Dr. Santiago Ramón y Cajal, a Spanish neuroscientist, pathologist, and histologist who specialized in neuroanatomy and the central nervous system (CNS). At that time, studies of the brain became more sophisticated with the use of the microscope and the development of the silver staining method developed by Dr. Camillo Golgi, an Italian biologist and pathologist (see Chapter 1). The research showed the intricate structures of single neurons, which led Dr. Cajal to the formation of the "neuron doctrine", the then revolutionary hypothesis that the neuron is the functional unit of the brain. Cajal also used microscopy to uncover many other cell types and propose functions for the cells he saw. His original investigations of the microscopic structure of the brain made him a pioneer of modern neuroscience. Since the mid-20th century, hundreds of his drawings illustrating the arborizations ("tree growing") of brain cells are still in use for educational and training purposes.

Personal life

Cajal was born on the 1st of May 1852 in the town of Petilla de Aragón, Navarre, Spain. His father was an anatomy teacher at the University of Zaragoza. As a child, he displayed talents as a painter, artist, and gymnast that served him well later in his career, but were neither appreciated nor encouraged by his father. At age 14, his father took him to graveyards to find human remains for his own anatomical studies. Cajal later decided to pursue medical studies and attended the University of Zaragoza Medical School, from which he graduated in 1873, at age 21, and then served as a medical officer in the Spanish Army. In 1874–75, he took part in an expedition to Cuba, where he contracted malaria and tuberculosis.

After returning to Spain, Cajal received his doctorate in medicine from the University of Madrid in 1877. Two years later, and until 1883, he became the director of his *alma mater,* the Zaragoza University. He married a certain Silveria Fañanás García, with whom he had seven daughters and five sons. He was subsequently offered the position of anatomy professor of the University of Valencia. His early work at these two universities focused on the pathology of inflammation, the microbiology of cholera, and the structure of epithelial cells and tissues. Cholera is an infection of the small intestine by a number of strains of the bacterium *Vibrio cholerae* with some types producing more severe disease than others. There were seven cholera pandemics that occurred successively during the periods: (1) 1817-24 (in the Bengal region of India, near Calcutta), (2) 1826-37 (in North America and Europe), (3) 1846-1860 (in North Africa, reaching North and South America), (4) 1863-75 (spreading from India to Naples and Spain, and reaching the United States), (5) 1881-96 (in India, spreading to Europe, Asia, and South America), (6) 1899-1923 (in Egypt, the Arabian peninsula, Persia, India, the Philippines, Germany and Italy), and (7) 1961-90 (in Indonesia and other developing countries). Cajal lived during the fourth through the sixth cholera pandemics, and this may have kindled his research interests.

Cajal died in Madrid on October 17, 1934, at the age of 82, continuing to work even on his deathbed.

Figure 2.1 – Photo of Santiago Ramón y Cajal (1852 - 1934)

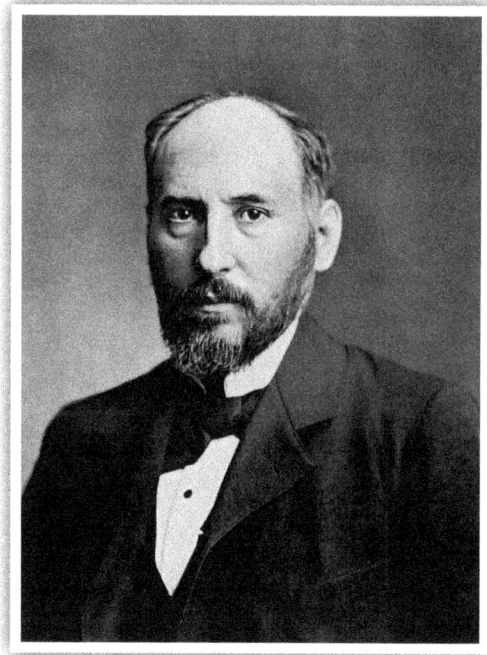

Source: Clark University in 1899. Restoration by Garrondo

Professional life

Figure 2.2 – Cajal drawings of the human sensory cortex area

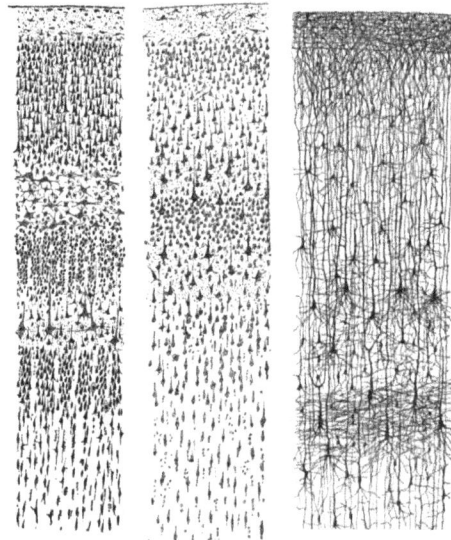

*Source: Cajal's book "Comparative study of the
sensory areas of the human cortex", 1899*

In 1887, Dr. Cajal moved to Barcelona for a professorship. There, he first learned about Golgi's cell staining method, which uses potassium dichromate and silver nitrate to (randomly) stain a few neurons a dark black color, while leaving the surrounding cells transparent. He improved on the method, used it as a central tool in his research on the CNS (brain and spinal cord) in which neurons are so densely intertwined that standard microscopic inspection would be nearly impossible. During this period, he made extensive detailed drawings of neural material, covering many species and most major regions of the brain.

In 1892, Cajal became professor at the University of Madrid, becoming in 1899 the director of the *Instituto Nacional de Higiene* (National Institute of Hygiene) and founder of the *Laboratorio de Investigaciones Biológicas* (Laboratory of Biological Investigations), later renamed the *Instituto Cajal* (Cajal Institute).

Scientific contributions

Cajal made several major contributions to neuroanatomy. In particular, he discovered that nerve cells are not continuous but rather contiguous with gaps between them. This provided definitive evidence for what **Heinrich Waldeyer** would name the "neuron theory", now widely considered the foundation of modern neuroscience. He was also the first to identify the origin of the **synaptic theory of memory,** stating the following in 1894 to the Royal Society of London: *"The ability of neurons to grow in an adult and their power to create new connections can explain learning"*. He was an advocate of the existence of dendritic spines, although he did not recognize them as the site of contact from presynaptic cells. He was a proponent of the polarization of nerve cell function. His student, **Rafael Lorente de Nó**, would continue this study of input-output systems into cabletheory and some of the earliest circuit analysis of neural structures.

By producing depictions of neural structures and their connectivity, and providing detailed descriptions of cell types, he discovered a new type of cell, which was subsequently named after him, the 'interstitial cell of Cajal' (ICC). This cell, found interleaved among neurons, is embedded within the smooth muscles lining the gut; it serves as the generator and pacemaker of the slow waves of contraction, which move material along the gastrointestinal tract, mediating neurotransmission from motor neurons to smooth muscle cells. In his 1894 Croonian Lecture, Cajal suggested (in an extended metaphor) that cortical pyramidal cells may become more elaborate with time, as a tree grows and extends its branches.

Cajal received many prizes, distinctions, and societal memberships during his scientific career, including honorary doctorates in medicine from Cambridge University and Würzburg University, and an honorary doctorate in philosophy from Clark University. As the founder with Camillo Golgi of twentieth century neuroscience, he was awarded the 1906 Nobel prize in Physiology or Medicine, which was shared with Golgi "*in recognition of their work on the structure of the nervous system*". He was the first person of Spanish origin to win a scientific Nobel Prize. This caused some controversy because Golgi, a staunch supporter of reticular theory, disagreed with Cajal in his view of the neuron doctrine. In addition, even before Cajal's work, Norwegian scientist **Fridtjof Nansen** had established the contiguous nature of nerve cells in his study of certain marine life (which Cajal failed to cite.)

Figure 2.3 - Ramón y Cajal's 1906 Nobel certificate.

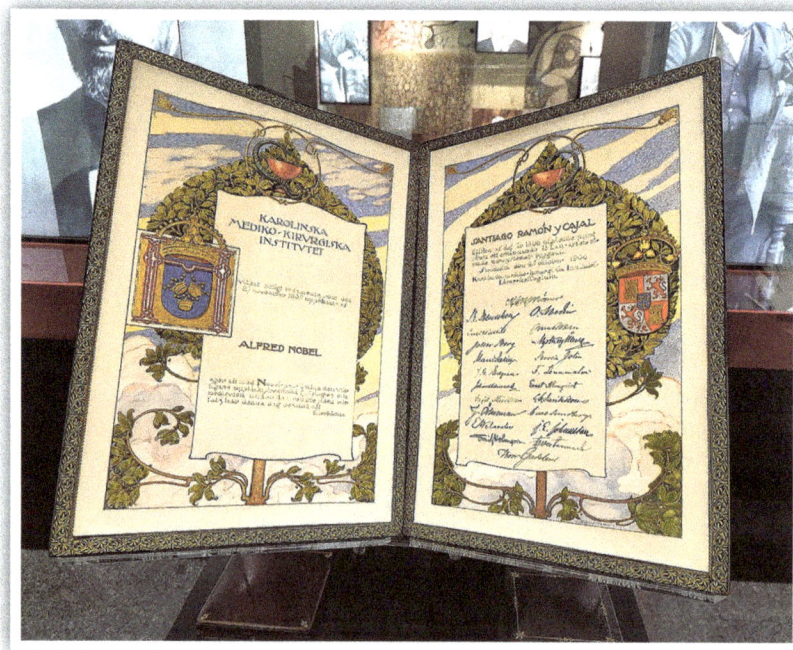

Reference: Museo Nacional de Ciencias Naturales
(National Museum of Natural Sciences), *Madrid*

Accomplishments and distinctions

Cajal was an International Member of both the (U.S) National Academy of Sciences (NAS) and the American Philosophical Society (APS). He was the recipient of many national and international prizes and distinctions. In particular, in 2014, the (U.S.) National Institutes of Health (NIH) initiated an ongoing exhibition of original Ramón y Cajal drawings in its John Porter Neuroscience Research Center. Further, from January 31 – May 29, 2016, Cajal's work was featured in the inaugural exhibition for the re-opening of the *Architecture of Life* at the University of California's Berkeley Art Museum and Pacific Film Archive. The catalog for the exhibition featured Cajal's drawing of the **Purkinje**'s cell on the front cover.

And so, after this cursory journey into the life and times of Dr. Santiago Ramón y Cajal, we bid him a fond farewell, paying him a grateful homage by employing his own signature to sign off this chapter (Figure 2.4).

Figure 2.4 – Signature of Dr. Santiago Ramón y Cajal

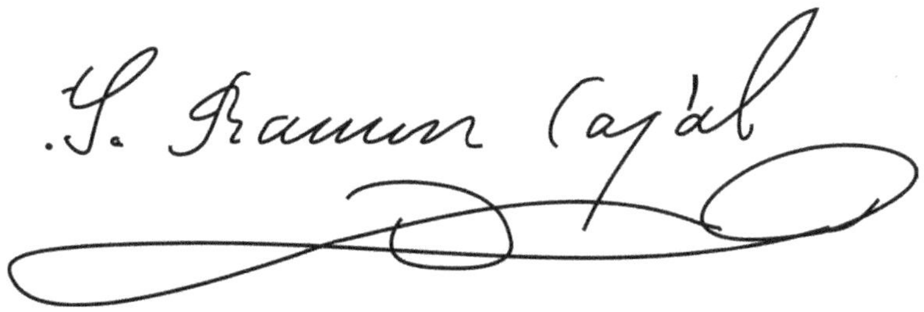

PART B
THE BRAIN IN HEALTH AND DISEASE

Acknowledgment: This Part B of the book is based in part on a Wikipedia copyrighted article (Human brain https://en.wikipedia.org/) and used under the Creative Commons Attribution-ShareAlike 3.0, (https://creativecommons. org/licenses/by-sa/3.0/) which permits unrestricted use, distribution, and reproduction in any medium, provided the original author and source are credited.

3

Wonders of the human brain - I. Gross anatomy and physiology

Contents

3

Wonders of the healthy brain - I. Gross anatomy

It is now time to explore the mysteries of the healthy human brain beginning from its early development. Special attention should be devoted to the several control functions exerted by the various brain ares to be described, and more particularly those concerned with **memory** and **cognitive functions**.

Gross anatomy of the healthy brain

The living brain is very soft, having a gel-like consistency similar to soft tofu. There is substantial individual variation in the adult human brain, the standard reference range for men being 1.18-1.62 kg (2.60–3.57 lb) and for women 1.03-1.40 kg (2.27–3.09 lb). The corresponding volume is approximately 1,260 cm³ in men and 1,130 cm³ in women. The cortical layers of neurons constitute much of the cerebral grey matter, while the deeper subcortical regions of myelinated axons make up the white matter. The white matter of the brain makes up about half of the total brain volume. Figure 3.1 pictures a brain bisected in the sagittal plane, showing the white matter of the *corpus callosum.*

Several important brain structures are implicated in playing key roles in stress response pathways. Let us take a quick grand tour of these major structures, each of which being responsible for a particular function(s), and of the central nervous system (CNS). This may be aided by studying Figures 3.1 through 3.6 all the while marveling at the varied functions and controls conducted by the several brain component structures.

The cerebral hemispheres

The cerebral hemispheres account for ~ 85% of the brain's weight. The neurons in them are connected by the *corpus callosum* (thick bundles of nerve cell fibers). The left hemisphere appears to focus on details whereas the right hemisphere focuses on the broad background.

Figure 3.1 - Human brain bisected in the sagittal plane, showing the white matter of the corpus callosum

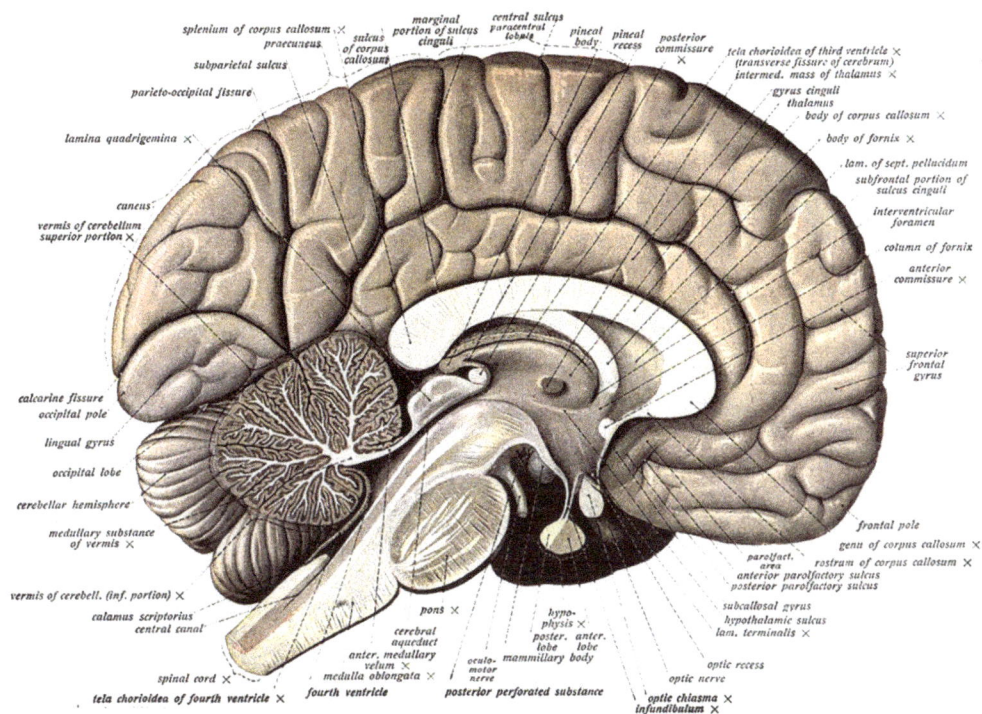

References: **Dr. Johannes Sobotta - Atlas and Text-book of Human Anatomy Volume III Vascular System, Lymphatic system, Nervous system and Sense Organs** *and an anatomical illustration from Sobotta's Human Anatomy 1908*

The cerebral cortex

The *cerebral cortex* is the outer layer of these hemispheres, controlling voluntary movement and regulating **cognitive** functions. The hemispheres have four lobes, each of which has different roles: the *frontal lobe* (for executive functions like thinking, organizing, planning, and problem-solving, as well as **memory**, attention, and movement); the *parietal lobe* sitting behind the frontal lobe (for perception and integration of stimuli from the senses); the *occipital lobe* at the back of the brain (for vision); and the *temporal lobe* running along the side of the brain under the frontal and parietal lobes (for senses of smell, taste, and sound, and the formation and storage of **memories**). (See Figures 3.2-3.6 below.)

The cerebrum

The *cerebrum* is the largest part of the brain, overlying the other brain structures (Figure 3.2). It is divided into nearly symmetrical left and right hemispheres by a deep groove, the *longitudinal fissure*. Asymmetry between the lobes is noted as a *petalia*. The hemispheres are connected by five commissures that span the longitudinal fissure, the largest of these is the *corpus callosum*. Each hemisphere is conventionally divided into four main lobes (*frontal, parietal, temporal, and occipital*), named according to the skull bones that overlie them. Each lobe is associated with one or two specialized functions though there is some functional overlap between them. Three other lobes are included by some sources (*central, limbic,* and *insular*). The central lobe comprises the pre-central gyrus and the post-central gyrus, the latter being included since it has a distinct functional role. The surface of the brain is folded into ridges (the *gyri*) and grooves (the *sulci*), many of which are usually named according to their position (such as the frontal gyrus of the frontal lobe or the central sulcus separating the central regions of the hemispheres). There are many small variations in the secondary and tertiary folds. The cerebrum contains the ventricles where the *cerebrospinal fluid* (CSF) is produced and circulated.

Figure 3.2 - Pictorial of the human brain

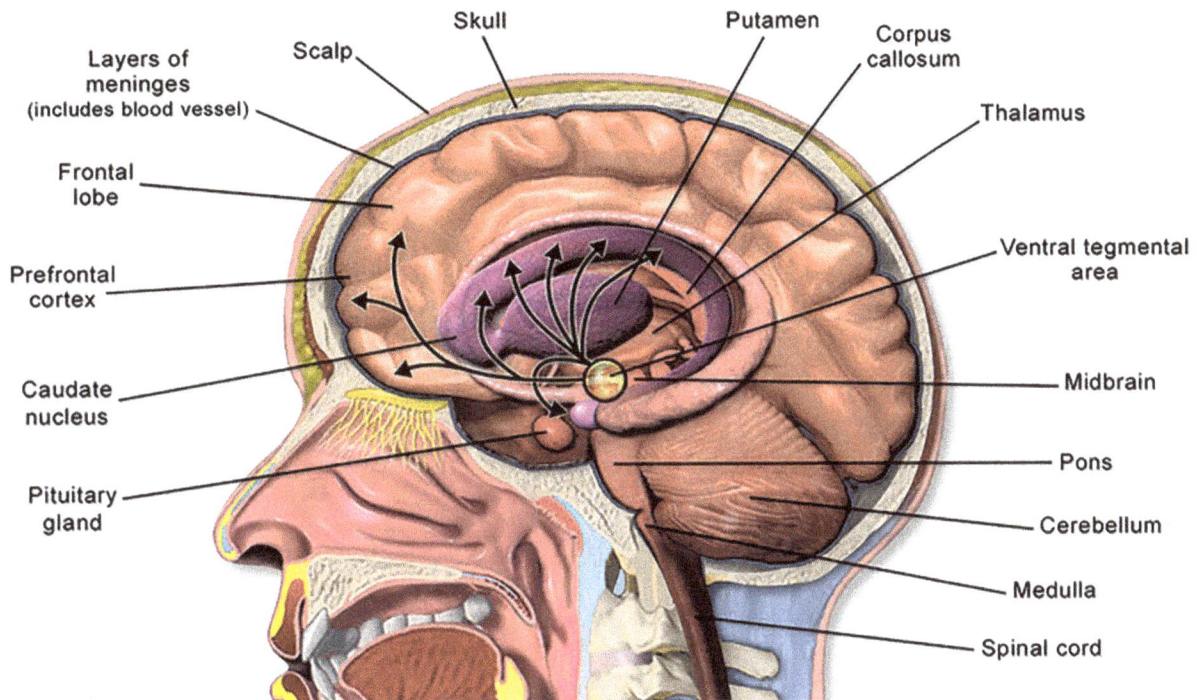

Source: Bruce Baus

Below the corpus callosum is the *septum pellucidum*, a membrane that separates the lateral ventricles. Beneath the lateral ventricles is the thalamus and to the front and below lies the hypothalamus. The hypothalamus leads on to the pituitary gland. At the back of the thalamus is the brainstem.

The prefrontal cortex

Located in the frontal lobe (Figure 3.2), the prefrontal cortex is the anterior-most region of the cerebral cortex. Its important function is to regulate **cognitive processes** including planning, attention, and problem-solving through extensive connections with other brain regions. The prefrontal cortex can become impaired during the stress response. This is the case among post-traumatically stressed mothers in response to video-stimuli depicting mother-child separation versus play. That observation points to a maternal epigenetic signature of the glucocorticoid receptor gene.

The cortex

The outer part of the cerebrum is the cerebral *cortex*, made up of grey matter arranged in layers. It is 2-4 millimeters (0.079 to 0.157 in) thick, and deeply folded to give a convoluted appearance. It is mapped by divisions into about 50 different functional areas known as *Brodmann's areas.* These areas are distinctly different when seen under a microscope. Beneath the cortex is the cerebral white matter. The largest part of the cerebral cortex is the *neocortex*, which has six neuronal layers. The rest of the cortex, the *allocortex*, has 3-4 layers.

The cortex is divided into two main functional areas – a *motor* cortex and a *sensory* cortex. The primary motor cortex, which sends axons down to motor neurons in the *brainstem* and *spinal cord*, occupies the rear portion of the frontal lobe, directly in front of the somatosensory area. The primary sensory areas receive signals from the sensory nerves and tracts by way of relaying nuclei in the *thalamus.*

Primary sensory areas include the visual cortex of the occipital lobe, the auditory cortex in parts of the temporal lobe, the insular cortex, and the somatosensory cortex in the parietal lobe. The remaining parts of the cortex are called the *association areas*. These areas receive input from the sensory areas and lower parts of the brain and are involved in the **complex cognitive processes** of perception, thought, and decision-making. The main functions of the frontal lobe are to control attention, abstract thinking, behavior, problem-solving tasks, and physical reactions and personality. The occipital lobe is the smallest lobe; its main functions are visual reception, visual-spatial processing, movement, and color recognition. There is a smaller occipital lobule in the lobe known as the *cuneus*. The temporal lobe controls **auditory and visual memories**, language, and some hearing and speech.

The brain stem

Located at the base of the brain, the *brainstem* connects the spinal cord with the rest of the brain. It resembles a stalk attached to, and leaving, the cerebrum at the start of the midbrain area. It includes the *midbrain*, the *pons*, and the *medulla oblongata*.

It lies in the back part of the skull, resting on the part of the base known as the *clivus*, and ends at the *foramen magnum*, a large opening in the occipital bone. The brainstem continues below this as the spinal cord, protected by the vertebral column.

Ten of the twelve pairs of cranial nerves emerge directly from the brainstem. The brainstem also contains many cranial nerve nuclei and nuclei of peripheral nerves, as well as nuclei involved in the regulation of many essential processes including breathing, control of eye movements, and balance. The *reticular formation*, a network of nuclei of ill-defined formation, is present within and along the length of the brainstem. Many nerve tracts, which transmit information to and from the cerebral cortex to the rest of the body, pass through the brainstem.

The brainstem functions are crucial to survival (heart rate, blood pressure, breathing, sleep, and dreaming).

Figure 3.3 - Functional areas of the human brain
(Dashed areas shown are commonly left hemisphere dominant)

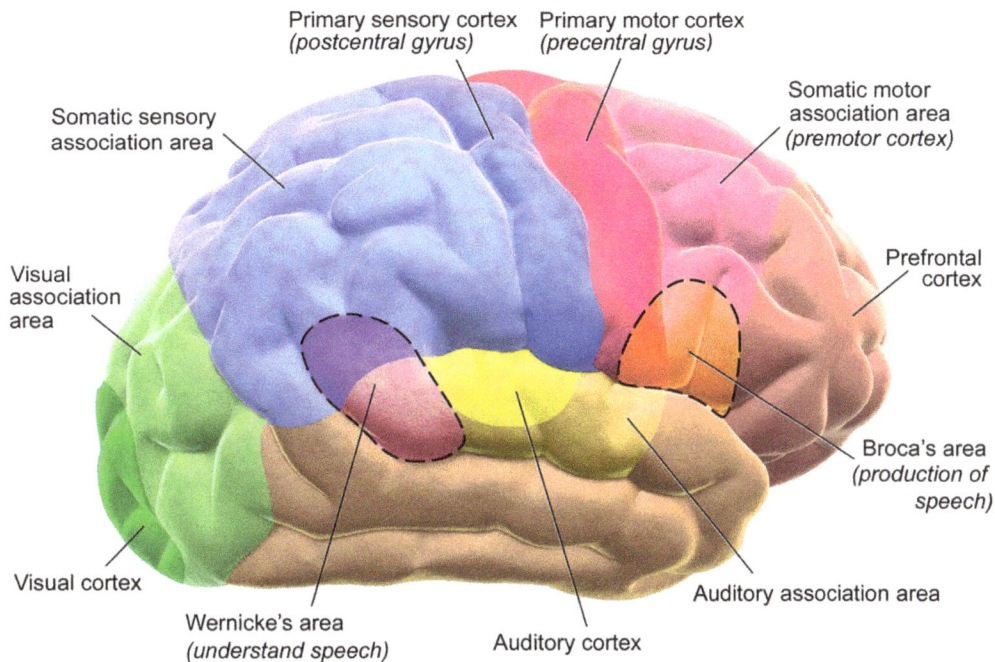

Source: "Medical gallery of Blausen Medical 2014 ". Blausen.com staff (2014).

The cerebellum

Behind the brainstem, located beneath the occipital lobe, is the *cerebellum* (or little brain). It has two hemispheres and is divided into 3 lobes (*anterior, posterior,* and *flocculonodular*). The anterior and posterior lobes are connected in the middle by the *vermis.* Compared to the cerebral cortex, the cerebellum has a much thinner outer cortex that is narrowly furrowed into numerous curved transverse fissures. Viewed from underneath between the two lobes is the third lobe the flocculonodular lobe. The cerebellum rests at the back of the cranial cavity, lying beneath the occipital lobes, and is separated from these by the *cerebellar tentorium,* a sheet of fiber.

It is connected to the midbrain of the brainstem by the superior cerebellar *peduncles,* to the *pons* by the middle cerebellar peduncles, and to the *medulla* by the inferior cerebellar peduncles. The cerebellum consists of an inner medulla of white matter and an outer cortex of richly folded grey matter. The cerebellum's anterior and posterior lobes appear to play a role in the coordination and smoothing of complex motor movements, and the flocculonodular lobe in the maintenance of balance although debate exists as to its **cognitive**, behavioral, and motor functions.The cerebellum plays roles in balance coordination and motor learning.

The meninges

The cerebrum, brainstem, cerebellum, and *spinal cord* are covered by three membranes called *meninges (the tough dura mater, the middle arachnoid mater, and the more delicate inner pia mater).* Between the latter two is the *subarachnoid space* and the *subarachnoid cisterns,* which contain the cerebrospinal fluid. The outermost membrane of the cerebral cortex is the basement membrane of the pia mater called the *glia limitans;* it is an important part of the blood-brain barrier (BBB).

The basal ganglia

Also called basal nuclei, the *basal ganglia* are a set of structures deep within the hemispheres involved in behavior and movement regulation. The largest component is the *striatum;* others are the *globus pallidus*, the *substantia nigra,* and the *subthalamic nucleus*. Part of the *dorsal striatum*, the *putamen*, and the *globus pallidus*, lie separated from the lateral ventricles and the *thalamus* by the internal capsule, whereas the *caudate nucleus* stretches around and abuts the lateral ventricles on their outer sides. At the deepest part of the lateral sulcus between the insular cortex and the striatum is a thin neuronal sheet called the *claustrum*.

Below and in front of the striatum are a number of basal forebrain structures. These include the *nucleus accumbens, nucleus basalis, Broca's diagonal band, substantia innominata, and the medial septal nucleus.* These structures are important in producing the neurotransmitter acetylcholine, which is then distributed widely throughout the brain. The basal forebrain, in particular the *nucleus basalis*, is considered to be the major cholinergic output of the central nervous system (CNS) to the striatum and neocortex.

The limbic system

The limbic system lies deep inside the cerebral hemispheres, linking the brainstem with the higher reasoning elements of the cerebral cortex. It plays a key role in **memory**, emotion, and instinctive behaviors. It includes: the *amygdalae* (for strong emotions such as fear), the *hippocampus* (for learning and **short-term memories** and their conversion into **long-term memories** for storage in other brain areas); the *thalamus* (for sensory and limbic information); and the *hypothalamus* (for monitoring activities such as body temperature, food intake, and the body's internal clock), the *pituitary gland,* the *locus coeruleus,* the *adrenal gland,* the *Raphe nucleus,* and the *spinal cord* (Figures 3.4-3.6).

- *The amygdalae* (in_**green** color in Figure 3.4): They consist of two small "almond"-shaped structures located bilaterally and deep within the medial temporal lobes of the brain. They are also part of the brain's limbic system, with projections to and from the hypothalamus, hippocampus, and locus coeruleus within the *pons* (gold color) among other areas. Thought to play a role in the processing of emotions, the amygdalae have been implicated in modulating stress response mechanisms, particularly when feelings of anxiety or fear are involved.

- **The hippocampus** (in **blue** color in Figure 3.4): It is a structure located bilaterally, deep within the medial temporal lobes of the brain, just below each amygdala. It is a part of the brain's limbic system thought to play an important role in **memory formation**. There are numerous connections to the hippocampus from the cerebral cortex, hypothalamus, and amygdalae, among other regions. During stress, the hippocampus is particularly important in that **cognitive processes such as prior memories** can have a great influence on enhancing, suppressing, or even independently generating a stress response. The hippocampus is also an area in the brain that is susceptible to damage brought upon by chronic stress.

- **The thalamus** (in **mid-rose** color in Figure 3.2).The thalamus is a large mass of gray matter located in the dorsal part of the diencephalon (a division of the forebrain). Nerve fibers project out of the thalamus to the cerebral cortex in all directions, allowing hub-like exchanges of information. It has several functions, such as the relaying of sensory signals, including motor signals to the cerebral cortex and the regulation of consciousness, sleep, and alertness. Anatomically, it is a paramedian symmetrical structure of two halves (left and right), within the vertebrate brain, situated between the cerebral cortex and the midbrain. It forms during embryonic development as the main product of the diencephalon, as first recognized in 1893 by the Swiss embryologist and anatomist Wilhelm His Sr.

- **The hypothalamus** (highlighted in **red** color in Figure 3.4): It is a small portion of the brain located below the *thalamus* and above the *brainstem*. One of its most important functions is to help link together the body's nervous and endocrine systems. This structure has many bidirectional neural inputs and outputs from and to various other brain regions. These connections help to regulate the hypothalamus' ability to secrete hormones into the body's bloodstream, having far-reaching and long-lasting effects on physiological processes such as metabolism. During a stress response, the hypothalamus secretes various hormones including the corticotropin-releasing hormone, which stimulates the body's pituitary gland and initiates a heavily regulated stress response pathway.

- **The pituitary gland** (**purple** color in Figure 3.4): It is a small organ that is located at the base of the brain just under the hypothalamus. This gland releases various hormones that play significant roles in regulating homeostasis. During a stress response, the pituitary gland releases hormones including the adrenocorticotropic hormone into the bloodstream, modulating a heavily regulated stress response system.
- **The locus coeruleus** (**gold** color in Figure 3.4): This is an area located in the pons of the brainstem that is the principal site of synthesis of the neurotransmitter norepinephrine, playing an important role in the fight-or-flight response of the sympathetic nervous system to stress. It receives input from the hypothalamus, amygdalae and the Raphe nucleus, among other regions, and projects widely across the brain as well as to the spinal cord.

Figure 3.4 - Brain cross-section showing the hypothalamus, amygdalae, hippocampus, pons, and pituitary gland

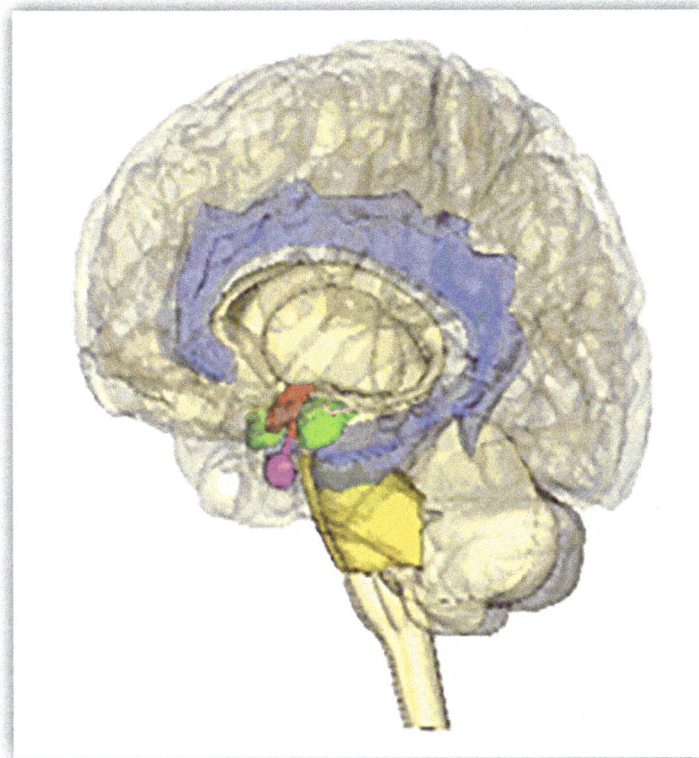

*(hypothalamus=__red__; amygdala=__green__; pituitary gland=__purple__;
hippocampus/fornix=__blue__;
pons and Raphe nucleus=__gold__)*

➤ **The adrenal gland** (Figure 3.5)**:** Although outside of the brain proper, the adrenal gland needs to be mentioned. It is a major organ of the endocrine system located directly on top of the kidneys. It is chiefly responsible for the synthesis of the stress hormones that are released into the bloodstream during a stress response. Cortisol is the major stress hormone it releases. In addition to the locus coeruleus, which exists as a source of the neurotransmitter norepinephrine within the central nervous system, during a stress response, the adrenal gland can also release norepinephrine into the body's blood stream, at which point norepinephrine acts as a hormone in the endocrine system.

➤ **The *Raphe nucleus:*** This is an area located in the pons of the brainstem (**gold** color) that is the principal site of the synthesis of the neurotransmitter serotonin. It plays an important role in mood regulation, particularly when stress is associated with depression and anxiety. Projections that extend from this region to widespread areas across the brain are thought to modulate an organism's circadian rhythm and sensation of pain among other processes.

➤ **The *spinal cord*** (Figure 3.6): Although not a part of the brain, it complements it in forming the CNS and must be indicated. It plays a critical role in transferring stress response neural impulses from the brain to the rest of the body. In addition to the neuroendocrine blood hormone signaling system initiated by the hypothalamus, the spinal cord communicates with the rest of the body by innervating the peripheral nervous system (PNS). Certain nerves that belong to the sympathetic branch of the central nervous system (CNS) exit the spinal cord and stimulate peripheral nerves, which in turn engage the body's major organs and muscles in a fight-or-flight manner.

Table 3.1 lists the brain structures and corresponding control(s) or function(s). Of particular importance to us are those structures that control or regulate memory and cognition, including the cerebral cortex, the prefrontal cortex, the cortex, the cerebellum (still under debate), and the limbic system (hypocampus, hypothalamus). It should be noted that there is not any single brain structure that is totally responsible for these functions. It is equally important to also note that the brain does not respond linearly to any stimulus. We still do not understand the particularities of this non-linear system, hindering us from truly fathoming the workings of the brain.

Table 3.1 – Brain structures and corresponding control(s) or function(s)

Brain structures	Associated control(s) or function(s)
Cerebral hemispheres	o Left hemisphere focuses on details o Right hemisphere focuses on the broad background
Cerebral cortex	o Controls voluntary movement and regulates **cognitive** functions o Frontal lobe: Controls executive functions (thinking, reasoning, organizing, planning, problem-solving, **memory**, attention, and movement), motor control, emotions, and language o Parietal lobe: Perception and integration of stimuli from the senses o Occipital lobe: Vision o Temporal lobe: Senses (smell, taste, and sound) and formation and storage of **memories**
Motor cortex	Involved in generation, planning, coordination, and control of movement
Prefrontal cortex	o Regulates higher-level **cognitive processes** (planning, attention, and problem-solving) o Broca's area, which is essential for language production.
Cortex	o Association areas involved in the **complex cognitive processes (**perception, thought, and decision-making) o Frontal lobe: Controls attention, abstract thinking, behavior, problem-solving tasks, physical reactions, and personality o Occipital lobe: Visual reception, visual-spatial processing, movement, and color recognition o Temporal lobe: Controls **auditory and visual memories**, language, and some hearing and speech
Brainstem	o Controls essential processes (breathing, eye movements, and balance) o Crucial to survival (heart rate, blood pressure, breathing, sleep, and dreaming)
Cerebellum	o Anterior and posterior lobes: Coordination and smoothing of complex motor movements, o Flocculonodular lobe: Maintenance of balance. Debate exists as to its **cognitive**, behavioral, and motor functions o Balance coordination and motor learning
Basal ganglia	o Produces neurotransmitter acetylcholine distributed widely throughout the brain o Major cholinergic output of the CNS to the striatum and neocortex o Behavior and movement regulation

Limbic system	o Key role in strong emotions and instinctive behaviors o Amygdalae: Processing of strong emotions (anxiety or fear), modulation of stress response mechanisms o Hippocampus: **Memory formation (**important role); learning and **short-term memories** and their conversion into **long-term memories** for storage in other brain areas. Important role in **memory formation** o Thalamus: Regulation of consciousness, sleep, and alertness; relay of sensory signals, including motor signals to the cerebral cortex; and regulation of consciousness, sleep, and alertness o Hypothalamus: Important since **cognitive processes (**such as **prior memories)** can have great influence on enhancing, suppressing, or even independently generating a stress response. Monitors metabolic activities (body temperature, food intake, and body's internal clock). Also, regulates stress response o Pituitary gland: Regulates homeostasis. During a stress response, releases hormones including the adrenocorticotropic hormone into the bloodstream, modulating a heavily regulated stress response system o Locus coeruleus: Principal site of synthesis of the neurotransmitter norepinephrine. Important role in fight-or-flight response of the sympathetic nervous system to stress
Adrenal gland	o Synthesis of stress hormones (major hormone: Cortisol) is the major stress hormone it releases o Additional source of neurotransmitter norepinephrine within the CNS and into the body's blood stream, at which point it acts as a hormone in the endocrine system.
Raphe nucleus	o Principal site of synthesis of neurotransmitter serotonin o Mood regulation (important role), particularly when stress is associated with depression and anxiety o Modulates circadian rhythm and sensation of pain among other processes
Spinal cord	o Transfers stress response neural impulses from the brain to the rest of the body o Communicates with the rest of the body by innervating the PNS

Figure 3.5 – The adrenal gland

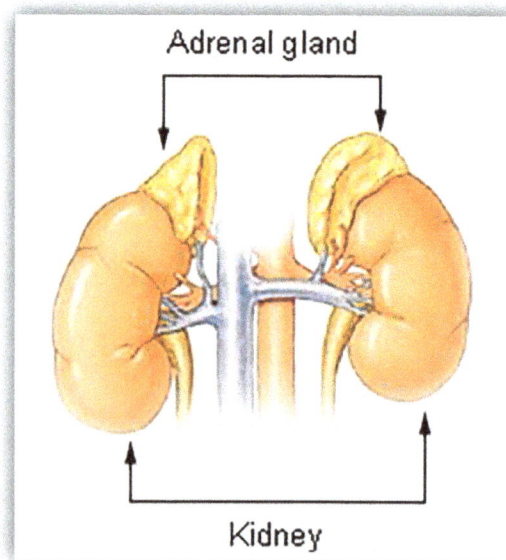

Lateralization

The cerebrum has a contralateral organization with each hemisphere of the brain, interacting primarily with one-half of the body: the left-side of the brain interacts with the right-side of the body and vice versa. The developmental cause for this is uncertain. Both the motor connections from the brain to the spinal cord and sensory connections from the spinal cord to the brain cross sides in the brainstem.

Visual input follows a more complex rule: the optic nerves from the two eyes come together at a point called the *optic chiasm*, and half of the fibers from each nerve split off to join the other. The result is that connections from the left-halves of the retina in both eyes go to the right-side of the brain, whereas connections from the right-half of the retina go to the left-side of the brain. Because each half of the retina receives light coming from the opposite half of the visual field, the functional consequence is that the visual input from the left-side of the world goes to the right-side of the brain, and *vice versa*. Thus, the right-side of the brain receives somatosensory input from the left-side of the body and visual input from the left-side of the visual field.

While the left- and right-sides of the brain appear symmetrical, they function asymmetrically. For example, the counterpart of the left-hemisphere motor area controlling the right-hand is the right-hemisphere area controlling the left-hand. There are, however, several important exceptions involving language and **spatial cognition**. The left frontal lobe is dominant for language. If a key language area in the left hemisphere is damaged, it can leave the victim unable to speak or understand whereas equivalent damage to the right hemisphere would cause only minor impairment to language skills.

Figure 3.6 - The human spinal cord

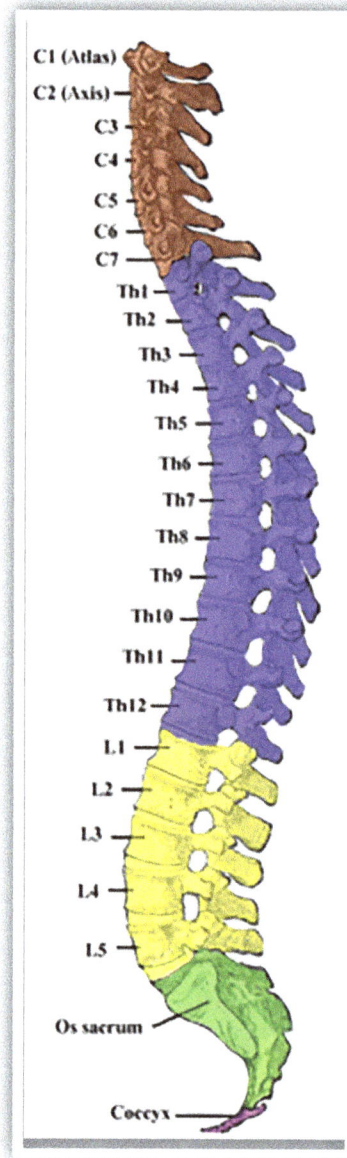

A substantial part of current understanding of the interactions between the two hemispheres has come from the study of "split-brain patients"—people who underwent surgical transection of the *corpus callosum* in an attempt to reduce the severity of epileptic seizures. These patients do not show unusual behavior that is immediately obvious but, in some cases, can behave almost like two different people in the same body, with the right-hand taking an action and then the left-hand undoing it. When briefly shown a picture on the right-side of the point of visual fixation, these patients are able to describe it verbally but, when the picture is shown on the left, they are unable to describe it although they may be able to give an indication with the left-hand of the nature of the object shown.

Comparative anatomy

Many features of the human brain are common to all mammalian brains, most notably a six-layered cerebral cortex and a set of associated structures including the hippocampus and amygdala.

As a primate brain, the human brain has a much larger cerebral cortex in proportion to body size than most mammals, and a highly developed visual system. As a hominid brain, the human brain is substantially enlarged even in comparison to the brain of a typical monkey. Humans have more association cortex, sensory, and motor parts than smaller mammals such as the rat and the cat.

The sequence of human evolution from *Australopithecus* (four million years ago) to *Homo sapiens* (modern humans) was marked by a steady increase in brain size. As brain size increased, this altered the size and shape of the skull from about 600 cm^3 in *Homo habilis* to an average of about 1,520 cm^3 in *Homo neanderthalensis*. Differences in DNA, gene expression, gene-environment, and gene-gene–environment interactions help explain the differences between the functions of the human brain and those of other primates.

The brain vasculature

To better understand what may happen to the brain in disease (the subject of the next chapter), it is also important to know a bit about its vasculature and what happens to it during aging. This is illustrated in Figure 3.7.

Figure 3.7 – The brain vasculature

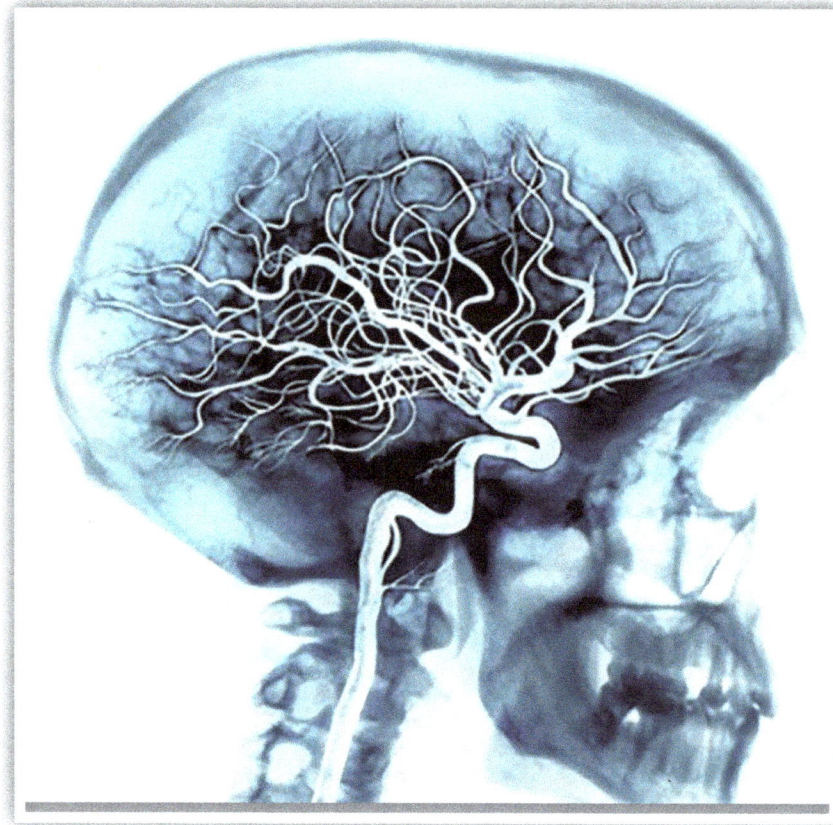

Take-aways

➤ The gross anatomy of the healthy brain was discussed. The living brain is very soft, having a gel-like consistency similar to soft tofu. There is substantial individual variation in the adult human brain. Several important brain structures are implicated in playing key roles in stress response pathways.

➤ The cerebral hemispheres account for ~ 85% of the brain's weight. The left hemisphere appears to focus on details whereas the right hemisphere focuses on the broad background.

➤ The cerebrum has a contralateral organization with each hemisphere of the brain, interacting primarily with one-half of the body: The left-side of the brain interacting with the right-side of the body and *vice versa*. Both motor connections from the brain to the spinal cord and sensory connections from the spinal cord to the brain cross sides in the brainstem. The cerebrum contains the ventricles where the *cerebrospinal fluid* is produced and circulated.

➢ A substantial part of current understanding of the interactions between the two hemispheres has come from the study of "split-brain patients"—people who underwent surgical transection of the *corpus callosum* in an attempt to reduce the severity of epileptic seizures. These patients do not show unusual behavior that is immediately obvious, but in some cases can behave almost like two different people in the same body, with the right-hand taking an action and then the left-hand undoing it.

➢ The prefrontal cortex has the important function of regulating **cognitive processes.** It can become impaired during the stress response.

➢ The cortex is divided into two main functional areas – a *motor* cortex and a *sensory* cortex. The primary motor cortex sends axons down to motor neurons in the *brainstem* and *spinal cord.* The primary sensory areas receive signals from the sensory nerves and tracts by way of relaying nuclei in the *thalamus.* The sensory areas and lower parts of the brain are involved in **complex cognitive processes.** The temporal lobe controls **auditory and visual memories,** language, and some hearing and speech.

➢ The brainstem functions are crucial to survival (heart rate, blood pressure, breathing, sleep and dreaming).

➢ The basal ganglia (nuclei) are involved in behavior and movement regulation. Their component structures are important in producing the neurotransmitter acetylcholine. In particular, the basal forebrain is the major cholinergic output of the central nervous system to the striatum and neocortex.

➢ The limbic system plays a key role in **memory**, emotion, and instinctive behaviors. It includes: the *amygdalae* (for strong emotions such as fear), the *hippocampus* (for learning and **short-term memories** and their conversion into **long-term memories** for residence in other brain areas); the *thalamus* (for sensory and limbic information); and the *hypothalamus* (for monitoring activities such as body temperature, food intake, and the body's internal clock), the *pituitary gland,* the *locus coeruleus,* the *adrenal gland,* the *Raphe nucleus,* and the *spinal cord.*

- The brain structures and their corresponding control(s) or function(s) have been tabulated. From them, the main structures of interst for **memory** and **cognition** can be evidenced.
- The cerebrum has a contralateral organization with each hemisphere of the brain, interacting primarily with one-half of the body: the left-side of the brain interacts with the right-side of the body and vice versa. The developmental cause for this is uncertain. Both the motor connections from the brain to the spinal cord and sensory connections from the spinal cord to the brain cross sides in the brainstem.
- Many features of the human brain are common to all mammalian brains, most notably a six-layered cerebral cortex and a set of associated structures including the hippocampus and amygdala.

Sidebar 3.1 - The developing brain

At the beginning of the third week of development, the embryonic ectoderm forms a thickened strip called the *neural plate*. By the fourth week, the neural plate has widened to give a broad cephalic end, a less broad middle part, and a narrow caudal end. These swellings are known as the *primary brain vesicles,* representing the beginnings of the forebrain, midbrain, and hindbrain.

Neural crest cells (derived from the ectoderm) populate the lateral edges of the plate at the neural folds. In the fourth week, during the *nurulation* stage, the neural folds close to form the neural tube, bringing together the neural crest cells at the neural crest. The neural crest runs the length of the tube with cranial neural crest cells at the cephalic end and caudal neural crest cells at the tail. Cells detach from the crest and migrate in a craniocaudal (head-to-tail) wave inside the tube. Cells at the cephalic end give rise to the brain, and cells at the caudal end give rise to the spinal cord. The tube flexes as it grows, forming the crescent-shaped cerebral hemispheres at the head.

On day 32, the cerebral hemispheres first appear. Early in the fourth week, the cephalic part bends sharply forward in a cephalic flexure. This flexed part becomes the forebrain (*prosencephalon*), the adjoining curving part becomes the midbrain (*mesencephalon*), and the part caudal to the flexure becomes the hindbrain (*rhombencephalon*). Formed as swellings, they are known as the three primary brain vesicles. In the fifth week of development, five secondary brain vesicles have formed. The forebrain separates into two vesicles (an anterior *telencephalon* and a posterior *diencephalon*). The telencephalon gives rise to the *cerebral cortex*, the *basal ganglia*, and related structures. The diencephalon gives rise to the *thalamus* and the *hypothalamus*. The hindbrain also splits into two areas (*metencephalon* and *myelencephalon*). The metencephalon gives rise to the *cerebellum* and the *pons*. The myelencephalon gives rise to the *medulla oblongata*.

Also, during the fifth week, the brain divides into repeating segments called *neuromeres*. In the hindbrain, these are known as *rhombomeres*.

A characteristic of the brain is the cortical folding known as *gyrification*. Why the cortex wrinkles and folds is not well-understood, but gyrification has been linked to intelligence and neurological disorders, and a number of gyrification theories have been proposed. These theories include those based on mechanical buckling, axonal tension, and differential tangential expansion. What is clear is that gyrification is not a random process, but rather a complex developmentally-predetermined process which generates patterns of folds that are consistent between individuals and most species. A gene present in the human genome (ArhGAP11B) may play a major role in gyrification and encephalization.

After just five months of prenatal development, the cortex is smooth.

By the gestational age of 24 weeks, the wrinkled morphology showing the fissures that begin to mark out the lobes of the brain is evident.

The first groove to appear in the fourth month is the *lateral cerebral fossa*. The expanding caudal end of the hemisphere has to curve over in a forward direction to fit into the restricted space. This covers the fossa and turns it into a much deeper ridge known as the *lateral sulcus,* marking out the temporal lobe.

By the sixth month, other sulci have formed that demarcate the frontal, parietal, and occipital lobes.

In summary:

- From 0-3 years old, babies do not form **explicit memories** (including **autobiographical memories**) but do form **implicit memories** (including **emotional, sensory,** and **motor memories**).
- **Lifelong memories** are encoded into the stress and emotional systems of the brain.

Sidebar 3.2 – Why the infant brain remembers?

One of the most pervasive myths about infancy, age 0-3 years old, is that infants do not remember anything so experience in infancy has (erroneously) been discarded. However, this myth stems from a lack of clarity around memory. **Memory means that an event occurs to permanently change brain cells and brain function.** As will be abundantly seen in the following chapters of this book, there are different forms of memory, including particularly **explicit** and **implicit** memories.

We tend to focus only on explicit memory, which includes **autobiographical** memories of conscious events in our lives—the "what," "where," "when," "who" memories. **In infancy, the brain does form autobiographical memories**, so infants have memories of events while they are infants. However, most adults experience infantile or childhood amnesia in which, years after infancy, they are unable to recall events in infancy from 0-3 years. This is thought to be due to a rapidly developing hippocampus in infancy. The reason might be that **long-term memories for events begin to form later around age 3-4**. However, a sizable amount of memory from infancy is stored in the brain as implicit memory, and this involves the unconscious mind.

The massive growth of the infant brain means that a considerable amount of memories and critical brain areas are formed in babyhood. Lifelong memories are encoded into the structure of the stress and emotional systems. **In infancy, the brain creates non-autobiographical implicit memories like sensory, motor, and emotional memory.** While babies may not remember discrete events from their infancy, they will remember how to eat, how to walk, and, importantly, their stress systems and emotional systems will remember how they were nurtured. Any amount of nurture benefits the baby.

While there is limited recollection of early life, nurturing experiences change DNA, stress systems, emotional systems, and stay in the brains. So, in fact, the reality is that **the infant brain has a huge capacity for memory.**

The parents' presence, relationship, communication, play, laughter, and responsiveness with their baby in their first three years is transformative to the brain and will remain with them for the rest of their life.

4

Wonders of the human brain – II. Microanatomy

Contents

4

Wonders of the healthy brain - II. Microanatomy

The human brain is primarily composed of neurons, glial cells, neural stem cells, and blood vessels as further detailed in the following sections. This chapter will also present the cerebrospinal fluid, the blood supply through the internal carotid and vertebral arteries. It further describes the blood drainage and the blood-brain barrier (BBB)

Cell types

The brain is made of about 100 billion nerve cells (called *neurons*) separated by about 100 trillion *synapses*, and several other cell types such as *glial cells* that help neurons survive and function. Glial cells hold neurons in place, provide them with nutrients, rid the brain of damaged cells and other cellular debris, and provide insulation to neurons in the brain and spinal cord...ideal housemaids! In fact, the brain has many more (~ 10 times more) glial cells than neurons. (Imagine ten mothers tending to any one child making sure it grows normally in a constantly cleaned environment!) Another essential feature of the brain is its enormous network of blood vessels, receiving ~ 20% of the body's blood supply even though it is only about 2% of the body's weight. Further, ~ 400 billion tiny blood vessels, or **capillaries**, carry oxygen, glucose (the brain's principal source of energy), nutrients, and hormones to brain cells so they can do their work and also carry away waste products.

Neurons

Neuron types include interneurons, pyramidal cells including Betz cells, motor neurons (upper and lower), and cerebellar Purkinje cells. By their body size, Betz cells are the largest cells in the nervous system. The adult human brain is estimated to contain 86 ± 8 billion neurons, with a roughly equal number (85 ± 10 billion) of non-neuronal cells. Out of these neurons, 16 billion (19%) are located in the cerebral cortex, and 69 billion (80%) are in the cerebellum.

A neuron consists of a cell body, an axon, and dendrites (Figure 4.1). Dendrites are often extensive branches that receive information in the form of signals from the axon terminals of other neurons. The signals received may cause the neuron to initiate an action potential (an electrochemical signal or nerve impulse) which is sent along its axon to the axon terminal to connect with the dendrites or with the cell body of another neuron.

An action potential is initiated at the initial segment of an axon, which contains a specialized complex of proteins. When an action potential reaches the axon terminal, it triggers the release of a neurotransmitter at a synapse, propagating a signal that acts on the target cell. These chemical neurotransmitters include dopamine, serotonin, gamma-aminobutyric acid (GABA), glutamate, and acetylcholine. GABA is the major inhibitory neurotransmitter in the brain, and glutamate is the major excitatory neurotransmitter. Neurons link at synapses to form neural pathways, neural circuits, and large elaborate network systems such as the salience network and the default mode network. The activity between them is driven by the process of neurotransmission.

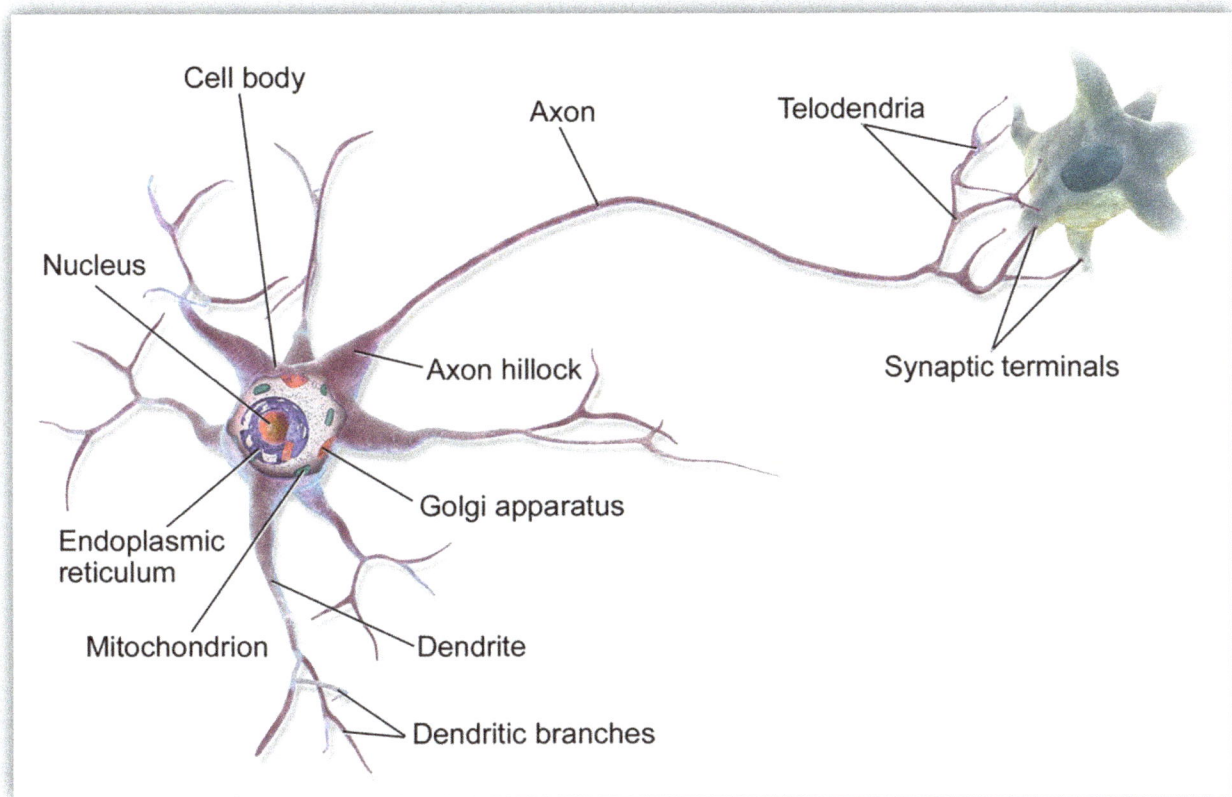

Figure 4.1 - A multipolar neuron

Cell body

Axon

Telodendria

Nucleus

Axon hillock

Synaptic terminals

Endoplasmic
reticulum

Golgi apparatus

Mitochondrion

Dendrite

Dendritic branches

Glial cells

Types of glial cell are astrocytes (including Bergmann glia), oligodendrocytes, ependymal cells (including tanycytes), radial glial cells, microglia, and a subtype of oligodendrocyte progenitor cells. Astrocytes are the largest of the glial cells. They are stellate cells with many processes radiating from their cell bodies. Some of these processes end as perivascular end-feet on capillary walls. The *glia limitans* of the cortex is made up of astrocyte foot processes that serve in part to contain the cells of the brain.

Mast cells

Mast cells are white blood cells that interact in the neuroimmune system in the brain. Mast cells in the central nervous system (CNS) are present in a number of structures including the meninges. They mediate neuroimmune responses in inflammatory conditions and help to maintain the BBB, particularly in brain regions where the barrier is absent. Mast cells serve the same general functions in the body and the CNS, such as effecting or regulating allergic responses, innate and adaptive immunity, autoimmunity, and inflammation. They also serve as the main effector cells through which pathogens can affect the biochemical signaling that takes place between the gastrointestinal tract and the CNS.

The cerebrospinal fluid

The cerebrospinal fluid (CSF) is a colorless trans-cellular fluid that circulates around the brain in the subarachnoid space, in the ventricular system, and in the central canal of the spinal cord. It also fills some gaps in the subarachnoid space, known as subarachnoid cisterns. The four ventricles (two lateral, a third, and a fourth ventricle) all contain the choroid plexus that produces the CSF. The third ventricle lies in the midline and is connected to the lateral ventricles. A single duct, the cerebral aqueduct between the *pons* and the *cerebellum*, connects the third ventricle to the fourth ventricle. Three separate openings, (one central and two lateral apertures) drain the CSF from the fourth ventricle to the *cisterna magnaone* of the major cisterns. From there, the CSF circulates around the brain and spinal cord in the subarachnoid space, between the *arachnoid mater* and the *pia mater*. At any one time, there is about 150 ml of CSF, mostly within the subarachnoid space. It is constantly being regenerated and absorbed, and is replaced about once every 5–6 hours.

A glymphatic system has been described as the lymphatic drainage system of the brain. The brain-wide glymphatic pathway includes drainage routes from the CSF and from the meningeal lymphatic vessels that are associated with the dural sinuses, and run alongside the cerebral blood vessels. The pathway drains interstitial fluid from the tissue of the brain.

Blood supply

The internal carotid arteries supply oxygenated blood to the front of the brain while the vertebral arteries supply blood to the back of the brain. These two circulations join together in the *circle of Willis*, a ring of connected arteries that lies in the inter-peduncular cistern between the midbrain and the pons.

Internal carotid arteries

The internal carotid arteries are branches of the common carotid arteries. They enter the *cranium* through the carotid canal, travel through the *cavernous sinus* and enter the *subarachnoid space*. They then enter the circle of Willis with two branches from which emerge the anterior cerebral arteries. These branches travel forward and then upward along the longitudinal fissure and supply the front and midline parts of the brain. One or more small anterior communicating arteries join the two anterior cerebral arteries shortly after they emerge as branches. The internal carotid arteries continue forward as the middle cerebral arteries. They travel sideways along the *sphenoid bone* of the eye socket, then upwards through the *insular cortex*, where final branches arise. The middle cerebral arteries send branches along their length.

Vertebral arteries

The vertebral arteries emerge as branches of the left and right subclavian arteries. They travel upward through the transverse foramina which are spaces in the cervical vertebrae. Each side enters the cranial cavity through the *foramen magnum* along the corresponding side of the medulla. They give off one of the three cerebellar branches. The vertebral arteries join in front of the middle part of the medulla to form the larger *basilar artery* (which sends multiple branches to supply the *medulla* and the *pons*) and the two other anterior and superior cerebellar branches. Finally, the basilar artery divides into two posterior cerebral arteries. These travel outwards, around the superior cerebellar peduncles, and along the top of the *cerebellar tentorium*, where it sends branches to supply the temporal and occipital lobes. Each posterior cerebral artery sends a small posterior communicating artery to join with the internal carotid arteries.

Blood drainage

Cerebral veins drain deoxygenated blood from the brain. The brain has two main networks of veins (exterior and interior), the exterior or superficial network on the surface of the cerebrum having three branches. These two networks communicate via anastomosing (joining) veins.

The veins of the brain drain into larger cavities of the dural venous sinuses usually situated between the *dura mater* and the covering of the skull. Blood from the cerebellum and midbrain drains into the great cerebral vein. Blood from the medulla and the pons of the brainstem have a variable pattern of drainage, either into the spinal veins or into adjacent cerebral veins. The blood in the deep part of the brain drains through a venous plexus into the cavernous sinus at the front, the superior and inferior petrosal sinuses at the sides, and the inferior sagittal sinus at the back. Blood drains from the outer brain into the large superior sagittal sinus, which rests in the midline on top of the brain. From there, it joins with the blood from the straight sinus at the confluence of sinuses. It then drains into the left and right transverse sinuses, draining into the sigmoid sinuses which receive blood from the cavernous sinus and superior and inferior petrosal sinuses. The sigmoid drains into the large internal jugular veins.

The blood–brain barrier

The larger arteries throughout the brain supply blood to smaller capillaries. These smallest of blood vessels in the brain are lined with cells joined by tight junctions so fluids do not seep-in or leak-out to the same degree as they do in other capillaries, creating the BBB. *Pericytes* play a major role in the formation of the tight junctions. The barrier is less permeable to larger molecules, but is still permeable to water, carbon dioxide, oxygen, and most fat-soluble substances (including anesthetics and alcohol). The BBB is not present in the circumventricular organs (these are structures in the brain that may need to respond to changes in body fluids) such as the *pineal gland*, the *area postrema*, and some areas of the *hypothalamus*. There is a similar blood–cerebrospinal fluid barrier B(CSF)B, which serves the same purpose as the BBB, but facilitates the transport of different substances into the brain due to the distinct structural characteristics between the two barrier systems.

Gross movement – such as locomotion and the movement of arms and legs – is generated in the motor cortex, divided into three parts: the primary motor cortex, found in the prefrontal gyrus with sections dedicated to the movement of different body parts. These movements are supported and regulated by two other areas lying anterior to the primary motor cortex: the premotor area and the supplementary motor area. The hands and mouth have a much larger area dedicated to them than other body parts, allowing finer movement; this has been visualized in a motor *homunculus*. Impulses generated from the motor cortex travel along the corticospinal tract along the front of the medulla and cross-over (decussate) at the *medullary pyramids*. They then travel down the spinal cord with most connecting to interneurons, in turn connecting to lower motor neurons within the grey matter that then transmits the impulse to move to muscles themselves. The *cerebellum* and the *basal ganglia*, play a role in fine, complex, and coordinated muscle movements. Connections between the cortex and the basal ganglia control muscle tone, posture, and movement initiation, and are referred to as the *extrapyramidal system*.

Take-aways

- The microanatomy of the human brain consists of neurons, glial cells, neural stem cells, and blood vessels.
- The cerebrospinal fluid, a colorless trans-cellular fluid, circulates around the brain in the subarachnoid space, in the ventricular system, and in the central canal of the spinal cord. It also fills some gaps in the subarachnoid space, known as subarachnoid cisterns. Three separate openings drain it. From there, the fluid circulates around the brain and spinal cord. It is constantly being regenerated and absorbed, and is replaced about once every 5–6 hours. The glymphatic system is the lymphatic drainage system of the brain.
- The internal carotid arteries supply oxygenated blood to the front of the brain while the vertebral arteries supply blood to the back of the brain. These two circulations join together in the *circle of Willis*, a ring of connected arteries.
- Cerebral veins drain the deoxygenated blood from the brain through two main networks of veins (exterior and interior) that communicate via anastomosing (joining) veins.

- The smallest blood vessels in the brain are lined with cells joined by tight junctions and so fluids do not seep-in or leak-out to the same degree as they do in other capillaries, creating the blood–brain barrier. The barrier is less permeable to larger molecules, but is still permeable to water, carbon dioxide, oxygen, and most fat-soluble substances (including anesthetics and alcohol). There is a similar blood–cerebrospinal fluid barrier, which serves the same purpose as the blood-brain barrier, but facilitates the transport of different substances into the brain due to the distinct structural characteristics between the two barrier systems.

- The brain allows us to carry out every element of our daily lives, manages our many body functions, and directs all the functions we carry out consciously because of the complicated mix of chemical and electrical processes that take place within it.

- The brain consumes up to 20% of the energy used by the human body, more than any other organ. In humans, blood glucose is the primary source of energy for most cells and is critical for normal function in a number of tissues, including the brain.

- Long-chain fatty acids cannot cross the blood–brain barrier, but the liver can break these down to produce ketone bodies. However, short-chain fatty acids (e.g., butyric acid, propionic acid, and acetic acid) and the medium-chain fatty acids, octanoic acid, and heptanoic acid can cross the barrier and be metabolized by brain cells.

- Although the human brain represents only 2% of the body weight, it receives 15% of the cardiac output, 20% of total body oxygen consumption, and 25% of total body glucose utilization. The brain mostly uses glucose for energy. Deprivation of glucose, as can happen in hypoglycemia, can result in loss of consciousness.

Sidebar 4.1 will briefly list a few of the 400 brain-specific genes.

Sidebar 4.1 - Brain-specific genes

Some 400 genes are shown to be brain-specific. In all neurons:

➢ ELAVL3 is expressed.

➢ In pyramidal neurons, NRGN and REEP2 are expressed.

➢ GAD1 (essential for the biosynthesis of the neurotransmitter GABA) is expressed in interneurons.

➢ Proteins expressed in glial cells are astrocyte markers for GFAP and S100B.

➢ Myelin basic protein is expressed in oligodendrocytes.

➢ The transcription factor, OLIG2, is also expressed in oligodendrocytes.

5

Wonders of the healthy brain – III. Functions

Contents

5

Wonders of the healthy brain – III. Functions

Special attention should be devoted to the several control functions exerted by the various brain structures. This chapter will discuss the healthy brain, its autonomic functions, and its physiology.

The healthy brain

The brain allows us to carry out every element of our daily lives, manages our many body functions, and directs all the functions we carry out consciously because of the complicated mix of chemical and electrical processes that take place within it.

The brain also plays a critical role in the body's perception of stress and its response to it. Stress is here considered in its most general sense (physical, chemical, physiological, emotional, etc.). However, pinpointing exactly which regions of the brain are responsible for particular aspects of a stress response is difficult and often unclear. The brain works not linearly but more in a network-like fashion, ferrying information about a stressful situation across several regions of the brain from cortical sensory areas to more basal structures and *vice versa.* This can help explain how stress and its negative consequences are heavily rooted in neural communication dysfunction.

The several functions of various brain areas and their mutual interactions are summarized in Table 5.1. However, the evidence for each one of them is variable and not always generally accepted. At the present time, the functions there displayed should therefore only be tentatively accepted.

Motor control

The frontal lobe is involved in reasoning, motor control, emotions, and language. It contains the motor cortex, which is involved in generation, planning, coordination, and control of movement; the prefrontal cortex, which is responsible for higher-level cognitive functioning; and Broca's area, which is essential for language production.

Generated movements pass from the brain through nerves to motor neurons in the body, which control the actions of muscles. The corticospinal tract carries movements from the brain, through the spinal cord, to the torso and limbs. The cranial nerves carry movements related to the eyes, mouth, and face.

Table 5.1 – Tentative brain areas functions and their interactions

Frontal lobe	Functions
	o Reasoning o Motor control o Emotions o Language
Motor cortex - Primary (prefrontal gyrus) - Pre-motor area - Supplementary area	o Generation, planning, coordination, and control of movement o Sections for movements of different body parts
Pre-frontal cortex	o Higher-level cognitive functioning
Lateral prefrontal cortex	o Generating emotions
Orbitofrontal cortex	o Generating emotions
Mid- and anterior insular cortex	o Generating emotions
Tuscaloosa cingulate cortex	o Sadness

Broca's, Knickers's areas (and a wider network of cortical regions)	o Language production
Cerebellum	o Fine, complex, and coordinated muscle movements
Basal ganglia	o Further controls muscle tone, posture, and movement initiation (extrapyramidal system) o Activation of happiness
Amygdala	o Elicitation of emotions such as fear
Ventral tegmental area	o Incentive salience
Ventral pallidum	o Incentive salience
Nucleus acumbens	o Incentive salience

Gross movement – such as locomotion and the movement of arms and legs – is generated in the motor cortex, divided into three parts: the primary motor cortex, found in the prefrontal gyrus with sections dedicated to the movement of different body parts. These movements are supported and regulated by two other areas lying anterior to the primary motor cortex: the premotor area and the supplementary motor area. The hands and mouth have a much larger area dedicated to them than other body parts, allowing finer movement; this has been visualized in a motor *homunculus*. Impulses generated from the motor cortex travel along the corticospinal tract along the front of the medulla and cross-over (decussate) at the *medullary pyramids*. They then travel down the spinal cord with most connecting to interneurons, in turn connecting to lower motor neurons within the grey matter that then transmits the impulse to move to muscles themselves. The *cerebellum* and the *basal ganglia*, play a role in fine, complex, and coordinated muscle movements. Connections between the cortex and the basal ganglia control muscle tone, posture, and movement initiation, and are referred to as the *extrapyramidal system*.

Sensory control

The sensory nervous system is involved with the reception and processing of sensory information. This information is received through the cranial nerves, through tracts in the spinal cord, and directly at centers of the brain exposed to the blood. The brain also receives and interprets information from the special senses of vision, smell, hearing, and taste. Mixed motor and sensory signals are also integrated.

From the skin, the brain receives information about fine touch, pressure, pain, vibration, and temperature. From the joints, the brain receives information about joint position. The sensory cortex is found just near the motor cortex and, like the motor cortex, has areas related to sensation from different body parts. Sensation collected by a sensory receptor on the skin is changed to a nerve signal that is passed up a series of neurons through tracts in the spinal cord. The dorsal column–*medial lemniscus* pathway contains information about fine touch, vibration, and position of joints. The pathway fibers travel up the back part of the spinal cord to the back part of the medulla, where they connect with second-order neurons that immediately send fibers across the midline. These fibers then travel upwards into the *ventrobasal complex* in the *thalamus* where they connect with third-order neurons, which send fibers up to the sensory cortex. The *spinothalamic tract* carries information about pain, temperature, and gross touch. The pathway fibers travel up the spinal cord and connect with second-order neurons in the reticular formation of the brainstem for pain and temperature, and also terminate at the *ventrobasal complex* of the *thalamus* for gross touch.

Vision

Vision is generated by light that hits the retina of the eye. Photoreceptors in the retina transduce the sensory stimulus of light into an electrical nerve signal that is sent to the visual cortex in the occipital lobe. Visual signals leave the retinas through the optic nerves. Optic nerve fibers from the retinas' nasal halves cross to the opposite sides joining the fibers from the temporal halves of the opposite retinas to form the optic tracts. The arrangements of the eyes' optics and the visual pathways mean vision from the left visual field is received by the right-half of each retina, is processed by the right visual cortex, and *vice versa*. The optic tract fibers reach the brain at the *lateral geniculate nucleus*, and travel through the optic nerve to reach the visual cortex.

Hearing and balance

Hearing and balance are both generated in the inner ear. Sound results in vibrations of the *ossicles*, which continue finally to the hearing organ and change in balance results in movement of liquids within the inner ear. This creates a nerve signal that passes through the *vestibulo-cochlear nerve*. From here, it passes through to the *cochlear nuclei*, the *superior olivary nucleus*, the *medial geniculate nucleus*, and finally the auditory radiation to the auditory cortex.

Smell

The sense of smell is generated by receptor cells in the epithelium of the olfactory mucosa in the nasal cavity. This information passes via the olfactory nerve which goes into the skull through a relatively permeable part. This nerve transmits to the neural circuitry of the *olfactory bulb* from where information is passed to the *olfactory cortex*.

Taste

Taste is generated from receptors on the tongue and passed along the facial and glossopharyngeal nerves into the solitary nucleus in the brainstem. Some taste information is also passed from the pharynx into this area via the vagus nerve. Information is then passed from there through the thalamus into the *gustatory complex*.

Autonomic functions of the brain

Autonomic functions of the brain include the regulation, or rhythmic control of the heart rate and rate of breathing, and maintaining homeostasis.

Regulation

Blood pressure and heart rate are influenced by the vasomotor center of the medulla, which causes arteries and veins to be somewhat constricted at rest. It does this by influencing the sympathetic and parasympathetic nervous systems via the vagus nerve. Information about blood pressure is generated by baroreceptors in aortic bodies in the aortic arch, and passed to the brain along the afferent fibers of the vagus nerve. Information about the pressure changes in the carotid sinus comes from carotid bodies located near the carotid artery and this is passed via a nerve joining with the glossopharyngeal nerve. This information travels up to the solitary nucleus in the medulla. Signals from there influence the vasomotor center to adjust vein and artery constriction accordingly.

The brain controls the rate of breathing mainly by respiratory centers in the medulla and the pons, which control respiration by generating motor signals that are passed down the spinal cord along the phrenic nerve to the diaphragm and other muscles of respiration. This is a mixed nerve that carries sensory information back to the centers. There are four respiratory centers, three with a more clearly defined function, and an *apneustic center* with a less clear function. In the medulla, a dorsal respiratory group causes the desire to breathe in, receiving sensory information directly from the body. Also in the medulla, the ventral respiratory group influences breathing out during exertion. In the pons, the *pneumotaxic center* influences the duration of each breath, and the apneustic center seems to have an influence on inhalation. The respiratory centers directly sense blood carbon dioxide and pH.

Information about blood oxygen, carbon dioxide, and pH levels are also sensed on the walls of arteries in the peripheral chemoreceptors of the aortic and carotid bodies. This information is passed via the vagus and glossopharyngeal nerves to the respiratory centers. High carbon dioxide, an acidic pH, or low oxygen stimulate the respiratory centers. The desire to breathe-in is also affected by pulmonary stretch receptors in the lungs which, when activated, prevent the lungs from over-inflating by transmitting information to the respiratory centers via the vagus nerve.

The hypothalamus in the diencephalon is involved in regulating many functions of the body. Functions include neuroendocrine regulation, regulation of the circadian rhythm, control of the autonomic nervous system, and the regulation of fluid, and food intake.

Sleep

The circadian rhythm is controlled by two main cell groups in the hypothalamus. The anterior hypothalamus includes the *suprachiasmatic nucleus* and the ventrolateral preoptic nucleus which, through gene expression cycles, generates a roughly 24-hour circadian clock. In the circadian day an ultradian rhythm takes control of the sleeping pattern. Sleep is an essential requirement for the body and brain; it allows the closing down and resting of the body's systems. There are also findings that suggest that the daily build-up of toxins in the brain are removed during sleep. Whilst awake the brain consumes a fifth of the body's total energy needs. Sleep necessarily reduces this use and gives time for the restoration of energy-giving adenosyne triphosphate (ATP). The effects of sleep deprivation show the absolute need for sleep.

Appetite

The lateral hypothalamus contains *orexinergic neurons* that control appetite and arousal through their projections to the ascending reticular activating system. The hypothalamus controls the pituitary gland through the release of peptides such as oxytocin, and vasopressin, as well as dopamine into the median eminence.

Language

While language functions were traditionally thought to be localized to the *Wernicke's* and *Broca's* areas, it is now mostly accepted that a wider network of cortical regions contributes to language functions.

The study on how language is represented, processed, and acquired by the brain is called neuro-linguistics, which is a large multidisciplinary field drawing from cognitive neuroscience, cognitive linguistics, and psycholinguistics.

Emotions

Emotions are generally defined as two-step multi-component processes involving (a) elicitation followed by (b) psychological feelings, appraisal, expression, autonomic responses, and action tendencies. Attempts to localize basic emotions to certain brain regions have been controversial. Some research found no evidence for specific locations corresponding to emotions but, instead, found circuitry involved in general emotional processes. The *amygdala*, orbitofrontal *cortex*, mid and anterior insular cortex and lateral prefrontal cortex, appeared to be involved in generating the emotions, while weaker evidence was found for the ventral tegmental area, ventral *pallidum* and *nucleus accumbens* in incentive salience. Others, however, have found evidence of activation of specific regions such as the basal ganglia in happiness, the subcallosal cingulate cortex in sadness, and amygdala in fear (see Table 5.1)..

Cognition

The brain is responsible for **cognition** (which operates through numerous processes) and **executive functions**. Executive functions include the ability to:

1. Filter information and tune-out irrelevant stimuli with attentional control and cognitive inhibition;
2. Process and manipulate information held in **working memory**;
3. Think about multiple concepts simultaneously and switch tasks with cognitive flexibility;
4. Inhibit impulses and prepotent responses with inhibitory control; and
5. Determine the relevance of information or appropriateness of an action.

Higher-order executive functions require the simultaneous use of multiple basic executive functions, including planning and fluid intelligence (i.e., reasoning and problem-solving). The prefrontal cortex plays a significant role in mediating executive functions. Planning involves activation of the dorsolateral prefrontal cortex (DLPFC), anterior cingulate cortex, angular prefrontal cortex, right prefrontal cortex, and supramarginal gyrus. **Working memory** manipulation involves the DLPFC, the inferior frontal gyrus, and areas of the parietal cortex. Inhibitory control involves multiple areas of the prefrontal cortex, as well as the caudate nucleus and subthalamic nucleus (see Table 5.2).

Other functions

Through the autonomic projections, the hypothalamus is involved in regulating functions such as blood pressure, heart rate, breathing, sweating, and other homeostatic mechanisms. The hypothalamus also plays a role in thermal regulation and, when stimulated by the immune system, is capable of generating a fever. The hypothalamus is influenced by the kidneys when blood pressure falls. The renin released by the kidneys stimulates a need to drink. The hypothalamus also regulates food intake through autonomic signals and hormone release by the digestive system.

Table 5.2 – Brain areas associated with executive functions

Brain areas	Function
	Executive functions: o Filter information and tune-out irrelevant stimuli with attentional control and cognitive inhibition o Process and manipulate information held in **working memory** o Think about multiple concepts simultaneously and switch tasks with cognitive flexibility o Inhibit impulses and prepotent responses with inhibitory control o Determine the relevance of information or appropriateness of an action.
Prefrontal cortex	o Mediates executive functions o Inhibitory control
Dorsolateral prefrontal cortex (DLPFC)	o Planning o **Working memory** manipulation
Anterior cingulate cortex	o Planning
Angular prefrontal cortex	o Planning
Right prefrontal cortex	o Planning
Supramarginal gyrus	o Planning
Inferior frontal gyrus	o **Working memory** manipulation
Parietal cortex	o **Working memory** manipulation
Caudate nucleus	o Inhibitory control
Subthalamic nucleus	o Inhibitory control

Neurotransmission

Brain activity is made possible by the interconnections of neurons that are linked together to reach their targets.

A neuron consists of a cell body, axon, and dendrites (see Figure 3.6). Dendrites are often extensive branches that receive information in the form of signals from the axon terminals of other neurons. The signals received may cause the neuron to initiate an action potential (an electrochemical signal or nerve impulse) which is sent along its axon to the axon terminal, to connect with the dendrites or with the cell body of another neuron.

An action potential is initiated at the initial segment of an axon, which contains a specialized complex of proteins. When an action potential reaches the axon terminal, it triggers the release of a neurotransmitter at a synapse, propagating a signal that acts on the target cell. These chemical neurotransmitters (five in number) include dopamine, serotonin, GABA, glutamate, and acetylcholine. GABA is the major inhibitory neurotransmitter in the brain, and glutamate is the major excitatory neurotransmitter. Neurons link at synapses to form neural pathways, neural circuits, and large elaborate network systems such as the salience network and the default mode network. The activity between them is driven by the process of neurotransmission.

Metabolism

As already stated, the brain consumes up to 20% of the energy used by the human body, more than any other organ. In humans, blood glucose is the primary source of energy for most cells and is critical for normal function in a number of tissues, including the brain. The human brain consumes approximately 25% of blood glucose in fasted, sedentary individuals. Brain metabolism normally relies upon blood glucose as an energy source, but during times of low glucose (such as fasting, endurance exercise, or limited carbohydrate intake), the brain uses ketone bodies for fuel with a smaller need for glucose. The brain can also utilize lactate during exercise. It stores glucose in the form of glycogen, *albeit* in significantly smaller amounts than that found in the liver or skeletal muscle. Long-chain fatty acids cannot cross the blood–brain barrier (BBB), but the liver can break these down to produce ketone bodies. However, short-chain fatty acids (e.g., butyric acid, propionic acid, and acetic acid) and the medium-chain fatty acids, octanoic acid, and heptanoic acid can cross the BBB and be metabolized by brain cells.

Although the human brain represents only 2% of the body weight, it receives 15% of the cardiac output, 20% of total body oxygen consumption, and 25% of total body glucose utilization. The brain mostly uses glucose for energy. Deprivation of glucose, as can happen in hypoglycemia, can result in loss of consciousness. The energy consumption of the brain does not vary greatly over time but active regions of the cortex consume somewhat more energy than inactive regions - this fact forms the basis for the functional brain imaging methods of positron emission tomography (PET) and functional magnetic resonance imaging (fMRI). These functional imaging techniques provide a three-dimensional image of metabolic activity. A preliminary study showed that brain metabolic requirements in humans peak at about five years old.

The function of sleep is not fully understood; however, there is evidence that sleep enhances the clearance of metabolic waste products, some of which are potentially neurotoxic, from the brain and may also permit repair. Evidence suggests that the increased clearance of metabolic waste during sleep occurs via increased functioning of the glymphatic system. Sleep may also have an effect on **cognitive** function by weakening unnecessary connections.

Take-aways

> Special attention should be devoted to the several control functions exerted by the various brain structures. The brain allows us to carry out every element of our daily lives, manages our many body functions, and directs all the functions we carry out consciously because of the complicated mix of chemical and electrical processes that take place within it. Brain activity is made possible by the interconnections of neurons that are linked together to reach their targets.

➤ The brain plays a critical role in the body's perception of stress (physical, chemical, physiological, emotional, etc.) and its response to it. Pinpointing exactly which regions of the brain are responsible for particular aspects of a stress response is difficult and often unclear. The brain works not linearly but more in a network-like fashion, ferrying information about a stressful situation across several regions of the brain from cortical sensory areas to more basal structures and *vice versa.* This can help explain, for example, how stress and its negative consequences are heavily rooted in neural communication dysfunction.

➤ The brain is responsible for **cognition**, which functions through numerous processes and executive functions. Executive functions include the ability to filter information and tune-out irrelevant stimuli. The brain also plays a critical role in the body's perception of stress and its response to it.

➤ Higher-order executive functions require the simultaneous use of multiple basic executive functions. **Working memory** manipulation involves the dorsolateral prefrontal cortex, the inferior frontal gyrus, and areas of the parietal cortex. Inhibitory control involves multiple areas of the prefrontal cortex, as well as the caudate nucleus and subthalamic nucleus.

➤ Autonomic functions of the brain include the regulation, or rhythmic control of the heart rate and rate of breathing, and maintaining homeostasis. Through the autonomic projections, the hypothalamus is involved in regulating functions such as blood pressure, heart rate, breathing, sweating, and other homeostatic mechanisms. It also plays a role in thermal regulation, and when stimulated by the immune system, is capable of generating a fever. Further, it is influenced by the kidneys. Lastly, it regulates food intake through autonomic signals and hormone release by the digestive system.

➤ The frontal lobe is involved in reasoning, motor control, emotions, and language. It contains the motor cortex, which is involved in generation, planning, coordination, and control of movement; the prefrontal cortex, which is responsible for higher-level cognitive functioning; and Broca's area, which is essential for language production.

➤ Gross movement – such as locomotion and the movement of arms and legs – is generated in the motor cortex supported and regulated by the premotor area and the supplementary motor area. The *cerebellum* and the *basal ganglia*, play a role in fine, complex, and coordinated muscle movements. Connections between the cortex and the basal ganglia control muscle tone, posture, and movement initiation, and are referred to as the *extrapyramidal system*.

➢ The sensory nervous system is involved with the reception and processing of sensory information. The brain also receives and interprets information from the special senses of vision, smell, hearing, and taste. Mixed motor and sensory signals are also integrated.

➢ From the skin, the brain receives information about fine touch, pressure, pain, vibration, and temperature. From the joints, the brain receives information about joint position. The sensory cortex is found just near the motor cortex and, like the motor cortex, has areas related to sensation from different body parts.

➢ Vision is generated by light that hits the retina of the eye.

➢ Hearing and balance are both generated in the inner ear.

➢ The sense of smell is generated by receptor cells in the epithelium of the olfactory mucosa in the nasal cavity.

➢ Taste is generated from receptors on the tongue and passed along the facial and glossopharyngeal nerves into the solitary nucleus in the brainstem.

➢ Information about blood oxygen, carbon dioxide, and pH levels are also sensed on the walls of arteries in the peripheral chemoreceptors of the aortic and carotid bodies.

➢ The hypothalamus in the diencephalon is involved in regulating many functions of the body, including neuroendocrine regulation, regulation of the circadian rhythm, control of the autonomic nervous system, and regulation of fluid, and food intake.

➢ The circadian rhythm is controlled by two main cell groups in the hypothalamus. Sleep is an essential requirement for the body and brain; it allows the closing down and resting of the body's systems. The daily build-up of toxins in the brain are removed during sleep. Sleep necessarily reduces this use and gives time for the restoration of energy-giving adenosyne triphosphate.

➢ The lateral hypothalamus contains *orexinergic neurons* that control appetite and arousal.

➢ While language functions were traditionally thought to be localized to the *Wernicke's* and *Broca's* areas, it is now mostly accepted that a wider network of cortical regions contributes to language functions.

➢ Attempts to localize basic emotions to certain brain regions have been controversial. Some research found no evidence for specific locations corresponding to emotions but, instead, found circuitry involved in general emotional processes.

PART C
DISORDERS OF THE NEURODEGENERATED BRAIN

6

The pathogenic brain

Contents

6

The neurodegenerated brain

It is not my intent to cover in detail all the brain diseases but rather give a synoptic overview of them so as to position those diseases of interest to this book within their proper context (in bold **red** font). That view is best charted in Tables 6.1 through 6.4 below, which present the constellation of brain diseases. I will begin with the diseases of the central nervous system (CNS), which can be due to inflammation, brain encephalopathy, diseases of the spinal cord, and those due to either/both encephalopathy or spinal cord/myelopathy, as presented below. The identified multiple possible contributors to memory impairments would theoretically need to be considered, as appropriate, for a correct diagnosis and treatment.

Diseases of the central nervous system - Inflammation

CNS diseases due to inflammation are shown in Table 6.1:

Table 6.1 – Diseases of the central nervous system: Inflammation

Pathology	Organ	Disorders/diseases
Inflammation	Brain	o Amoebic brain abscess (ABA) o Cavernous sinus thrombosis (CST) - Septic - Aseptic o **Encephalitis:** - Herpes viral - Lethargica - Limbic - Viral
	Spinal cord	o Epidural abscess o **Myelitis:** - Polio - Transverse o Tropical spastic paraparesis
	Either/both	Acute/disseminated Myalgic o **Myelitis:** - Encephalo- - Meningo-

Brain

➢ **Amoebic brain abscess (ABA):** An affliction caused by the anaerobic parasitic protist *Entamoeba histolytica*. It is extremely rare, the first case having been reported in 1849. These abscesses are difficult to diagnose and very few case reports suggest complete recovery even after the administration of appropriate treatment regimen. (Figure 6.1 is a copy of a brain MRI scan in a patient with lung cancer, +RT for brain metastasis: red T1; green PD tse; blue T2 tse.)

Figure 6.1 – MRI scan of an amoebic brain abscess (ABA)

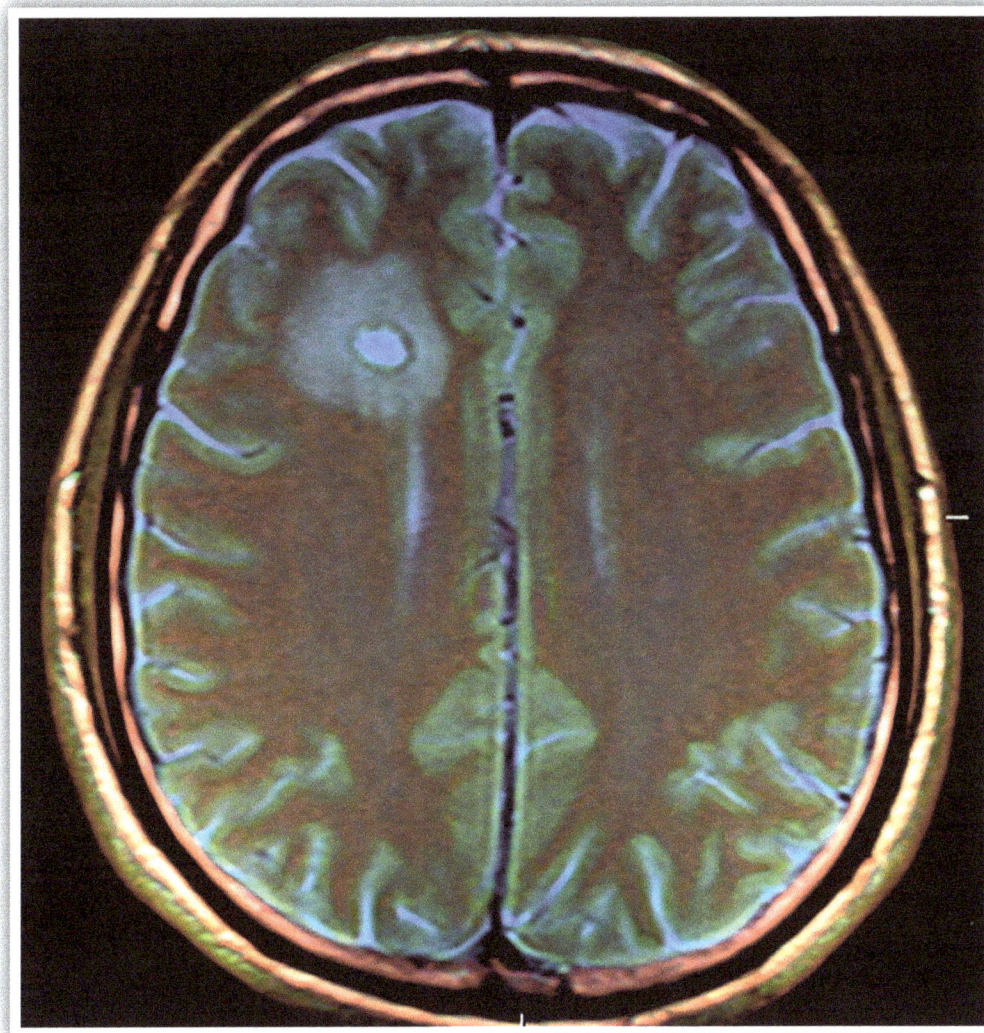

Reference: Nevit Dilmen

> **Cavernous sinus thrombosis (CST):** The formation of a blood clot within the cavernous sinus, which is a cavity at the base of the brain which drains deoxygenated blood from the brain back to the heart. This is a rare disorder and can be of two types–septic and aseptic. The most common form is the septic one; its cause is usually from a spreading infection in the nose, sinuses, ears, or teeth. *Staphylococcus aureus* and *Streptococcus* are often the associated bacteria. CST symptoms include: Decrease or loss of vision, chemosis, exophthalmos (bulging eyes), headaches, and paralysis of the cranial nerves. This infection is life-threatening and requires immediate treatment, which usually

includes antibiotics and sometimes surgical drainage. The cause of the aseptic form is usually associated with trauma, dehydration, anemia, and other disorders (see Figure 6.2).

Figure 6.2 – Cavernous sinus thrombosis (CST)

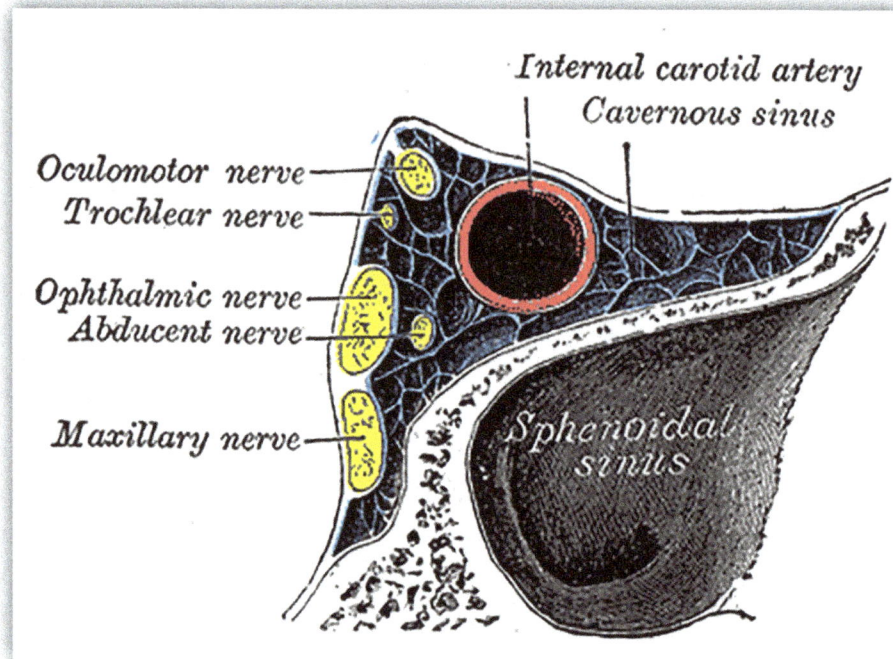

Reference: Henry Vandyke Carter and Henry Gray's Anatomy of the Human Body (Plate 571)

➤ **Encephalitis:** Inflammation of the brain. The severity can be variable with symptoms including **reduction or alteration in consciousness, memory problems**, and other symptoms (headache, fever, confusion, a stiff neck, and vomiting). Complications may include seizures, hallucinations, trouble speaking, and problems with hearing. Causes of encephalitis include viruses such as herpes simplex virus (HSV) and rabies virus as well as bacteria, fungi, or parasites. Other causes include autoimmune diseases and certain medications. However, in many cases the cause remains unknown. Risk factors include a weak immune system. Diagnosis is typically based on symptoms and supported by blood tests, medical imaging, and analysis of cerebrospinal fluid. Certain types are preventable with vaccines, antiviral medications (such as *Acyclovir*), anticonvulsants, and corticosteroids.

Spinal cord

- ➢ **Epidural abscess:** Refers to a collection of pus and infectious material located in the epidural space superficial to the *dura mater* which surrounds the CNS. Due to its location adjacent to brain or spinal cord, these abscesses have the potential to cause weakness, pain, and paralysis.

- ➢ **Myelitis:** Inflammation of the spinal cord which can disrupt the normal responses from the brain to the rest of the body, and from the rest of the body to the brain. It can cause the myelin and axon to be damaged resulting in symptoms such as paralysis and sensory loss. Myelitis is classified in several categories depending on the area or the cause of the lesion; however, any inflammatory attack on the spinal cord is often referred to as transverse myelitis. (Figure 6.3 is a coronal T2-weighted MR image showing high signal in the temporal lobes including hippocampal formations and parahippocampal gyrae, insulae, and right inferior frontal gyrus.)

Figure 6.3 – MRI image of an encephalitis

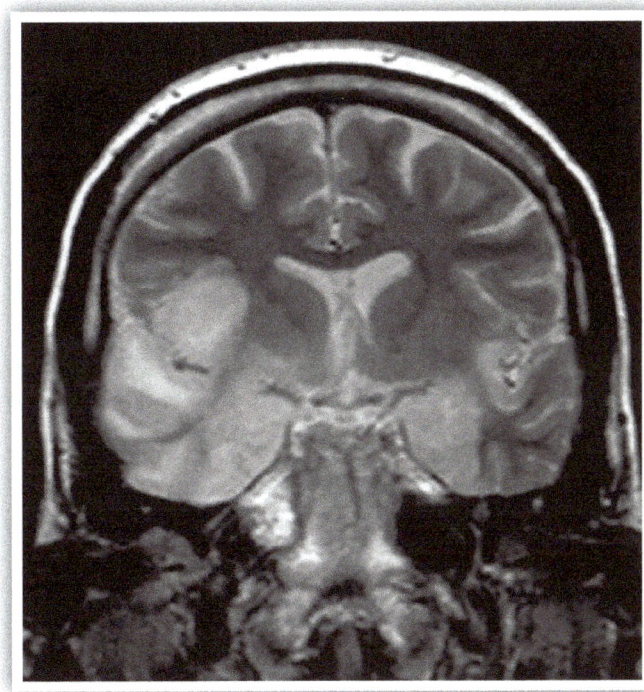

Reference: Laughlin Dawes - http://www.radpod. org/2007/03/24/herpes-simplex-encephalitis/

When it comes to brain inflammation, only encephalitis would be of concern regarding **memory** and **cognition.**

Diseases of the central nervous system - Brain encephalopathy

Likewise, Table 6.2 lists the disorders/diseases due to brain encephalopathy whether degenerative, demyelinating, episodic/paroxysmal, cerebrospinal fluid, or other causes:

Table 6.2 - Diseases of the central nervous system: Brain encephalopathy

Pathology	Characteristics	Disease category	Disorders/diseases
Encephalopathy	**A. Degenerative**	**Extrapyramidal & movement disorders**	o Akathisia o Athetosis o Basal ganglia disease o Blepharospasm o Chorea o Choreoathetosis o Dyskinesia o Dystonia o Epilepsy - Myoclonic o Hemiballismus o **Huntington's disease (HD)** o Meige's syndrome (MS) o **Myoclonus** - **Alzheimer's disease (AD)** - Gaucher's disease (GD), - **Creutzfeldt–Jakob disease (CJD)** - Subacute sclerosing panencephalitis, o Neuroleptic malignant syndrome (NMS)

			o Osteoarthritis (OA)
			o **Parkinson's disease (PD)**
			o **Parkinsonism**
			o **Pantothenate kinase-associated neurodegeneration (PKAN)**
			o **Progressive supranuclear palsy(PSP)**
			o Restless legs syndrome (RLS)
			o Spasmodic torticollis (ST)
			o Status dystonicus (SD)
			o Stiff person syndrome (SPS)
			o Striatonigral degeneration (SND) or multiple system atrophy (MSA)
			o Tauopathy
			o Tremor - Essential - Intentional
		Dementia	o **Alzheimer's disease (AD)**
			o **Aphasia: Primary progressive (PPA)**
			o **Atrophy: Posterior cortical (PCA)**
			o **Degeneration: frontotemporal lobar (FLD)**
			o **Dementia:** - **Early onset** - **Frontotemporal (or Pick's disease)** - **HIV** - **Juvenile**

			- **Lewy body dementias (LBD)**
			    - **with Lewy bodies**
			  - **Late onset**
			  - **Pugilistica**
			  - **Vascular**
			o **Parkinson's disease (PD)**
			o **Synucleinopathies**
			o **Tauopathy**
			o Leigh's syndrome (LS)

		Mitochondrial DNA disease	o Mitochondrial DNA depletion syndrome (MDS or MDDS) or Alpers' disease (AD)

	B. Demyelinating		o Autoimmune:
			  - **Multiple sclerosis (MS)**
			  - Neuromyelitis optica (NMO) and NMO spectrum disorder (NMOSD)
			  - Schilder's disease (SD): May include adrenoleukodystrophy (ALD) or diffuse myelinoclastic sclerosis (DMS).
			o Hereditary:
			  - Alexander's disease (AD)
			  - CAMFAK syndrome
			  - **Canavan's disease (CD)** or Canavan–Van Bogaert–Bertrand disease (CBBD)
			  - Krabbe's disease (KD) or globoid cell leukodystrophy (GCL) or galactosylceramide lipidosis (GSL)
			  - Marchiafava–Bignami disease (MBD)

			- MFC
			- ML
			- Myelinolysis: central pontine
			- PMD
			- VWM
	C. Episodic/ paroxysmal	**Seizure/epilepsy**	o **Dravet's syndrome (DS)** - Focal - Generalized o Epilepsy: - Myoclonic - Status *epilepticus* o **Lennox-Gastaut syndrome (LGS)** - West's syndrome (WS)
		Headache	o Migraine - Cluster - Familial - Tension
		Cerebrovascular	o ACA o **Aphasia: acute** o Amaurosis *fugax* o Foville's syndrome (FS) o MCA o Medullary: - Lateral - Medial o Millard–Gubler disease (MGD) o PCA o **Stroke** - Lacunar - Transient ischemic attack (TIA) o **Transient global amnesia (TGA)** - **Anterograde amnesia** o Weber's syndrome (WS)

		Sleep disorders	o Cataplexy
			o Circadian rythm
			o Insomnia
			- Hyper
			- Hypo
			o Klein-Levin disease (KLD)
			o Narcolepsy
			o **Sleep apnea**
			- Hypoventilation syndrome:
			- Congenital Central
			o Sleep disorder:
			- Advanced phase
			- Delayed phase
			- Non-24 hour wake
			- Jet lag
	D. Cerebrospinal fluid	o Cerebral edema	
		o Choroid plexus papilloma (CPP)	
		o Hydrocephalus: Normal pressure (NPH)	
		o Hyper/hypotension: Intracranial idiopathic	
	E. Others	o Brain herniation	
		o **Encephalopathy:**	
		- **Wernicke's (WE)**	
		- **Anti-NMDA receptor**	
		- **HIV encephalopathy**	
		- Hashimoto's encephalopathy (HE)	
		o Reye's encephalopathy (RE)	

A. Encephalopathy - Degenerative

Extrapyramidal and movement disorders

- **Akathisia:** A movement disorder characterized by a subjective feeling of inner restlessness accompanied by mental distress and an inability to sit still. The most severe cases may result in aggression, violence, and/or suicidal thoughts. Akathisia is also associated with threatening behavior and physical aggression. Antipsychotic medications are a leading cause. It may also occur upon stopping antipsychotics. Diagnosis differs from restless leg syndrome (RLS) – see below - in that akathisia is not associated with sleeping although the two conditions may share symptoms in individual cases.

- **Athetosis:** A symptom characterized by slow, involuntary, convoluted, writhing movements of the fingers, hands, toes, and feet and in some cases, arms, legs, neck, and tongue. Lesions to the brain are most often the direct cause of the symptoms, particularly to the *corpus striatum*. Athetosis is often accompanied by the symptoms of cerebral palsy, as it is often a result of this physical disability.

- **Basal ganglia disease (BGD):** A group of physical problems caused by the failure of the basal ganglia (nuclei) to properly suppress unwanted movements or to properly prime upper motor neuron circuits to initiate motor function. (The diagram in Figure 6.4 illustrates the basal ganglia in red and related structures in blue within the brain.) These disorders are known as hypokinetic disorders, which can leads to the inability to suppress unwanted movements. One possible causal factor could be the natural accumulation of iron in the basal ganglia, causing neurodegeneration due to its involvement in toxic, free-radical reactions. Basal ganglia disorders can lead to other dysfunctions such as obsessive–compulsive disorder (OCD) and Tourette's syndrome (TS).

- **Blepharospasm:** Any abnormal contraction of the orbicularis oculi muscle. In most cases, symptoms last for a few days and then disappear without treatment, but in some cases the twitching is chronic and persistent, causing life-long challenges. In these cases, the symptoms are often severe enough to result in functional blindness.

➢ **Chorea:** An abnormal involuntary movement disorder, one of a group of neurological disorders called dyskinesias. The quick movements of the feet or hands are comparable to dancing.

Figure 6.4 - Diagram of the basal ganglia and related structures within the brain

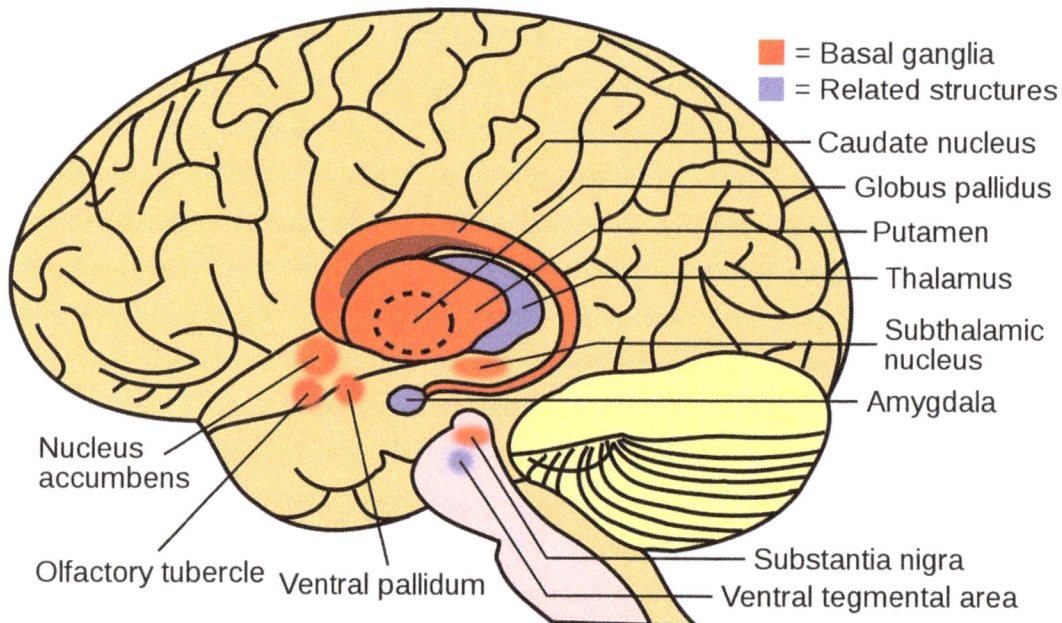

- = Basal ganglia
- = Related structures

Caudate nucleus
Globus pallidus
Putamen
Thalamus
Subthalamic nucleus
Amygdala
Nucleus accumbens
Olfactory tubercle
Ventral pallidum
Substantia nigra
Ventral tegmental area

➢ **Choreoathetosis:** The occurrence of involuntary movements in a combination of chorea (irregular migrating contractions) and athetosis (twisting and writhing). It is caused by many different diseases and agents. It is a symptom of several diseases, including Lesch–Nyhan syndrome (LNS), phenylketonuria (PKU), and Huntington's disease (HD) – see below - and can be a feature of kernicterus (rapidly increasing unconjugated bilirubin that cross the blood-brain-barrier in infants). It is also a common presentation of dyskinesia as a side effect of *Levodopa-Carbidopa* in the treatment of Parkinson's disease (PD).

➢ **Dyskinesia:** Refers to a category of movement disorders that are characterized by involuntary muscle movements, including movements similar to tics or chorea and diminished voluntary movements. It can be anything from a slight tremor of the hands to an uncontrollable movement of the upper body or lower extremities.

➢ **Dystonia:** A neurological hyperkinetic movement disorder in which sustained or repetitive muscle contractions result in twisting and repetitive movements or abnormal fixed postures. The movements may resemble a tremor. Dystonia is often intensified or exacerbated by physical activity, and symptoms may progress into adjacent muscles. The disorder may be hereditary or caused by other factors such as birth-related or other physical trauma, infection, poisoning (e.g., lead poisoning) or reaction to pharmaceutical drugs, particularly neuroleptics, or stress.

> **Epilepsy:** A group of non-communicable neurological disorders characterized by recurrent epileptic seizures. An epileptic seizure is the clinical manifestation of an abnormal, excessive, purposeless, and synchronized electrical discharge in the brain cells called neurons. Epileptic seizures can vary from brief and nearly undetectable periods to long periods of vigorous shaking due to abnormal electrical activity in the brain, tend to recur, and may have no immediate underlying cause. These episodes can result in physical injuries (e.g., broken bones, causing accidents). The underlying mechanism is excessive and abnormal neuronal activity in the brain cortex. The cause is unknown but may occur as the result of brain injury, stroke, brain tumors, infections of the brain, or birth defects through a process known as epileptogenesis. Known genetic mutations are directly linked to a small proportion of cases.

> **Hemiballismus** (or hemiballism): A basal ganglia syndrome resulting from damage to the subthalamic nucleus in the basal ganglia. It is a rare hyperkinetic movement disorder characterized by violent involuntary limb movements on one side of the body, which can cause significant disability. Ballismus affects both sides of the body and is much rarer. Hemiballismus differs from chorea in that the movements occur in the proximal limbs whereas in chorea the limb movements are in the distal limbs. Also in chorea the movements are more dance-like, flowing from one region to another.

> **Huntington's disease (HD)** or **Huntington's chorea (HC):** An incurable neurodegenerative disease that is mostly inherited. The earliest symptoms are often subtle problems with mood or mental/psychiatric abilities. (Figure 6.5 is a study using a robotic microscope to show how mutant HD's protein affects neurons.) A general lack of coordination and an unsteady gait often follow. It is also a basal ganglia

disease causing a hyperkinetic movement disorder known as chorea. As the disease advances, uncoordinated, involuntary body movements of chorea become more apparent. Physical abilities gradually worsen until coordinated movement becomes difficult and the person is unable to talk. Mental abilities generally decline into **dementia**, depression, apathy, and impulsivity at times.

➢ **Meige's syndrome (MS)** or **Brueghel's syndrome (BS)** or **oral facial dystonia OFD):** A type of dystonia. It is actually a combination of two forms of dystonia, blepharospasm and oromandibular dystonia (OMD). The combination of upper and lower dystonia is sometimes called cranial-cervical dystonia.

➢ **Myoclonus:** A brief, involuntary, irregular (lacking rhythm) twitching of a muscle, a joint, or a group of muscles, different from clonus, which is rhythmic or regular. It describes a medical sign and, generally, is not a diagnosis of a disease. These myoclonic twitches, jerks, or seizures are usually caused by sudden muscle contractions (positive myoclonus) or brief lapses of contraction (negative myoclonus). The most common circumstance under which they occur is while falling asleep (hypnic jerk). They can be a sign of various neurological disorders. They may occur alone or in sequence, in a pattern or without pattern. They may occur infrequently or many times each minute.

Figure 6.5 – Mutant Huntington's disease (HD) proteins affecting neurons

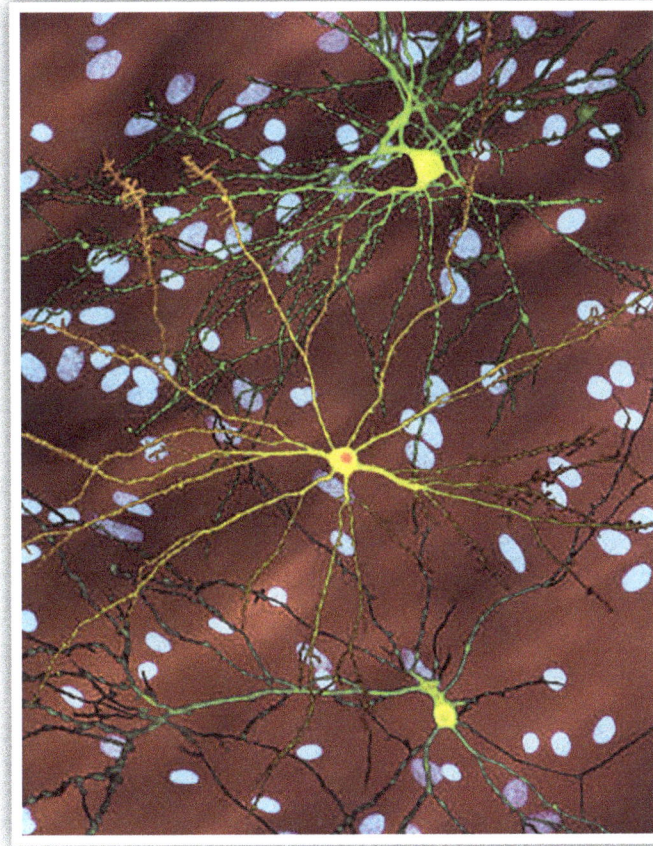

Source: Steven Finkbeiner, Gladstone Institute of Neurological Disease, The Taube-Koret Center for Huntington's Disease Research, and the University of California San Francisco.

Most often, myoclonus is one of several signs in a wide variety of nervous system disorders such as multiple sclerosis (MS), **Parkinson's disease (PD)**, dystonia, cerebral palsy, **Alzheimer's disease (AD)**, Gaucher's disease (GD), **Creutzfeldt–Jakob disease (CJD)**, subacute sclerosing panencephalitis, serotonin toxicity, some cases of Huntington's disease, some forms of epilepsy, and occasionally in intracranial hypotension.

Figure 6.6 – MRI of sporadic Creutzfeldt-Jakob disease

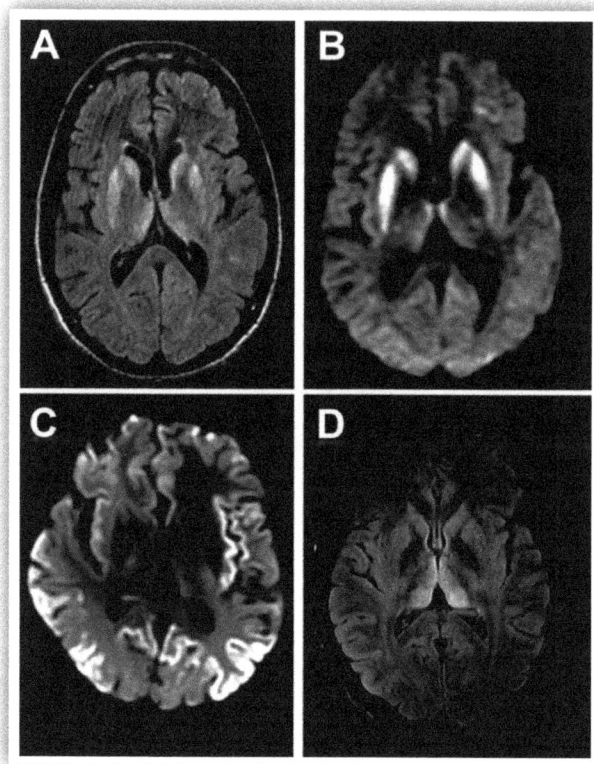

Reference: Pract Neurol - https://www.ncbi.nlm.nih.gov/pmc/articles/PMC5520355/figure/F2/

In almost all instances in which myoclonus is caused by CNS disease, it is preceded by other symptoms; for instance, in CJD it is generally a late-stage clinical feature that appears after the patient has already started to exhibit gross neurological deficits. Anatomically, myoclonus may originate from lesions of the cortex, subcortex or spinal cord.

○ **Gaucher's disease (GD):** A genetic disorder in which the enzyme glucocerebroside (a sphingolipid, also known as glucosylceramide) accumulates in cells and certain organs. The disorder is characterized by bruising, fatigue, anemia, low blood platelet count, and enlargement of the liver and spleen. The enzyme can collect in the spleen, liver, kidneys, lungs, brain, and bone marrow. Manifestations may include enlarged spleen and liver, liver malfunction, skeletal disorders or bone lesions that may be painful, severe neurological complications, swelling of lymph nodes and (occasionally) adjacent joints, distended abdomen, a brownish tint to the skin, anemia, low blood platelet count, and yellow fatty deposits on the white of the eye (sclera).

- **Creutzfeldt-Jakob disease (CJD),** also known as **subacute spongiform encephalopathy** or **neurocognitive disorder due to prion disease.** It is an invariably fatal degenerative brain disorder. Early symptoms include **memory** problems, behavioral changes, poor coordination, and visual disturbances. Later symptoms include **dementia**, involuntary movements, blindness, weakness, and coma. About 70% of people die within a year of diagnosis. CJD is caused by a type of abnormal protein known as a prion. Infectious prions are misfolded proteins that can cause normally folded proteins to also become misfolded.

- **Subacute sclerosing panencephalitis** (**SSPE**) also known as **Dawson's disease (DD):** It is a rare form of progressive brain inflammation caused by a persistent infection with the measles virus. The condition primarily affects children, teens, and young adults. It is almost always fatal and should not be confused with acute disseminated encephalomyelitis (ADE), which can also be caused by the measles virus, but has a very different timing and course.

- **Neuroleptic malignant syndrome (NMS):** A rare but life-threatening reaction that can occur in response to neuroleptic or antipsychotic medication. Symptoms include high fever, confusion, rigid muscles, variable blood pressure, sweating, and fast heart rate. Complications may include rhabdomyolysis, high blood potassium, kidney failure, or seizures.

- **Osteoarthritis (OA):** A type of degenerative joint disease that results from breakdown of joint cartilage and underlying bone. The most common symptoms are joint pain and stiffness. Other symptoms may include joint swelling, decreased range of motion, and, when the back is affected, weakness or numbness of the arms and legs. Causes include previous joint injury, abnormal joint or limb development, and inherited factors. OA is believed to be caused by mechanical stress on the joint and low grade inflammatory processes.

- **Parkinson's disease (PD):** A chronic degenerative disorder of the CNS that mainly affects the motor system. The symptoms usually emerge slowly, and as the disease worsens, non-motor symptoms become more common. Early symptoms are tremor, rigidity, slowness of movement, and difficulty with walking. Problems may also arise with **cognition**, behavior, sleep, and sensory systems. Parkinson's disease **dementia** becomes common in advanced stages of the disease. The motor symptoms of the disease result from the death of nerve cells in the substantia nigra, a region of the midbrain that supplies dopamine to the basal ganglia. The cause of this cell death is poorly understood, but involves the aggregation of the protein alpha-synuclein into Lewy bodies within the neurons. The cause of PD is unknown, but a combination of genetic and environmental factors are believed to play a role.

Figure 6.7 – MRI of the pantothenate kinase-associated neurodegeneration

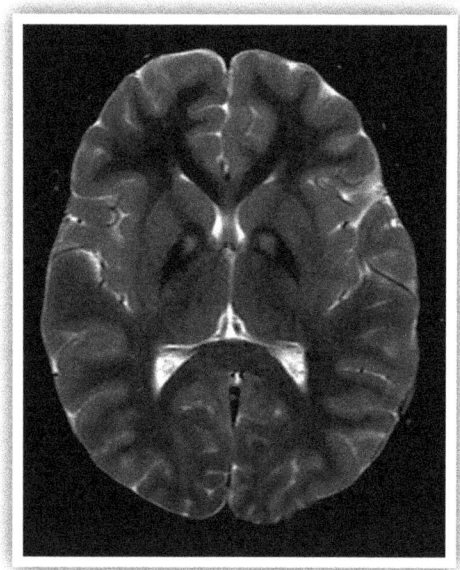

> **Parkinsonism:** A clinical syndrome characterized by tremor, bradykinesia (slowed movements), rigidity, and postural instability. It usually leads to **dementia with Lewy bodies (DLB), Parkinson's disease dementia (PDD)**, and many other conditions. This set of symptoms occurs in a wide range of conditions and may have many causes, including neurodegenerative conditions, drugs, toxins, metabolic diseases, and other conditions than PD.

> **Pantothenate kinase-associated neurodegeneration (PKAN)** also known as **Hallervorden-Spatz syndrome (HSS)** is a genetic degenerative disease of the brain that can lead to **parkinsonism**, dystonia, **dementia**, and ultimately death. Neurodegeneration in PKAN is accompanied by an excess of iron that progressively builds up in the brain. (The MRI image of Figure 6.7 used a T2-weighed GRASE sequence to shows iron deposits in the basal ganglia, the so-called eye-of-the-tiger sign.)

> **Progressive supranuclear palsy (PSP):** A late-onset neurodegenerative disease involving the gradual deterioration and death of specific volumes of the brain. The condition leads to symptoms including loss of balance, slowing of movement, difficulty moving the eyes, and **cognitive impairment**. PSP may be mistaken for other types of neurodegeneration such as PD, frontotemporal dementia (FTD), and Alzheimer's disease (AD). The cause of the condition is uncertain, but involves the accumulation of the tau-protein within the brain. (Figure 6.8 is a sagittal T1-weigted MRI image showing atrophy of the midbrain, with preservation of the volume of the pons. This appearance has been called the "penguin sign")

> **Restless legs syndrome (RLS)** or **Willis–Ekbom disease (WED):** Generally, a long-term disorder that causes a strong urge to move one's legs. This is often described as aching, tingling, or crawling in nature. Due to the disturbance in sleep, people with RLS may have daytime sleepiness, low energy, irritability and a depressed mood. Additionally, many have limb twitching during sleep, a condition known as periodic limb movement disorder. Risk factors for RLS include low iron levels, kidney failure, **PD**, diabetes mellitus, rheumatoid arthritis, pregnancy and celiac disease.

> **Spasmodic torticollis (ST)** or **cervical dystonia (CD):** An extremely painful chronic neurological movement disorder causing the neck to involuntarily turn to the left, right, upwards, and/or downwards. Both agonist and antagonist muscles contract simultaneously. Causes of the disorder are predominantly idiopathic.

> **Status dystonicus** (SD): A serious and potentially life-threatening disorder which occurs in people who have primary or secondary dystonia. Symptoms consist of widespread severe muscle contractions.

- **Stiff-person syndrome (SPS)** or **stiff-man syndrome (SMS):** A rare neurologic disorder of unclear cause characterized by progressive muscular rigidity and stiffness. The stiffness primarily affects the truncate muscles and is superimposed by spasms, resulting in postural deformities. Chronic pain, impaired mobility, and lumbar hyperlordosis are common symptoms.

Figure 6.8 – Showing atrophy of the midbrain in progressive supranuclear palsy

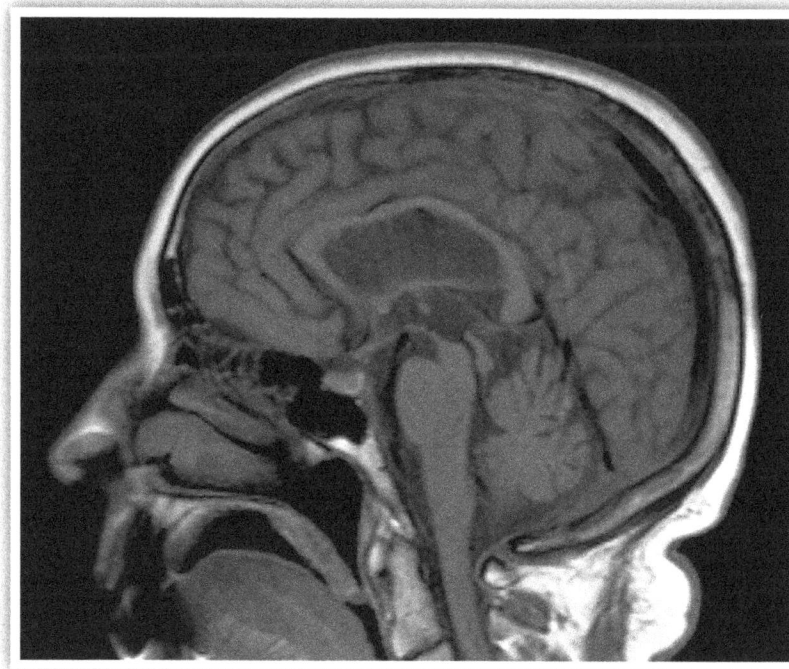

Reference: Laughlin Dawes - radpod.org

- **Striatonigral degeneration (SND)** or **multiple system atrophy (MSA):** A rare neurodegenerative disorder characterized by autonomic dysfunction, tremors, slow movement, muscle rigidity, and postural instability (collectively known as parkinsonism) and ataxia. This is caused by progressive degeneration of neurons in several parts of the brain including the basal ganglia, inferior olivary nucleus, and cerebellum. It commonly manifests as orthostatic hypotension, impotence, loss of sweating, dry mouth, and urinary retention and incontinence. Palsy of the vocal cords is an important and sometimes initial clinical manifestation of the disorder. MSA often presents with some of the same symptoms as **PD**. MSA is distinct from multisystem proteinopathy, a more common muscle-wasting syndrome. It is also different from multiple organ dysfunction syndrome, sometimes referred to as multiple organ failure, and from multiple organ system failures, an often-fatal complication of septic shock and other severe illnesses or injuries.

> **Tauopathy:** It belongs to a class of neurodegenerative diseases involving the aggregation of tau protein into neurofibrillary or gliofibrillary tangles in the human brain. Tangles are formed by hyperphosphorylation of the microtubule protein known as tau, causing the protein to dissociate from microtubules and form insoluble aggregates.The mechanism of tangle formation is not well understood, and whether tangles are a primary cause of **AD** or play a peripheral role is unknown.

> **Tremor:** An involuntary, somewhat rhythmic, muscle contraction and relaxation involving oscillations or twitching movements of one or more body parts. It is the most common of all involuntary movements and can affect the hands, arms, eyes, face, head, vocal folds, trunk, and legs. Most tremors occur in the hands. In some people, a tremor is a symptom of another neurological disorder.

Dementias

> **Alzheimer's disease (AD):** A neurodegenerative disease that usually starts slowly and progressively worsens. It is the cause of 60%–70% of cases of **dementia**. The most common early symptom is progressive **memory** loss and difficulty in remembering recent events. As the disease advances, symptoms can include problems with language, disorientation (including easily getting lost), mood swings, loss of motivation, self-neglect, and behavioral issues. As a person's condition declines, they often withdraw from family and society. Gradually, bodily functions are lost, ultimately leading to death. Although the speed of progression can vary, the typical life expectancy following diagnosis is three to nine years. The cause of AD is poorly understood. There are many environmental and genetic risk factors associated with its development. The strongest genetic risk factor is from an allele of APOE. Other risk factors include a history of head injury, clinical depression, and high blood pressure. A probable diagnosis is based on

the history of the illness and cognitive testing, with medical imaging and blood tests to rule out other possible causes. Initial symptoms are often mistaken for normal brain aging. Good nutrition, physical activity, and engaging socially are known to be of benefit generally in aging, and may help in reducing the risk of **cognitive decline.** No current treatments can stop or reverse its progression, though some may temporarily improve symptoms.

➢ **Primary progressive aphasia** (**PPA**): A type of neurological syndrome in which language capabilities slowly and progressively become impaired. As with other types of aphasia, the symptoms that accompany PPA depend on what parts of the left hemisphere are significantly damaged. However, unlike most other aphasias, PPA results from continuous deterioration in brain tissue, which leads to early symptoms being far less detrimental than later symptoms. Those with PPA slowly lose the ability to speak, write, read, and generally comprehend language. Eventually, almost every patient becomes mute and completely loses the ability to understand both written and spoken language. Many, if not most of those with PPA experience impairment of **memory, short-term memory formation** and **loss of executive functions**. (Figure 6.9 shows regions of the left hemisphere that can give rise to aphasia when damaged.)

Figure 6.9 – Primary progressive aphasia

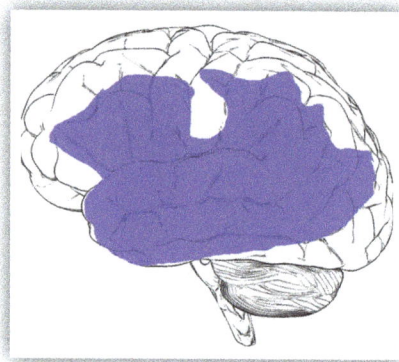

Reference: I. Henseler, F. Regenbrecht, and H. Obrig, 2014). doi: 10.1093/brain/awt374

➢ **Posterior cortical atrophy (PCA)** or **Benson's syndrome (BS):** A rare form of **dementia** which is considered a visual variant or an atypical variant of Alzheimer's disease (**AD**). The disease causes atrophy of the posterior part of the cerebral cortex, resulting in the progressive disruption of complex visual processing. PCA usually affects people at an earlier age than typical AD cases. In rare cases, PCA can be caused by dementia with Lewy bodies (**DLB**) and Creutzfeldt–Jakob disease (**CJD**). (Figure 6.10 shows brain lobes, main sulci, and boundaries.)

➤ **Frontotemporal lobar degeneration** (**FTLD**): A pathological process that occurs in **frontotemporal dementia (FTD)**. It is characterized by atrophy in the frontal lobe and temporal lobe of the brain, with sparing of the parietal and occipital lobes.

Figure 6.10 – Posterior cortical atrophy (PCA)

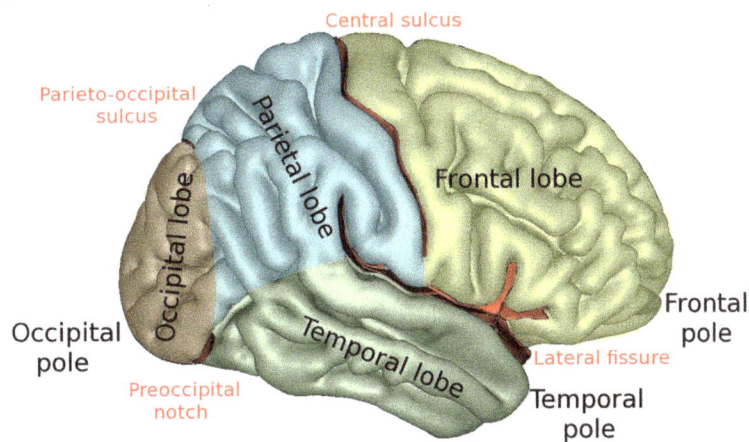

Reference: Sebastian023

➤ **Dementia:** The general name for a decline in cognitive abilities that impacts a person's ability to do everyday activities. This typically involves problems with **memory**, thinking, and behavior. Aside from memory impairment and a disruption in thought patterns, the most common symptoms include emotional problems, difficulties with language, and decreased motivation. The symptoms may be described as occurring in a continuum over several stages. A diagnosis of dementia requires the observation of a change from a person's usual mental functioning and a greater cognitive decline than what is caused by normal aging. Several diseases and injuries to the brain such as a stroke can give rise to dementia. However, the most common cause is **Alzheimer's disease**. Dementia is listed as an acquired brain syndrome, marked by a **decline in cognitive function**, and is contrasted with neurodevelopmental disorders. It is also described as a spectrum of disorders with causative subtypes of dementia based on a known disorder, such as Parkinson's disease for **Parkinson's disease dementia (PDD)**; Huntington's disease for **Huntington's disease dementia (HDD)**; vascular disease, for **vascular disease dementia (VDD)**; HIV infection causing **HIV dementia (HIVD)**; frontotemporal lobar degeneration for **frontotemporal dementia (FTLD)**; Lewy body disease for **dementia with Lewy bodies (DLB);** and prion diseases. Subtypes of neurodegenerative dementias may also be based on the underlying pathology of misfolded proteins such as synucleinopathies, and tauopathies. More than one type of dementia existing together is known as **mixed dementia (MD).**

Figure 6.11 - Illustrating the dopamine pathways throughout the brain

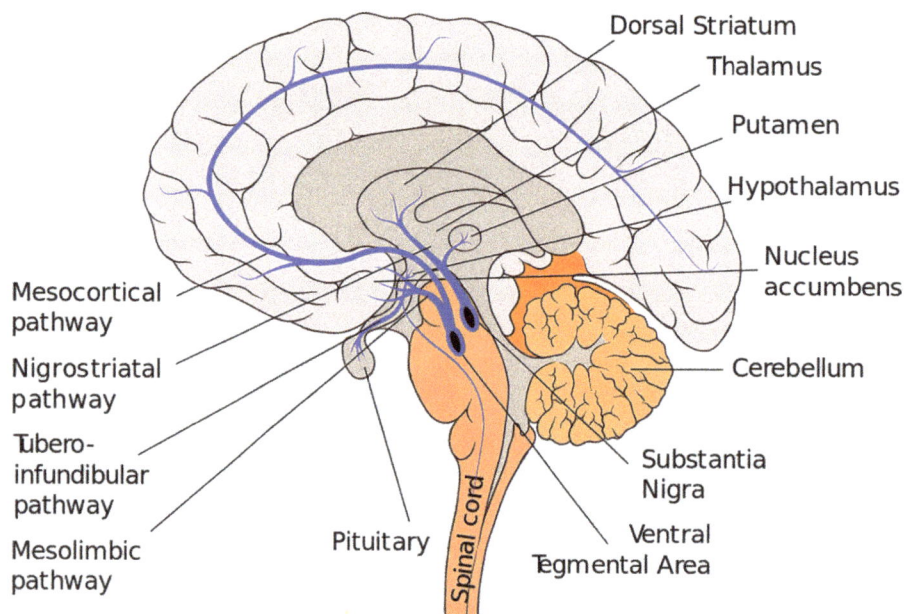

Source: Patrick J. Lynch

> **Synucleinopathies** (or **α-synucleinopathies**): Neurodegenerative diseases characterized by the abnormal accumulation of aggregates of alpha-synuclein protein in neurons, nerve fibers or glial cells. There are three main types: **Parkinson's disease (PD), dementia with**

Lewy bodies (DLB), and **multiple system atrophy (MSA)**. Other rare disorders, such as various neuroaxonal dystrophies, also have α-synuclein pathologies. [Figure 6.11 illustrates the main dopaminergic pathways of the human brain: the mesocortical pathway, connecting the ventral tegmental area (VTA) with the frontal cortex; the mesolimbic pathway, connecting the VTA with the nucleus accumbens; the nigrostriatal pathway, connecting the substantia nigra with the dorsal striatum; and the tuberoinfundibular pathway, connecting hypothalamus with pituitary.]

➢ **Leigh syndrome (LS)** or **Leigh disease (LD)** or **subacute necrotizing encephalomyelopathy (SANE):** An inherited neurometabolic disorder that affects the CNS. Normal levels of thiamine, thiamine monophosphate, and thiamine diphosphate are commonly found, but there is a reduced or absent level of thiamine triphosphate. This is thought to be caused by a blockage in the enzyme thiamine-diphosphate kinase.

Mitochondrial DNA

➢ **Mitochondrial DNA depletion syndrome (MDS or MDDS)** or **Alper's disease (AD):** Any of a group of autosomal recessive disorders that cause a significant drop in mitochondrial DNA in affected tissues. Symptoms can be any combination of myopathic, hepatopathic, or encephalomyopathic. These syndromes affect tissue in the muscle, liver, or both the muscle and brain, respectively. The condition is typically fatal in infancy and early childhood, though some have survived to their teenage years with the myopathic variant and some have survived into adulthood with the SUCLA2 encephalomyopathic variant.

B. Demyelinating

➢ **Autoimmune - Multiple sclerosis (MS) or multiple cerebrospinal sclerosis (MCSS):** The most common demyelinating disease in which the insulating covers of nerve cells in the brain and spinal cord are damaged. This damage disrupts the ability of parts of the nervous system to transmit signals, resulting in a range of signs and symptoms, including physical, **mental**, and sometimes **psychiatric problems**. Specific symptoms can include double vision, visual loss, muscle weakness, and trouble with sensation or coordination. MS takes several forms, with new symptoms either occurring in isolated attacks (relapsing forms) or building up over time (progressive forms).While the cause is unclear, the underlying mechanism is thought to be either destruction by the immune system or failure of the myelin-producing cells. Proposed causes for this include genetics and environmental factors, such as viral infections. No cure for MS is known. MS is the most common immune-mediated disorder affecting the CNS. (Figure 6.12 above schematically describes the main symptoms of MS. Note the **cognitive impairment.**)

➢ **Autoimmune - Neuromyelitis optica (NMO) and NMO spectrum disorders (NMOSD):** Autoimmune diseases characterized by acute inflammation of the optic nerve: optic neuritis (ON) and spinal cord (myelitis). Episodes of ON and myelitis can be simultaneous or successive. A relapsing disease course is common, especially in untreated patients.The etiology remains unknown (idiopathic NMO). NMO can be similar to MS in clinical and radiological presentation, and MS may very rarely present with an NMO-like phenotype. However, NMO is not related to MS in the vast majority of cases and differs from MS substantially in terms of pathogenesis, clinical presentation, magnetic resonance imaging, cerebrospinal fluid findings, disease course, and prognosis.

➢ **Autoimmune - Schilder's disease (SD):** May refer to two different diseases – **Adrenoleukodystrophy (ALD)** and **diffuse myelinoclastic sclerosis (DMS).**

Figure 6.12 – Main symptoms of multiple sclerosis

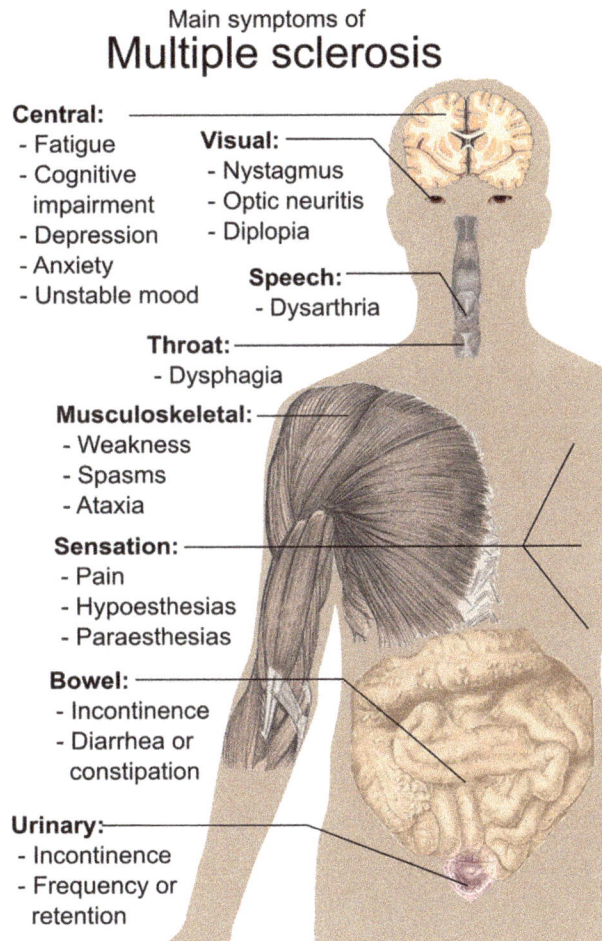

Source: Mikael Haggstrom

(a) **ALD:** A disease linked to the X chromosome. It is a result of fatty acid buildup caused by failure of peroxisomal fatty acid beta oxidation which results in the accumulation of very long chain fatty acids in tissues throughout the body. The most severely affected tissues are the myelin in the CNS, the adrenal cortex, and the Leydig cells in the testes.

(b) **DMS:** A very infrequent neurodegenerative disease that presents clinically as pseudotumoral demyelinating lesions, making its diagnosis difficult. It is considered one of the borderline forms of MS. Other diseases in this group are:

- Balo concentric sclerosis (BCS) also formerly known as **leuko-encephalitis periaxialis concentrica (LEPC):** BCS is a disease in which the white matter of the brain appears damaged in concentric layers, leaving the axis cylinder intact. It is a demyelinating disease similar to standard MS, but with the particularity that the demyelinated tissues form concentric layers. The concentric ring appearance is not specific to Baló's MS. Concentric lesions have also been reported in patients with neuromyelitis optica, standard MS, progressive multifocal leukoencephalopathy, cerebral autosomal dominant arteriopathy with subcortical infarcts, leukoencephalopathy, concomitant active hepatitis C and human herpes virus 6.

- **Marburg multiple sclerosis (MMS)** or **acute fulminant multiple sclerosis (AFMS):** MMS is considered one of the MS borderline diseases, which is a collection of diseases classified by some as MS variants and by others as different diseases. Other diseases in this group are neuromyelitis optica (NMO), Balo concentric sclerosis (BCS), and Schilder's disease (SD), and for some as tumefactive multiple sclerosis (TMS).

- **Hereditary - Alexander's disease (AD):** A very rare autosomal dominant leukodystrophy, which is a neurological condition caused by anomalies in the myelin which protects nerve fibers in the brain. The most common type is the infantile form that usually begins during the first two years of life. Symptoms include **mental** and physical developmental delays, followed by the loss of developmental milestones, an abnormal increase in head size and seizures. Adult-onset forms of AD are less common than the juvenile ones. The symptoms sometimes mimic those of PD or MS, or may present primarily as a psychiatric disorder. AD is a progressive and often fatal disease. Neuropathology of Alexander's disease. (Figure 6.13 is an archival image of the brain of a 4-year-old boy showing macroencephaly and periventricular demyelinization as noted by the brownish discoloration around the cerebral ventricles.)

- **Hereditary - CAMFAK (or CAMAK syndrome):** (The aconym "CAMFAK" comes from the first letters of the characteristic findings of the disease: **ca**taracts, **m**icrocephaly, **fa**ilure to thrive, and kyphoscoliosis.) A rare inherited neurologic disease, characterized by peripheral and central demyelination of nerves, similar to that seen in Cockayne's syndrome. The disease may occur with or without failure to thrive and arthrogryposis. Severe intellectual deficit and death within the first decade are typical.

○ **Cockayne's syndrome** (**CS**) or **Neill-Dingwall syndrome (NDS):** A rare and fatal autosomal recessive neurodegenerative disorder characterized by growth failure, impaired development of the nervous system, abnormal sensitivity to sunlight (photosensitivity), eye disorders and premature aging. Problems with any or all of the internal organs are possible. It is associated with a group of disorders called leukodystrophies, which are conditions characterized by **degradation of neurological white matter**. There are two primary types of Cockayne syndrome: Cockayne syndrome type A (CSA), arising from mutations in the ERCC8 gene, and Cockayne syndrome type B (CSB), resulting from mutations in the ERCC6 gene. It result in death within the first or second decade of life.

Figure 6.13 – Neuropathology of Alexander's disease

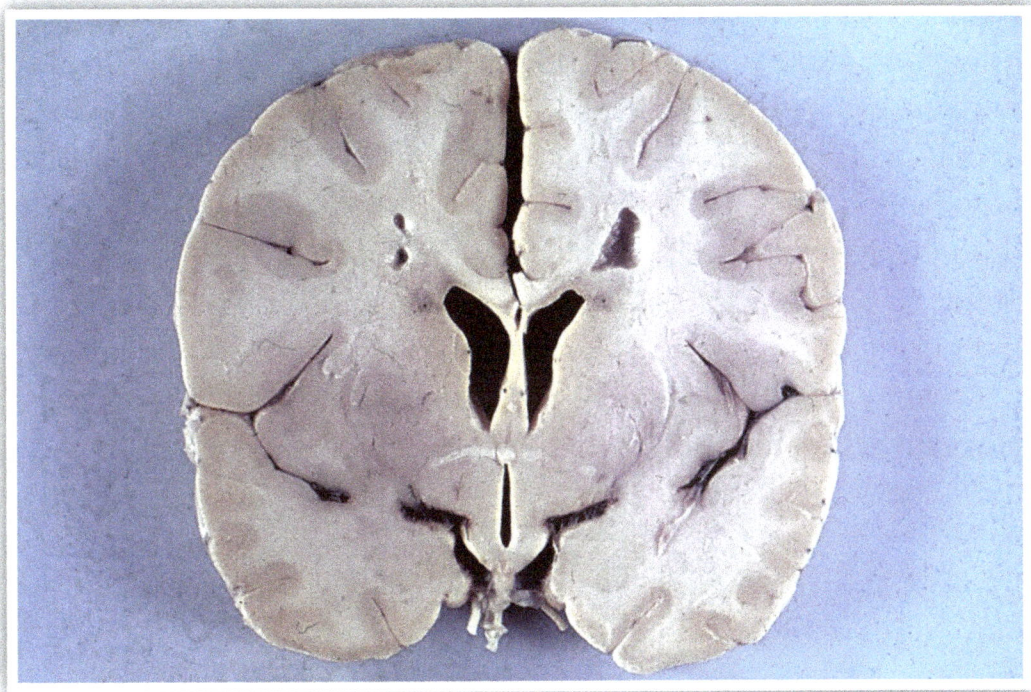

Reference: Marvin 101

➢ **Hereditary – Canavan's disease (CD) or Canavan–Van Bogaert–Bertrand (CBBD) disease:** A rare and fatal autosomal recessive degenerative disease that causes progressive damage to nerve cells and loss of white matter in the brain. It is one of the most common degenerative cerebral diseases of infancy. It is caused by a deficiency of the enzyme aminoacylase 2 and is one of a group of genetic diseases referred to as leukodystrophies. It is characterized by degeneration of myelin in the phospholipid layer insulating the axon of a neuron and is associated with a gene located on human chromosome 17. Symptoms of the most common (and most serious) form of CD typically appear in early infancy usually between the first three to six months of age. CD then progresses rapidly from that stage, with typical cases involving **intellectual disability**, loss of previously acquired motor skills, feeding difficulties, abnormal muscle tone (i.e., initial floppiness - hypotonia - that may eventually translate into spasticity), poor head control, and megalocephaly (abnormally enlarged head). Paralysis, blindness, or seizures may also occur.

➢ **Hereditary - Krabbe's disease (KD) or globoid cell leukodystrophy (GCL) or galactosylceramide lipidosis (GSL):** A rare and often fatal lysosomal storage disease that results in progressive damage to the nervous system. KD involves dysfunctional metabolism of sphingolipids and is inherited in an autosomal recessive pattern. The buildup of unmetabolized lipids adversely affects the growth of the nerve's protective myelin sheath (the covering that insulates many nerves) resulting in demyelination and severe progressive degeneration of motor skills. As part of a group of disorders known as leukodystrophies, KD results from the imperfect growth and development of myelin.

➢ **Hereditary - Marchiafava–Bignami disease (MBD):** A progressive neurological disease of alcohol use disorder, characterized by corpus callosum demyelination and necrosis and subsequent atrophy. Here, the middle two-thirds of the corpus callosum becomes necrotic. It is very difficult to diagnose and there is no specific treatment.

Figure 6.14 – Corpus callosum in Marchiafava–Bignami disease (MBD)

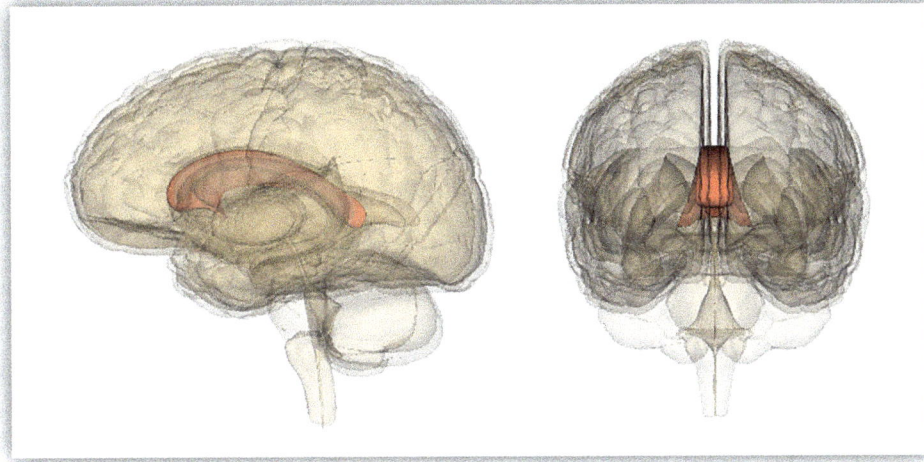

Source: Anatomography maintained by Life Science Databases(LSDB)

> **Hereditary – Myelinolysis - central pontine (MCP):** A neurological condition involving severe damage to the myelin sheath of nerve cells in the pons (an area of the brainstem). It is predominately iatrogenic (treatment-induced), and is characterized by acute paralysis, dysphagia (difficulty swallowing), dysarthria (difficulty speaking), and other neurological symptoms. It was described as a disease of alcoholics and malnutrition. It is distinct from demyelinating conditions such as multiple sclerosis and other neuroinflammatory disorders. Central pontine myelinolysis, and osmotic demyelination syndrome, present most commonly as a complication of treatment of patients with profound hyponatremia (low sodium), which can result from a varied spectrum of conditions, based on different mechanisms. It occurs as a consequence of a rapid rise in serum tonicity following treatment in individuals with chronic, severe hyponatremia who have made intracellular adaptations to the prevailing hypotonicity.

C. Episodic/paroxysmal

Seizures, Epilepsy

> **Dravet's syndrome (DS)** previously known as **severe myoclonic epilepsy of infancy (SMEI):** An autosomal dominant genetic disorder

which causes a catastrophic form of epilepsy. It is characterized by prolonged febrile and non-febrile seizures within the first year of a child's life. The disease progresses to other seizure types like myoclonic and partial seizures, psychomotor delay, and ataxia. It is characterized by **cognitive impairment**, behavioral disorders, and motor deficits. Behavioral deficits often include hyperactivity and impulsiveness, and in more rare cases, autistic-like behaviors. DS is also associated with sleep disorders including somnolence and insomnia. The associated seizures become worse as the patient ages. Children with DS typically experience a lagged development of language and motor skills, hyperactivity and sleep difficulties, chronic infection, growth and balance issues, and difficulty relating to others.

> **Epilepsy:** A group of non-communicable neurological disorders characterized by recurrent epileptic seizures. (An epileptic seizure is the clinical manifestation of an abnormal, excessive, purposeless and synchronized electrical discharge in the brain cells called neurons.) Epileptic seizures can vary from brief and nearly undetectable periods to long periods of vigorous shaking due to abnormal electrical activity in the brain. These episodes can result in physical injuries, either directly such as broken bones or through causing accidents. Seizures tend to recur and may have no immediate underlying cause. The cause of epilepsy is unknown (cryptogenic); some cases occur as the result of brain injury, stroke, brain tumors, infections of the brain, or birth defects through a process known as epileptogenesis. Known genetic mutations are directly linked to a small proportion of cases.

> **Lennox-Gastaut syndrome (LGS):** A complex, rare, and severe childhood-onset epilepsy. It is characterized by multiple and concurrent seizure types including tonic seizure, cognitive dysfunction, and abnormal aspect on electroencephalogram (EEG) such as slow spike waves. Typically, it presents in children aged 3–5 years and most of the time persists into adulthood with slight changes in the electroclinical phenotype. It has been associated with perinatal injuries, congenital infections, brain malformations, brain tumors, genetic disorders such as tuberous sclerosis and several gene mutations. Sometimes, LGS

is observed after infantile epileptic spasm syndrome formerly called West's syndrome (WS).

Headache

> **Migraine:** A genetically-influenced complex neurological disorder characterized by episodes of moderate-to-severe headache, most often unilateral, and generally associated with nausea and light and sound sensitivity. Other characterizing symptoms may include vomiting, cognitive dysfunction, allodynia, and dizziness. Exacerbation of headache symptoms during physical activity is another distinguishing feature.Up to one-third of migraine sufferers experience 'aura': a premonitory period of sensory disturbance widely accepted to be caused by cortical spreading depression at the onset of a migraine attack. Although primarily considered to be a headache disorder, migraine is highly heterogenous neurological disease in its clinical presentation and is better thought of as a spectrum disease rather than a distinct clinical entity.The currently accepted theory suggests that multiple primary neuronal impairments lead to a series of intracranial and extracranial changes, triggering a physiological cascade that leads to migraine symptomatology. Migraine is associated with psychiatric disorders (major depression, bipolar disorder, anxiety disorders, and obsessive–compulsive disorder).

Cerebrovascular

> **Aphasia (see also above primary progressive aphasia, PPA): Aphasia is related to the individual's language cognition.** In aphasia, a person may be unable to comprehend or unable to formulate language because of damage to specific brain regions. It can be due to stroke, head trauma, epilepsy, brain tumors, brain damage and brain infections, or neurodegenerative diseases (such as dementias). In the case of progressive aphasia, the four aspects of communication (spoken language production and comprehension, and written language production and comprehension) must have significantly declined over a short period of time. Impairments in any of these aspects can impact on functional communication. Intelligence, however, is unaffected.

Aphasia also affects visual language such as sign language. In contrast, the use of formulaic expressions in everyday communication is often preserved. One prevalent deficit in the aphasias is a difficulty in finding the correct word (anomia).

➤ **Amaurosis _fugax;_** A painless temporary loss of vision in one or both eyes that appears as a "black curtain coming down vertically into the field of vision", monocular blindness, dimming, fogging, or blurring. Total or sectorial vision loss typically lasts only a few seconds, but may last minutes or even hours. Duration depends on the cause of the vision loss. Obscured vision due to papilledema may last only seconds, while a severely atherosclerotic carotid artery may be associated with a duration of one to ten minutes.

➤ **Foville's syndrome (FS):** It is caused by the blockage of the perforating branches of the basilar artery in the region of the brainstem known as the pons. It is most frequently due to lesions such as vascular disease and tumors involving the dorsal pons.

➤ **Stroke:** A medical condition in which poor blood flow to the brain causes cell death. There are two main types: ischemic (due to lack of blood flow) or hemorrhagic (due to bleeding). Both cause parts of the brain to stop functioning properly. Signs and symptoms may include an inability to move or feel on one side of the body, **problems understanding or speaking**, dizziness, or loss of vision to one side. They often appear soon after the stroke has occurred.

Figure 6.15 - Illustration of embolic stroke showing blockage lodged in blood vessel

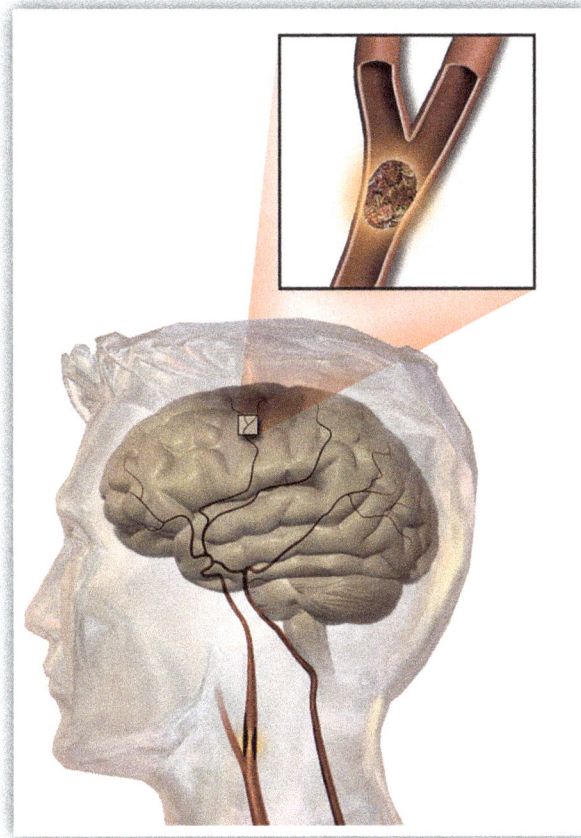

Reference: Blausen Medical Communications

If symptoms last less than one or two hours, the stroke is a 'transient ischemic attack' (TIA), also called a 'mini-stroke'. A hemorrhagic stroke may also be associated with a severe headache. The symptoms of a stroke can be permanent. Long-term complications may include pneumonia and loss of bladder control. Bleeding may occur due to a ruptured brain aneurysm. The biggest risk factor for stroke is high blood pressure. Other risk factors include high blood cholesterol, tobacco smoking, obesity, diabetes mellitus, a previous TIA, end-stage kidney disease, and atrial fibrillation. (Figure 6.15 illustrates an embolic stroke showing a blockage lodged in a blood vessel.)

➢ **Transient global amnesia (TGA):** A neurological disorder whose key defining characteristic is a temporary but almost total disruption of **short-term memory** with a range of problems accessing **older**

memories. A person in a state of TGA exhibits no other signs of impaired cognitive functioning but recalls only the last few moments of consciousness, as well as possibly a few deeply encoded facts of the individual's past, such as their childhood, family, or home perhaps.

- ○ **Anterograde amnesia:** Both TGA and anterograde amnesia deal with disruptions of **short-term memory**. However, a TGA episode generally lasts no more than 2 to 8 hours before the patient returns to normal with the ability to form new memories.

- ➤ **Weber's syndrome (WS)** also known as **midbrain stroke syndrome** (MSS) or **superior alternating hemiplegia (SAH):** A form of stroke that affects the medial portion of the midbrain. It involves oculomotor fascicles in the interpeduncular cisterns and cerebral peduncle so it characterizes the presence of an ipsilateral lower motor neuron type oculomotor nerve palsy and contralateral hemiparesis or hemiplegia.

Sleep disorders

- ➤ **Cataplexy:** A sudden and transient episode of muscle weakness accompanied by full conscious awareness. It is, typically triggered by emotions such as laughing, crying, or terror. It is caused by an autoimmune destruction of hypothalamic neurons that produce the neuropeptide hypocretin (also called orexin), which regulates arousal and has a role in stabilization of the transition between wake and sleep states. Cataplexy without narcolepsy is rare and the cause is unknown.
- ➤ **Narcolepsy:** A chronic neurological syndrome of hypothalamic disorder that involves a decreased ability to regulate sleep–wake cycles. Symptoms often include periods of excessive daytime sleepiness and brief involuntary sleep episodes, vivid hallucinations or an inability to move (sleep paralysis) while falling asleep or waking up. Narcolepsy paired with cataplexy is an autoimmune disorder. There are two main characteristics of narcolepsy: excessive daytime sleepiness and abnormal REM sleep. A person with narcolepsy is likely to become drowsy or fall asleep, often at inappropriate or undesired times and places, or just be very tired throughout the day.
- ➤ **Sleep apnea (SA):** A sleep disorder in which pauses in breathing or periods of shallow breathing during sleep occur more often than

normal. SA may be either obstructive sleep apnea (OSA), the most common form in which breathing is interrupted by a blockage of air flow, or

Figure 6.16 – Weber's syndrome

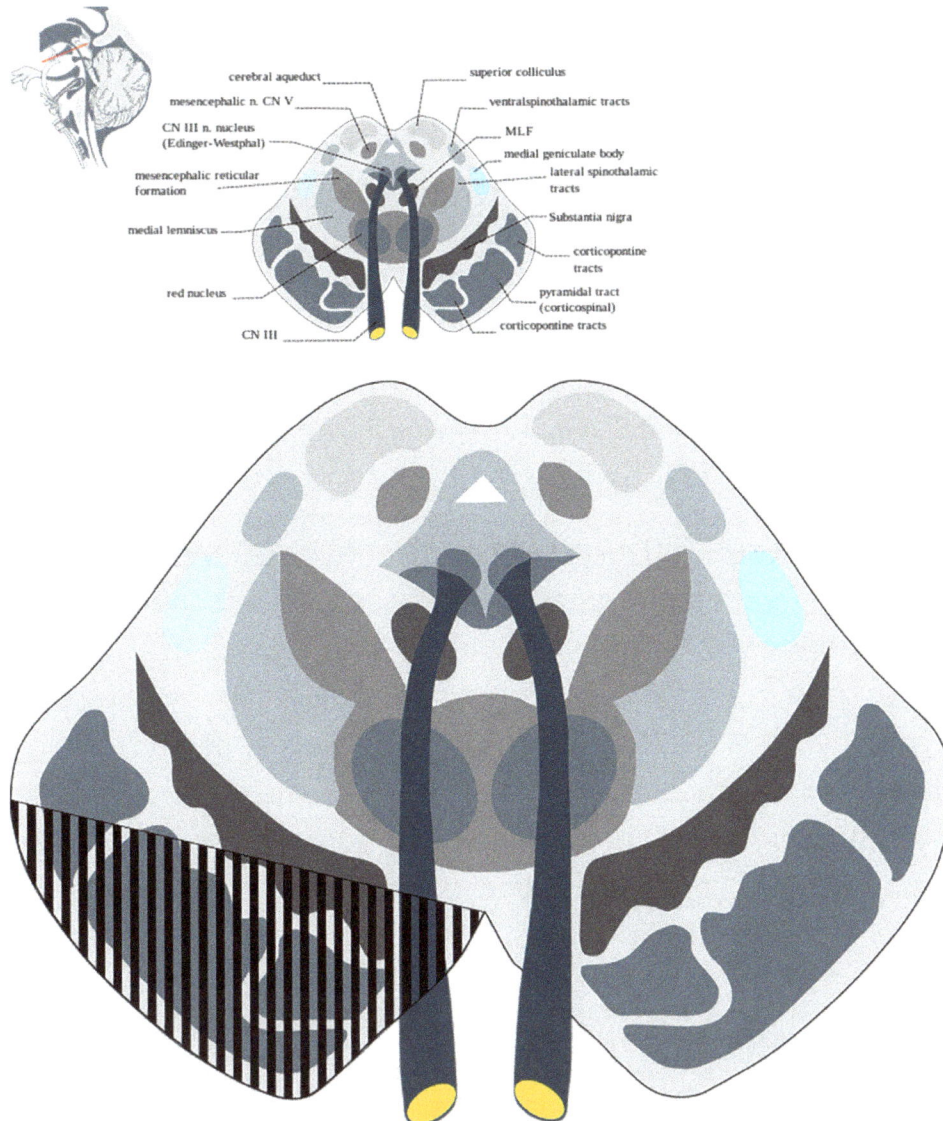

central sleep apnea (CSA) in which regular unconscious breath simply stops, or a combination of the two. OSA has four key contributors (a narrow, crowded, or collapsible upper airway; an ineffective pharyngeal dilator muscle function during sleep; airway narrowing during sleep; and unstable control of breathing). It is often a chronic condition. Episodes of hypoxemia (drop in the percentage of oxygen in the circulation to a lower than normal level) and hypercapnia (concentration of carbon dioxide higher than normal level) will trigger additional effects on the body.

Further, if the level of blood oxygen goes low enough for long enough, brain damage and even death can occur. A systemic disorder, sleep apnea is associated with a wide array of effects, including increased risk of car accidents, hypertension, cardiovascular disease, myocardial infarction, stroke, atrial fibrillation, insulin resistance, higher incidence of cancer, and neurodegeneration. **Alzheimer's disease** (AD) and severe obstructive sleep apnea are connected because there is an increase in the protein beta-amyloid as well as white-matter damage. AD in this case comes from the lack of proper rest or poorer sleep efficiency resulting in neurodegeneration. Having sleep apnea in mid-life brings a higher likelihood of developing AD in older age, and if one has AD then one is also more likely to have sleep apnea.

> **Hypoventilation (or respiratory depression) syndrome (RDS):** It occurs when ventilation is inadequate to perform needed respiratory gas exchange. It causes an increased concentration of carbon dioxide (hypercapnia) and respiratory acidosis. Hypoventilation is not synonymous with respiratory arrest, in which breathing ceases entirely and death occurs within minutes due to hypoxia and leads rapidly into complete anoxia, however, both are medical emergencies. Hypoventilation can be considered a precursor to hypoxia and its lethality is attributed to hypoxia with carbon dioxide toxicity.

D. Cerebrospinal fluid

> **Cerebral edema (CE):** The excess accumulation of fluid (edema) in the intracellular or extracellular spaces of the brain. This typically causes impaired nerve function and increased pressure within the skull, and can eventually lead to direct compression of brain tissue and blood vessels. Symptoms vary based on the location and extent of edema and generally include headaches, nausea, vomiting, seizures, drowsiness, visual disturbances, dizziness, and in severe cases, coma and death. CE is commonly seen in a variety of brain injuries including:

Ischemic stroke; subarachnoid hemorrhage; traumatic brain injury (TBI); subdural, epidural, or intracerebral hematoma; hydrocephalus; brain cancer; brain infections; low blood sodium levels; and acute liver failure. CE is a major cause of brain damage and contributes significantly to the mortality of ischemic strokes and TBIs. (Figure 6.17 is a skull MRI (T2 flair) scan of a brain metastasis with accompanying edema.)

➤ **Choroid plexus papilloma (CPP):** A rare benign neuroepithelial intraventricular lesion found in the choroid plexus. It leads to increased cerebrospinal fluid production, thus causing increased intracranial pressure and hydrocephalus. CPP occurs in the lateral ventricles of children and in the fourth ventricle of adults. This is unlike most other pediatric tumors and adult tumors, in which the locations of the tumors is reversed. In children, brain tumors are usually found in the infratentorial region and in adults, brain tumors are usually found in the supratentorial space. The relationship is reversed for choroid plexus papillomas (Figure 6.18).

Figure 6.17 – MRI image of a brain metastasis with accompanying edema

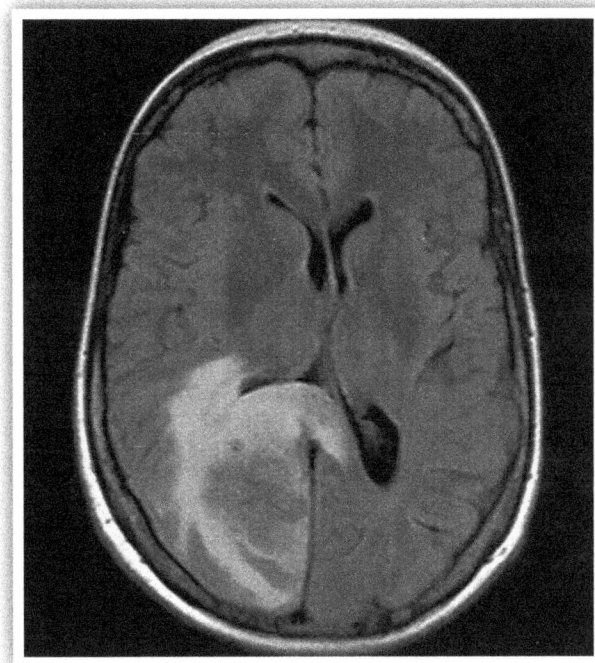

Reference: Dragher01

> **Normal pressure hydrocephalus (NPH):** A condition in which an accumulation of cerebrospinal fluid (CSF) occurs within the brain. This typically causes increased pressure inside the skull. Older people may have headaches, double vision, poor balance, urinary incontinence, personality changes, or **mental impairment.** In babies, it may be seen as a rapid increase in head size. Other symptoms may include vomiting, sleepiness, seizures, and downward pointing of the eyes. The four types of hydrocephalus are communicating, non-communicating, *ex vacuo*, and normal pressure. Hydrocephalus can occur due to birth defects or be acquired later in life. Causes include meningitis, brain tumors, traumatic brain injury, intraventricular hemorrhage, and subarachnoid hemorrhage. (Figure 6.19 is a brain-CT scan with hydrocphalus.)

Figure 6.18 - Choroid plexus papilloma

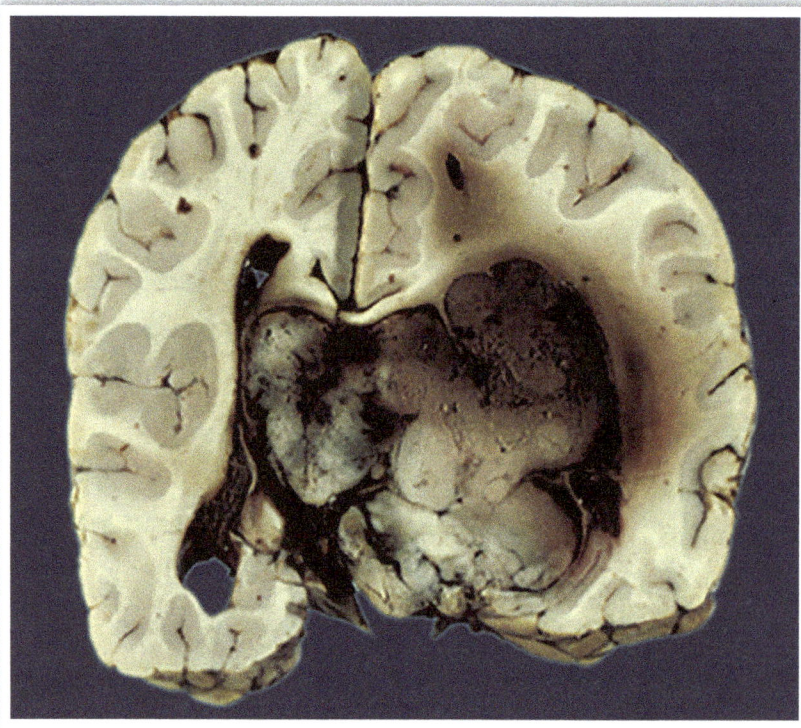

Figure 6.19 – CT scan of the brain with hydrocephalus

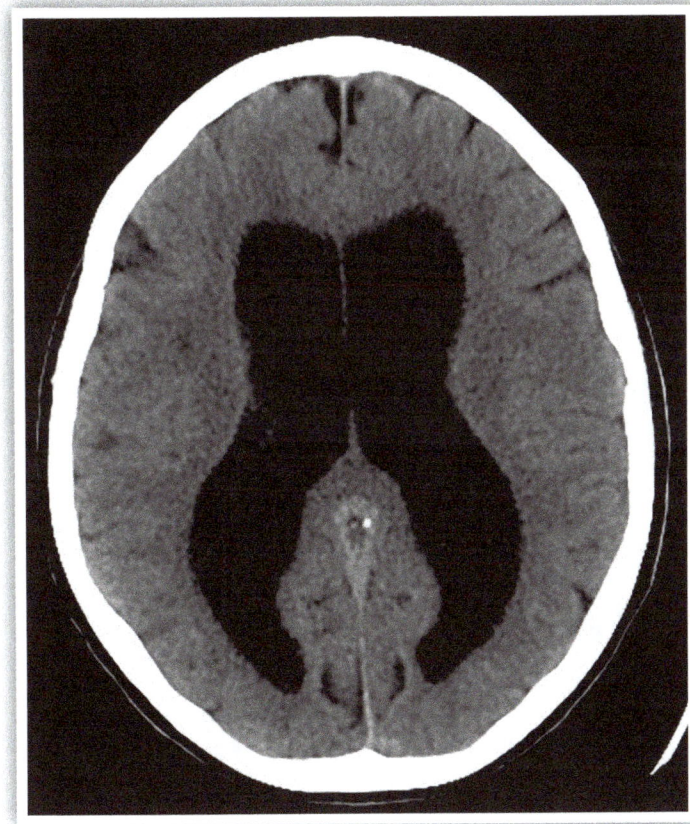

Reference: Lucien Monfils

E. Others

> **Brain herniation:** A potentially deadly side effect of very high pressure within the skull that occurs when a part of the brain is squeezed across structures within the skull. The brain can shift across such structures as the falx cerebri, the tentorium cerebelli, and even through the foramen magnum (the hole in the base of the skull through which the spinal cord connects with the brain). Herniation can be caused by a number of factors that cause a mass effect and increase intracranial pressure (ICP): these include traumatic brain injury (TBI), intracranial hemorrhage, or brain tumor.

Herniation can also occur in the absence of high ICP when mass lesions such as hematomas occur at the borders of brain compartments. In such cases local pressure is increased at the place where the herniation occurs, but this pressure is not transmitted to the rest of the brain, and therefore does not register as an increase in ICP. Because herniation puts extreme pressure on parts of the brain and thereby cuts off the blood supply to various parts of the brain, it is often fatal. (Figure 6.20 is an MRI image showing injury due to brain herniation in a patient with choriocarcinoma.)

Figure 6.20 – Coronal MRI showing brain herniation injury

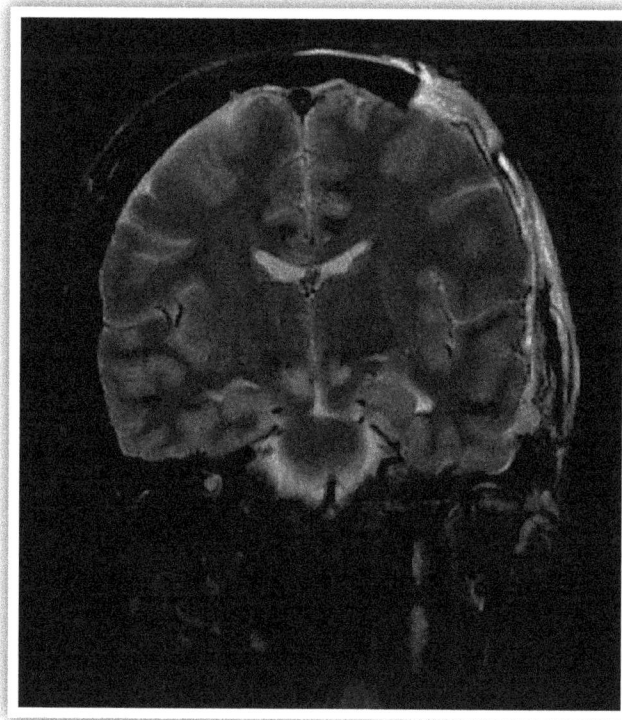

Reference: Rocque BG, Başkaya MK (2008).
"Spontaneous acute subdural hematoma as an initial presentation of choriocarcinoma: A case report". J Med Case Reports **2:**211. doi:10.1186/1752-1947-2-211.

> **Encephalopathy:** Any disorder or disease of the brain, especially chronic degenerative conditions. It does not refer to a single disease, but rather to a syndrome of overall brain dysfunction. It has many possible organic and inorganic causes. The hallmark of encephalopathy is an altered mental state or delirium. Characteristic of the altered mental state is impairment of the **cognition**, attention, orientation, sleep–wake

cycle and consciousness. An altered state of consciousness may range from failure of selective attention to drowsiness. Hypervigilance may be present; with or without: cognitive deficits, headache, epileptic seizures, myoclonus (involuntary twitching of a muscle or group of muscles) or asterixis ("flapping tremor" of the hand when wrist is extended). Depending on the type and severity of encephalopathy, common neurological symptoms are **loss of cognitive function**, subtle personality changes, and an inability to concentrate. Other neurological signs may include dysarthria, hyponimia, problems with movements (they can be clumsy or slow), ataxia, tremor. Other neurological signs may include involuntary grasping and sucking motions, nystagmus (rapid, involuntary eye movement), jactitation (restlessness while in bed), and respiratory abnormalities such as Cheyne-Stokes respiration (cyclic waxing and waning of tidal volume), apneustic respirations and post-hypercapnic apnea. Focal neurological deficits are less common.

- o **Wernicke's encephalitis (WE):** It can co-occur with Korsakoff's alcoholic syndrome, characterized by amnestic-confabulatory syndrome: retrograde amnesia, anterograde amnesia, confabulations (**invented memories**), **poor recall,** and disorientation.
- o **Anti-NMDA receptor encephalitis:** The most common autoimmune encephalitis. It can cause paranoid and grandiose delusions, agitation, hallucinations (visual and auditory), bizarre behavior, fear, **short-term memory loss**, and confusion.
- o **HIV encephalopathy:** It can lead to **dementia.**
- o **Hashimoto's encephalitis (HE):** A steroid-responsive encephalopathy associated with autoimmune thyroiditis (SREAT). It is a neurological condition characterized by encephalopathy, thyroid autoimmunity, and good clinical response to corticosteroids. It is associated with Hashimoto's thyroiditis.

➢ **Reye's syndrome (RS)**: A rapidly worsening brain disease. Symptoms may include vomiting, personality changes, confusion, seizures, and loss of consciousness. While liver toxicity typically occurs in the syndrome, jaundice usually does not. The cause is unknown.

Diseases of the central nervous system due to the spinal cord are charted in Table 6.3.

Table 6.3 - Diseases of the central nervous system: Spinal cord

Organ	Disorders/diseases
Spinal cord/Myelopathy	o Foix-Alajouanine syndrome (FAS) o Morvan's syndrome (MS) o Spinal cord compressiom (SCC) o Syringobulbia o Syringomyelia o Vascular myelopathy (VM)

➤ **Morvan's syndrome (MS) or fibrillary chorea (FC)** (in French: *la chorée fibrillaire*): A rare, life-threatening autoimmune disease describing patients with multiple, irregular contractions of the long muscles, cramping, weakness, pruritus, hyperhidrosis, insomnia, and delirium. This rare disorder is characterized by severe insomnia, amounting to no less than complete lack of sleep (agrypnia) for weeks or months in a row, and associated with autonomic alterations consisting of profuse perspiration with characteristic skin miliaria (also known as sweat rash), tachycardia, increased body temperature, and hypertension. Patients display a remarkable hallucinatory behavior, and peculiar motor disturbances, which are best described as neuromyotonic discharges. The association of the disease with thymoma, tumor, autoimmune diseases, and autoantibodies suggests an autoimmune or paraneoplastic etiology. Besides an immune-mediated etiology, it is also believed to occur in gold, mercury, or manganese poisoning.

➤ **Spinal cord compressiom (SCC):** A form of myelopathy in which the spinal cord is compressed. Causes can be bone fragments from a vertebral fracture, a tumor, abscess, ruptured intervertebral disc or other lesion.

➤ **Syringobulbia:** A medical condition in which syrinxes, or fluid-filled cavities, affect the brainstem (usually the lower brainstem). The exact cause is often unknown, but may be linked to a widening of the central canal of the spinal cord. This may affect one or more cranial nerves, resulting in various kinds of facial palsies. Sensory and motor nerve pathways may be affected by interruption or compression of nerves.

> **Syringomyelia:** A generic term referring to a disorder in which a cyst or cavity (called syrinx) forms within the spinal cord. This cyst can expand and elongate over time, destroying the spinal cord. The damage may result in loss of feeling, paralysis, weakness, and stiffness in the back, shoulders, and extremities. Syringomyelia may also cause a loss of the ability to feel extremes of hot or cold, especially in the hands. It may also lead to a cape-like bilateral loss of pain and temperature sensation along the upper chest and arms.

> **Vascular myelopathy (VM):** Refers to an abnormality of the spinal cord in regard to its blood supply. The blood supply is complicated and supplied by two major vessel groups: the posterior spinal arteries and the anterior spinal arteries; both arteries running the entire length of the spinal cord and receiving anastomotic (conjoined) vessels in many places. The anterior spinal artery has a less efficient supply of blood and is therefore more susceptible to vascular disease. Whilst atherosclerosis of spinal arteries is rare, necrosis (death of tissue) in the anterior artery can be caused by disease in vessels originating from the segmental arteries such as atheroma (arterial wall swelling) or aortic dissection (a tear in the aorta).

> **Foix-Alajouanine syndrome (FAS)** or **subacute ascending necrotizing myelitis (SANM):** A disease caused by an arteriovenous malformation of the spinal cord. Most cases involve dural arteriovenous malformations that present in the lower thoracic or lumbar spinal cord. Patients can present with symptoms indicating spinal cord involvement such as (paralysis of arms and legs, numbness and loss of sensation and sphincter dysfunction) and disseminated nerve cell death in the spinal cord.

Diseases of the central nervous system - Encephalopathy or/and spinal cord myelopathy

CNS diseases that are either or both encephalopathy and spinal cord/myelopathy are summarized in Table 6.4:

Table 6.4 - Diseases of the central nervous system: Either/both encephalopathy, spinal cord/myelopathy

Characteristic	Disease category	Diseases
Degenerative	**A. Ataxia**	o Ataxia telangectasia (AT) o Friedreich's ataxia (FA)
	B. Motor Neuron Diseases (MND)	_LMN only:_ o Atrophy: 　- Progressive muscular (PMA) 　- Spinal Muscular (SMA) 　- Congenital Distal Spinal Muscular (cdSMA) 　- DSMA1 　- SMA-LED 　- SMA-PCH 　- SMA-PME 　- SMAX1 　- SMAX2 o Distal hereditary motor neuropathies _UMN only:_ o Palsy: 　- Progressive bulbar (PBP) 　- Fazio-Lande infantile (IFLP) 　- Pseudobulbar (PBP) o Paraplegia: 　- Hereditary spastic (HSP) o Sclerosis: Primary lateral _Both LMN, UMN:_ o **Amyotrophic lateral sclerosis (ALS)**

Degenerative

A. Ataxia

> **Ataxia telangectasia (AT) or** ataxia–telangiectasia syndrome **(ATS) or Louis–Barre syndrome (LBS):** A rare, neurodegenerative,

autosomal recessive disease causing severe disability. Ataxia refers to poor coordination and telangiectasia to small dilated blood vessels, both of which are hallmarks of the disease. It impairs certain areas of the brain including the cerebellum, causing difficulty with movement and coordination. It weakens the immune system, causing a predisposition to infection. Lastly, it prevents repair of broken DNA, increasing the risk of cancer.

> **Friedreich's ataxia (FA):** An autosomal-recessive genetic disease that causes difficulty walking, a loss of coordination in the arms and legs, and impaired speech that worsens over time. Many develop hypertrophic cardiomyopathy and require a mobility aid. As the disease progresses, some affected people lose their sight and hearing. Other complications may include scoliosis and diabetes mellitus.

B. Motor neuron diseases (MND)

Atrophies

> **Progressive muscular atrophy (PMA) or Duchesne–Aran disease (DAD) or Duchesne –Aran muscular atrophy (DAMA):** A disorder characterized by the degeneration of lower motor neurons, resulting in generalized, progressive loss of muscle function. This is to be contrasted with amyotrophic lateral sclerosis (ALS), the most common MND, which affects both the upper and lower motor neurons, or primary lateral sclerosis (PLS), another MND, which affects only the upper motor neurons. The distinction is important because PMA is associated with a better prognosis than ALS.

> **Spinal muscular atrophy (SMA):** A genetically and clinically heterogeneous group of rare debilitating disorders characterized by the degeneration of lower motor neurons (neuronal cells situated in the anterior horn of the spinal cord) and subsequent atrophy (wasting) of various muscle groups in the body.

> **Congenital distal spinal muscular atrophy (cdSMA):** A hereditary condition characterized by muscle wasting (atrophy), particularly of distal muscles in legs and hands, and by early-onset contractures (permanent shortening of a muscle or joint) of the hip, knee, and

ankle. The condition is a result of a loss of anterior horn cells localized to lumbar and cervical regions of the spinal cord early in infancy, which in turn is caused by a mutation of the TRPV4 gene. The disorder is inherited in an autosomal dominant manner.

Neuropathies

➤ **Distal hereditary motor neuropathies (dHMN):** A genetically and clinically heterogeneous group of motor neuron diseases that result from genetic mutations in various genes and are characterized by degeneration and loss of motor neuron cells in the anterior horn of the spinal cord and subsequent muscle atrophy.

➤ **Palsy:** A medical term referring to various types of paralysis or paresis, often accompanied by weakness and the loss of feeling and uncontrolled body movements such as shaking. Specific kinds of palsy include:
  - Bell's palsy: Partial facial paralysis.
  - Bulbar palsy: Impairment of cranial nerves;.
  - Cerebral palsy: A neural disorder caused by intracranial lesions.
  - Conjugate gaze palsy: A disorder affecting the ability to move the eyes.
  - Erb's palsy (or brachial palsy): It involves paralysis of an arm.
  - Fazio-Lande infantile palsy.
  - Spinal muscular atrophy (or wasting palsy).
  - Progressive supranuclear palsy: A degenerative disease.
  - Squatter's palsy: A bilateral peroneal nerve palsy that may be triggered by sustained squatting.
  - Third nerve palsy: Involves the cranial nerve III.

Paraplegia

➤ **Hereditary spastic paraplegia (HSP) or hereditary spastic paraparesis (HSP), or familial spastic paraplegia (FSP), or French settlement disease (FSD), or Strumpell disease (SD), or Strumpell-Lorrain disease.(SLD):** A group of inherited diseases whose main feature is a progressive gait disorder. The disease presents with progressive stiffness (spasticity) and contraction in the lower limbs. It is different from cerebral palsy.

> **<u>Primary lateral sclerosis (PLS):</u>** A very rare neuromuscular disease characterized by progressive muscle weakness in the voluntary muscles. It belongs to a group of disorders known as motor neuron diseases (MND, discussed earlier) which develop when the nerve cells that control voluntary muscle movement degenerate and die, causing weakness in the muscles they control. It only affects upper motor neurons with no evidence of the degeneration of spinal motor neurons or muscle wasting (amyotrophy) that occurs in amyotrophic lateral sclerosis (ALS).

> **<u>Amyotrophic lateral sclerosis (ALS)</u>** also known as **Lou Gehrig's disease:** A rare neurodegenerative disease that results in the progressive loss of motor neurons that control voluntary muscles. It is the most common form of the motor neuron diseases. Around half of people with ALS develop at least mild difficulties with thinking and behavior, and about 15% develop **frontotemporal dementia**. Motor neuron loss continues until the abilities to eat, speak, move, or, lastly, breathe are lost.

Sidebar 6.1 discusses the presence of pathogens in the brain.

Take-aways

> A synoptic overview of the brain diseases/disorders was provided for a proper contextual clinical background of the contributions reported in this book.
> Pathologies due to inflammation, include:
> - Encephalopathy: Degenerative, demyelinating, episodic/paroxysmal, cerebrospinal fluid, and other causes.
> - Spinal cord/myelopathy, and/or
> - Degenerative encephalopathy and spinal cord/myelopathy.
> Among the CNS diseases due to inflammation, only encephalitis is of interest. Its severity can be variable with symptoms including reduction or alteration in consciousness and memory problems.

➤ Among the CNS diseases due to encephalopathies, one must distinguish between:
  ○ Degenerative diseases, including:
    ▪ Extrapyramidal & movement disorders: Particularly Huntington's disease; myoclonus (Alzheimer's disease, Creutzfeldt-Jakob disease); Parkinson's disease and parkinsonism; panthotenate kinase-associated degeneration; and progressive supranuclear palsy.
    ▪ Dementias: Including Alzheimer's disease; primary progressive aphasia; posterior cortical atrophy; frontotemporal lobar degeneration, and the various dementias (early onset; frontotemporal; HIV; juvenile; Lewy bodies; late onset; pugilistica; and vascular); Parkinson's disease; synucleinopathies; and tauopathy.
    ▪ Seizures/epilepsy: Dravet's syndrome; Lennox-Gastaud syndrome.
  ○ Demyelinating diseases, including:
    ▪ Multiple sclerosis; and
    ▪ Canavan's disease.
  ○ Episodic paroxysmal diseases, including:
    ▪ Seizures;
    ▪ Cerebrovascular diseases (acute aphasia; stroke; transcranial global amnesia and anteretrograde)
    ▪ Sleep disorders, especially sleep apnea.
  ○ Other related diseases including the encephalopathies of:
    ▪ Wernicke's;
    ▪ Anti-MDS receptor; and
    ▪ HIV.
➤ Among the CNS neurodegenerative diseases:
  ○ Motor neuron diseases, including particularly:
    ▪ Amyotrophic lateral sclerosis.
➤ The above multiple possible contributors to memory impairments would theoretically need to be considered, as appropriate, for a correct diagnosis and treatment.

Sidebar 6.1 – On the origin of neurodegenerative diseases

A core neuroscience dogma is that the soma of each neuron communicates simultaneously with thousands of other neurons connected to it through the long dendrites. These dendritic trees were posited to function like electrical cables collecting signals from the connecting neurons, thus allowing electrical communications between them. Recently (October 2023), the validity of this hypothesis has been questioned by researchers at the Bar-Ilan University (BIU) and the Gonda (Goldschmied) Multidisciplinary Brain Research Center in Ramat Gan, Israel.

According to the lead researcher (Prof. Ido Kanter), "…neuronal features are independent of these physiological conditions – a finding that strongly pinpoints dendrites as the segments controlling neuronal plasticity features such as the neuronal firing frequency and the stimulation threshold of the neuron".

If corroborated, the above results would call for a re-examination of the origin of degenerative diseases because the origin of many neuron functions are beyond the traditional framework and must be attributed to the dendrites instead of the soma. In addition, these results also question the origin of the brain's awake-and-sleep states.

Sidebar 6.2 – Pathogens …in the brain?

The connection between influenza infection and psychosis has been reported in Europe as early as 1835. It became more apparent during the Spanish flu epidemic of 1918. As we recall, that epidemic, caused by the H1N1 virus (a subtype of the H1N5 virus), correlated with an epidemic of Parkinson's disease (PD) a few decades later. In the U.S., between the 1940s and early 1950s, the diagnosis of PD increased abruptly from 1%-2% to 2.5%-3% (that is, about 50% more people were diagnosed with the disease) before falling back to its previous rate of 1%-2%. However, because of the unexplained, geographically distant, and delayed onset of PD by several decades, that connection was cast aside.

Bacteria, viruses, fungi, and other microbes are part of a growing list of pathogens found in the brains of patients with neurodegenerative diseases (NDDs). Generally, brain infections by pathogens can lead to transient or permanent neurologic or psychiatric dysfunctions. Microbes in the brain may indicate **meningitis** or **encephalitis**, two diseases that are active infections with inflammation. For NDDs like **Parkinson's**, **Alzheimer's**, and other diseases that were not thought to be infectious, finding pathogens in the brain is both surprising and concerning.

Evidence has continued to accumulate linking the brain to various pathogens. But, how do these organisms get into the brain since it is protected by the blood brain barrier (BBB)? They do so when the barrier looses some of its impermeability. Other avenues for reaching directly the brain are the intra-nasal and sinus access, the mouth through the lingual nerve, the gut through the vagus nerve, and even the eye through the olfactory bulbs, all of which connect to the brain by replicating and spreading. Thus, in 1974, Gamboa., et al. found viral antigens in the brains of deceased people affected by encephalitis lethargica. It was associated with (and some thought caused by) the 1918 Spanish flu epidemic and it was even speculated that the condition could be a precursor to PD. Other scientists had also noted the connection between influenza and neural dysfunction. In 1997, Ogata., et al. reported that rats exposed to the Japanese encephalitis virus developed symptoms similar to human PD. At that time, this connection between viral infection and brain disease had been hotly contested because of other conflicting experiments. In 2001, utilizing the technology known as polymerase chain reaction (PCR) to look for the genome of the H1N1 virus in the preserved brain tissue of victims of encephalitis lethargica, researchers at the (U.S.) Armed Forces Institute of Pathology (AFIP) found no sign of the virus. In 2003, Heiko Braak proposed the widely accepted hypothesis that PD starts in the gut and moves into the brain, a process that may take place over 25-30 years over the life of the infected individual. However, in 2006, researchers at the (U.S.) Centers for Disease Control & Prevention (CDC&P) studying the effects of the influenza strain that caused the 1918 Spanish flu epidemic did not see any signs of inflammation in the brains of infected mice. The above conflicting results suggested that more work was needed to link viral infection and NDDs.

Then, seminal experiments were conducted by Richard Smeyne. In 2008, observing ducks infected by the H5N1 virus, he wondered whether a connection existed between the viral infection and the extensive neurodegeneration he observed (devastation of the substantia nigra, which is often damaged in Parkinson patients, and obliteration of all the neurons). The virus was inducing inflammation and death into the parts of the brain that degenerate in Parkinson's. He further remarked that in rodents, which have a much shorter lifetime than humans, the same travel from the gut to the brain as hypothesized by Braak, may take only a few weeks as opposed to decades in humans. Even if they cannot reach the brain, the viruses can still play a role in neurodegeneration by triggering severe inflammation. In 2009, in other mice experiments, Smeyne also observed that H5N1 not only is not blocked by the BBB from entering the brain but it can easily infiltrate nerve cells in the brain and kill them, especially targeting the dopamine-producing neurons in the substantia nigra.

While H1N1 could not penetrate the barrier, it still caused central nervous system immune cells (the microglia) to flow into the substantia nigra and the hippocampus, causing inflammation and cell death in the area. Interestingly, we have here two different flus, two different mechanisms, but the same effect - inflammation and death in that part of the brain that degenerates in PD. Other experiments than Smeyne's suggested that viral infections can contribute to NDDs. The connection is not limited to influenza but extended to several different viruses, including measles and herpes that can give rise to symptoms of multiple sclerosis (MS) in rodents. In addition, levels of herpes virus were found to be higher in the brains of people who died from Alzheimer's than in those without the disease. Also, some HIV patients developed dementia that appears to be associated with the infection. Lately, in 2017, after administering the toxin MPTP (a byproduct of a bad batch of synthetic heroin that led users to develop Parkinson's), Smeyne et al. additionally observed that the treated mice developed signs of Parkinson's, losing 25% more neurons in the substantia nigra than uninfected mice treated with the toxin. He, then, concluded that whereas the H1N1 viral infection alone may not cause PD, it primed the nervous system to be sensitive to other things that would. All of the above experiments are prompting a reconsideration of the pathogen connection to the brain.

Now, infections of the brain often also involve other parts of the CNS including the spinal cord. They can cause inflammation of the brain (encephalitis) and of the layers of tissue (meninges) that cover the brain and the spinal cord (meningitis). Often, bacterial meningitis spreads to the brain itself, causing encephalitis. Similarly, viral infections that cause encephalitis often also cause meningitis. Usually in encephalitis and meningitis, infection is not confined to one area but may occur throughout the brain, within the meninges, along the entire length of the spinal cord and over the entire brain. Infection may also be confined to one area (empyema in an existing space in the body; abscess). Bacteria and other infectious organisms can reach the brain and meninges in several ways by being carried by the blood, entering the brain directly from the outside (for example, through a skull fracture or during surgery on the brain), or spreading from nearby infected structures (for example, sinuses or middle ear). Sometimes a brain infection, a vaccine, cancer, or another disorder may trigger an autoimmune reaction as a result of which the brain becomes inflamed. Encephalitis is most commonly due to viruses (herpes simplex, herpes zoster, cytomegalovirus, West Nile virus, HIV and prion disease).

However, the flu-Parkinson connection is not the only link between viruses and neurological problems. The broader link between viruses and neurodegeneration can be seen from the following developments that took place in the late 1980s-early 1990s. Mice infected with viruses such as measles and herpes suffered the same kind of damage to their oligodendrocytes as patients with multiple sclerosis do. It is unclear whether the viruses invaded the oligodendrocytes directly or simply provoked the mice's immune systems to attack the cells (an autoimmune reaction), but the end result was demyelination of neurons. One of the viruses that induced MS symptoms in mice was herpes virus 6 which has also been tentatively associated with the onset and development of AD. Indeed, over the past few decades, tentative links have been documented between viral infections and AD. From a review of data from brain banks and published studies, Joel Dudley et al. found that AD patients had elevated levels of viruses such as human herpes viruses 6 and 7 in four key brain regions. Based on genetic and proteomic data, they also found that human herpes virus 6 may induce gene expression that spurs the development of the protein amyloid β which forms plaques – one of the hallmarks of Alzheimer's.

While viruses may not cause the disease, their presence suggests that pathogens may play a part in neurodegenerative diseases after all. Compared to previous musings on the pathogen hypothesis, we now have more powerful genetic and other sequencing methods that can take a more unbiased look at the microbial DNA/RNA landscape of brain tissue. Further, in the case of HIV, beginning in the 1990s, it was shown that it could traverse the blood brain barrier, infiltrate the brain, and spur neuronal death and a loss of synaptic connections. In late 2010, it was further shown that patients with HIV developed dementia and loss of brain matter that mirrors what is seen in Alzheimer's. More recently, other studies showed that HIV patients develop plaques of amyloid β (like in Alzheimer's) and can also develop slowness in movement and tremors (like in Parkinson's). Lastly, in 2019, Korte et al. reported that the brains of mice infected with certain strains of the flu virus suffered memory deficits even after they seemingly recovered. It turned out their brains were full of microglia even 30-60 days after the infection first took hold and can remain high for up to 120 days (equivalent to more than 10 years in human time).

More recently, Smeyne et al. conducted another experiment on mice in which (a) one group of mice received an H1N1 vaccine 30 days before infecting the animal with the virus and (b) another group of mice were treated with Tamiflu for the week after they were infected. Both groups were allowed to recover before being given a low dose of a toxic material (MPTP), and (c) a control group received neither the vaccine nor the flu treatment. They determined that while (c) developed Parkinson-like symptoms, (a) and (b) developed no neurodegenerative effects. In other words, mice were protected against Parkinson-like symptoms by either prophylactic treatment (with a vaccine) or by early treatment (with Tamiflu). Extrapolating these results from mice to humans, if valid, the logical conclusion would be that if a person gets a pathogen infection, vaccination or at least treatment with Tamiflu may treat the influenza but also help prevent the complications of influenza infection.

In summary, the long time lag between viral infection and the development of neurodegenerative diseases is exactly the reason why scientists have had (and continue to have) trouble accepting that viruses could cause the diseases. The link is difficult to demonstrate except perhaps in rodent studies. We need to better understand how the brain responds to viral infection long after our immune system has cleared the infection from our bodies. This will help us develop ways to mitigate the neurological effects. Further, understanding how infections trigger the immune system could lead to ways to down-regulate glia-driven inflammation in hope of preventing long-term damage.

The pathogenic hypothesis remains a hypothesis whose rigorous testing is long overdue. Not with standing the several instances of the link between viruses and neurodegenerative diseases, even if a definitive link were established, it may only be correlative not causal. While the cause(s) of the major neurodegenerative disorders (Alzheimer's, Parkinson's, epilepsy, and others) remain unknown, I have posited earlier that they are the consequence of a runaway brain autoimmune system that is unable to maintain homeostasis between opposing synaptoblastic and synaptoclastic pressures. At this juncture, this runaway autoimmune disease explanation remains the only plausible one and the root cause of neurodegenerative diseases, everything else amounting to consequences of risks and correlations.

PART D
THE AGING BRAIN

7

Alzheimer's disease - A primer

Contents

7

Alzheimer's disease - A primer

In 1901, Dr. Alois Alzheimer, a German psychiatrist and neuropathologist, first described the disease that now bears his name in a 46-year-old woman whose name Frau Auguste Deter has since remained in the medical annals. It is associated with progressive memory loss accompanied by confusion, language problems, and an unpredictable behavior. Five years later, after she died, he examined her brain and saw that it was full of unusual clumps known as *plaques*. Over a century later, it was determined that these plaques are full of a protein called beta-amyloid, one of the hallmarks of the disease. While other features of Alzheimer's disease (AD) have since been discovered, the theory that beta-amyloid is the main cause of this as yet incurable disease has (erroneously) dominated.

Over the past few decades, once considered a rare disorder, AD has emerged from obscurity to become a major public health problem impacting millions of older Americans and their families, and others worldwide. Year-2018 estimates vary, but experts suggest that as many as 5.5 million Americans and 55 million worldwide age 65 and older are living with AD and other dementias. According to the Alzheimer's Association (AA), the number of Americans is anticipated to increase to 13 million by 2050. Many others under age 65 also have the disease. Currently, AD is ranked as the sixth leading cause of death in the U.S., but **recent estimates** indicate that the disorder may actually rank third just behind **heart disease** and **cancer** as a cause of death for older people. With increased life expectancy, the disease will become even more prevalent, resulting in an extremely heavy financial burden on society and its resources. Unless it can be effectively treated or prevented, the number of people with the disease will increase significantly if current population trends continue. This is because increasing age is the most important known risk factor for AD. It behooves me to join others (patients and their families, physicians, scientists, and even politicians) in stressing the urgency and importance of finding a cure for it.

The National Institute on Aging (NIA), the lead agency for AD research at the (U.S.) National Institutes of Health (NIH), launched its AD program in 1978, and since then the study of the disease has become one of its top priorities. Several other research organizations, both in the U.S. and abroad, also conduct and sponsor studies on AD. Many private-sector research, education, and advocacy groups contribute to these efforts in the hope that the study of AD would move ahead rapidly. Our knowledge of the disease is continuously increasing and refined as we better understand its biology and begin to have some inkling of its root cause(s). But, after more than 45 years of such efforts, I must sadly note that we have not yet found a cure. Nonetheless, as a researcher in the field, with the strong conviction built over several decades of scientific research, I can affirm that, sooner rather than later, science will conquer this disease like other diseases, stop it in its tracks, minimize its effects, and make it reversible and preventable.

A brief history of the disease

In ancient times, old age was associated with dementia, a broad term referring to a decline in cognitive function to the extent that it interferes with daily life and activities. As indicated earlier, in 1901, Dr Alzheimer identified the first case of what later became known as Alzheimer's disease (AD) and reported publicly on the case. In the period 1901-1906, eleven cases similar to the one presented by Alzheimer were reported in the medical literature. In the following year, after suppressing some of the clinical features (delusions and hallucinations) and pathological characteristics (arteriosclerotic changes) contained in the original Alzheimer's report, Emil Kraepelin described the disease as a distinctive one. He named it as *presenile dementia* (a subtype of *senile dementia)*. For the next seventy years, the diagnosis of AD was reserved only for individuals between the ages of 45 and 65 who developed symptoms of dementia. It is only in 1977 that AD was diagnosed as independent of age when patients presented with a characteristically common symptom pattern, disease course, and neuropathology. It took seven additional years for the (U.S.) National Institute of Neurological Disorders and Stroke (NINDS) and the Alzheimer's Disease and Related Disorders Association (ADRDA) - now known as the Alzheimer's Association (AA) - to issue in 1984 a set of diagnostic criteria. In 1991, the amyloid hypothesis (I stress hypothesis) was first proposed and has remained with us ever since.

Closer to us, the prevalence of AD in the U.S. in 2000 was estimated to be 1.6% both overall and in the 65–74 age group. This rate increased to 19% in the 75–84 group and 42% in the older than 84 group. In less developed regions of the world, these prevalence rates are lower, perhaps pointing to lifestyle as a contributor to the disease or/and to insufficient diagnostic capabilities. In 2000-2010, of the **244** (yes, 244!) **experimental Alzheimer drugs tested**, **only one** (*Memantine*) **was approved in 2003** by the (U.S.) Food & Drug Administration (FDA), In 2005, the World Health Organization (WHO) estimated that 0.379% of people worldwide had dementia, the prevalence would increase to 0.441% in 2015 and to 0.556% in 2030, and would triple by 2050 while the absolute number would quadruple by that date. In **2009, a new disease theory suggested that a close relative of the β-amyloid protein, and not necessarily the β -amyloid itself, may be a major culprit in the disease.** In 2015, the number of people worldwide diagnosed with AD was approximately 29.8 million. Up till the present time, without the required biological understanding of the disease and its root cause(s), and like for other diseases (multiple sclerosis, diabetes, etc.), we had declared AD as incurable and had been content to treat its symptoms, manage its risks, and consider its correlation(s) with other medical observations.

Then, in 2017, following a Eureka moment, I then posited that the disruption of the blood-brain barrier (BBB) is part of the etiology of the disease (not a consequence of it) and that **AD is but an autoimmune disease having gone rogue** in its attempt to maintain brain homeostasis. I am convinced that this is the root cause of the disease, have published it in several, peer-reviewed, learned medical/scientific Journals, and lectured on it at several international symposia and congresses on brain disorders. That conclusion has not been challenged so far and it is unceasingly being supported by other researchers. Figure 7.1 is a reproduction of the cover of my book on this disease.

Figure 7.1 – Alzheimer's disease – Demystifying the disease and what you can do about it

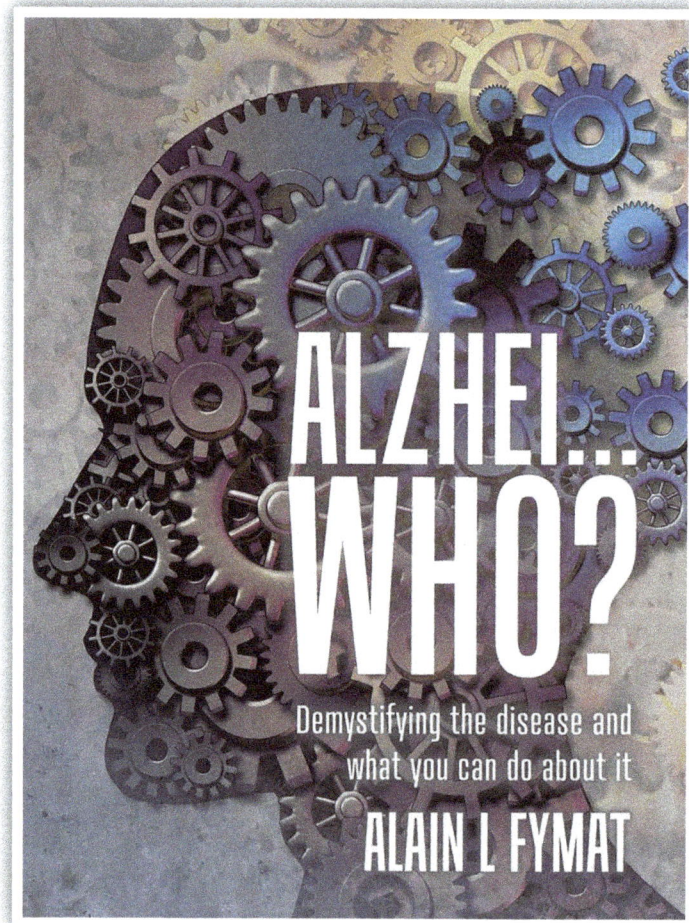

(Reference: Fymat A.L., Tellwell Talent Publishers, 2017)

What is AD?

Over the past few decades, once considered a rare disorder, AD has emerged from obscurity to become a major public health problem. Based on a lack of treatment, it has been generally considered as an irreversible, progressive brain disease that slowly destroys **memory and thinking**

skills, eventually even the ability to carry out the simplest tasks. It is a chronic neurodegenerative disorder (NDD) of poorly (or not) understood cause(s).

In healthy people, all sensations, movements, thoughts, **memories**, and feelings are the result of signals that pass through billions of nerve cells (or neurons) in the brain. Neurons constantly communicate with each other through electrical charges that travel down axons, causing the release of chemicals across tiny gaps to neighboring neurons. Other cells in the brain, such as astrocytes and microglia, clear away debris and help keep neurons healthy.

In a person with AD, toxic changes in the brain destroy this healthy balance over years, even decades. Researchers believe that this process involves two proteins called **beta-amyloid** and **tau**, which somehow become toxic to the brain. It appears that abnormal tau accumulates, eventually forming **tangles** inside neurons. Also, beta-amyloid clumps into **plaques**, which slowly build up between neurons. As the level of amyloid reaches a tipping point, there is a rapid spread of tau throughout the brain.

But tau and beta-amyloid may not be the only factors involved in AD. Other changes that affect the brain may also play a role over time. Thus, the vascular system may fail to deliver sufficient blood and nutrients to the brain; the brain may lack the glucose needed to power its activity; chronic inflammation sets in as microglial cells fail to clear away debris, and astrocytes react to distressed microglia. Eventually, neurons lose their ability to communicate and as they die, the brain shrinks. This decay process begins in the hippocampus, that part of the brain that is important to learning and **memory**. People may begin to experience **memory** loss, impaired decision-making, and language problems. As more neurons die throughout the brain, a person with AD gradually loses the ability to think, remember, make decisions, and function independently.

In brief, according to current knowledge, AD is an age-related, progressive, irreversible neurological disorder in which brain cells die slowly, destroying **memory** and thinking skills, eventually even the ability to carry out the simplest tasks. In most people with AD, symptoms first appear after age 60.

The **memory loss and the associated cognitive decline** had developed over a period of years or decades. When it appears in persons aged in their 30s and mid-60s, it is called *early onset AD* but the more prevalent form occurs in the mid-60s and older and is called *late onset AD*. By contrast, in the absence of disease, the human brain often can function well into the 10th decade of life. It is time to review the hallmarks of the disease.

The four major hallmarks of AD

There are four major hallmarks in the brain that are associated with the disease processes of AD. Again, these are hallmarks, *not* causes of the disease. They are: Amyloid (beta) plaques, neurofibrillary (tau) tangles, loss of connections between nerve cells (neurons) in the brain, and chronic inflammation. Whereas these hallmarks are still considered the main features of AD, many other complex brain changes are thought to play a role in AD, too. **The damage initially appears to take place in the hippocampus but, as neurons die, additional parts of the brain are affected**. By the final stage of the disease, damage is widespread and brain tissue has shrunk significantly. Let us now consider each hallmark separately, what are they made of, and what are their respective contributions to AD:

- *Amyloid plaques:* The beta-amyloid protein involved in AD comes in several different molecular forms that collect between neurons. It is formed from the breakdown of a larger protein, called **amyloid precursor protein** (APP), an amyloid peptide. One form, **beta-amyloid 42**, is thought to be especially toxic. In the Alzheimer's brain, abnormal levels of this naturally occurring protein clump together to form plaques that collect between neurons and disrupt cell function. APP is also mixed with a collection of additional proteins, remnants of neurons, and bits and pieces of other nerve cells. They are contrasted with healthy cells in Figure 7.2.

Figure 7.2 - Microscope slides of healthy and Alzheimer-diseased cells showing plaques and neurofibrillary tangles

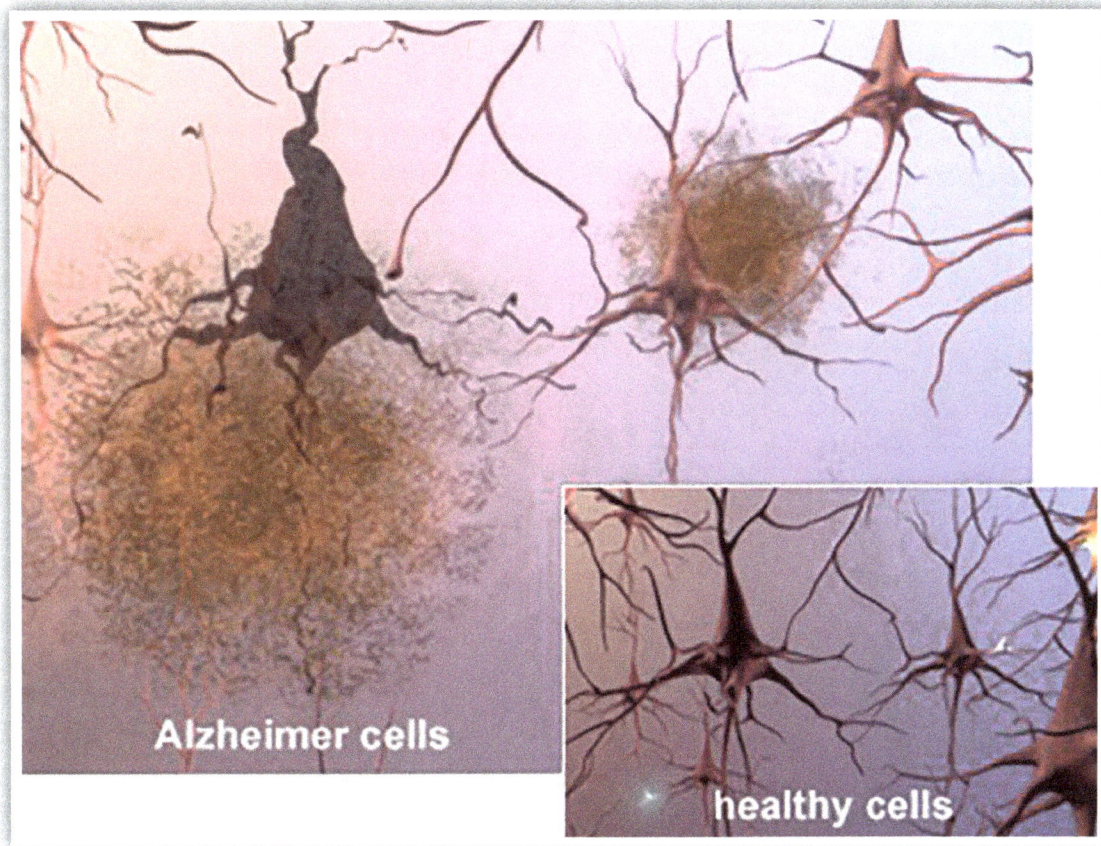

The senile plaques of the cerebral cortex and cerebral blood vessels shown in Figure 7.3 were obtained after an immunostaining process of a micrograph plate. Amyloid beta (Aβ or Abeta) denotes peptides of 36–43 amino acids that are crucially involved in AD as the main component of the amyloid plaques found in the brains of Alzheimer patients. The peptides derive from APP. Research is ongoing to better understand how, and at what stage of the disease, the various forms of beta-amyloid influence AD.

> ➤ **Neurofibrillary (tau) tangles:** Neurofibrillary tangles are abnormal accumulations of a hyperphosphorylated protein called "tau" that collect inside neurons. (Phosphorylation is the addition of a chemical group to any protein, which affects its activity levels in biochemical reactions.) Normal tau is required for healthy neurons. Healthy neurons are in part supported internally by structures called microtubules, which help guide nutrients and molecules from the cell body to the axon and

dendrites. The pictorial in Figure 7.4 illustrates how microtubules within healthy neurons are stabilized by tau molecules whereas, in diseased neurons, they disintegrate and fall apart to produce tangled clamps of tau proteins.

Figure 7.3 - Micrograph showing amyloid beta in senile plaques of the cerebral cortex and cerebral blood vessels

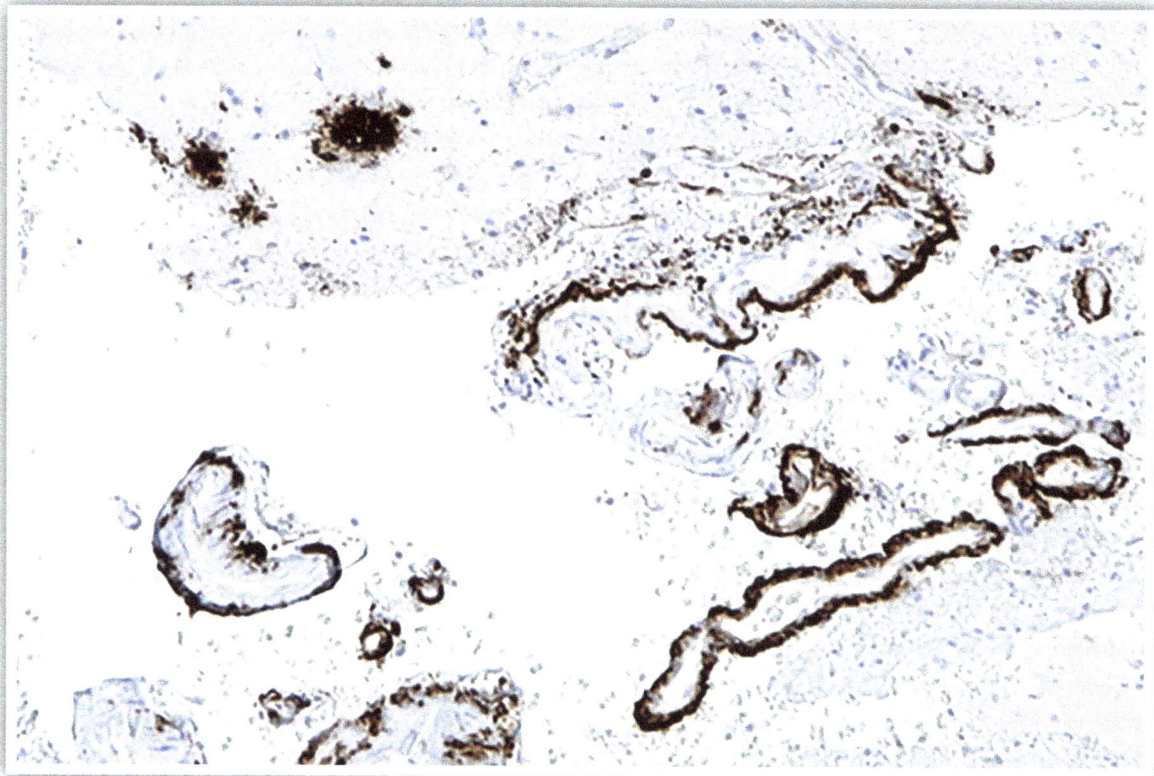

In Figure 7.3, amyloid beta is shown in brown color in senile plaques of the cerebral cortex (upper left of image) and cerebral blood vessels (lower left and right of the image).

In healthy neurons, tau normally binds to and stabilizes microtubules. However, in AD, the tau proteins clump together to form prion-like misfolded oligomers like in Aβ plaques, and there is evidence that misfolded Aβ can induce tau to misfold. Abnormal chemical changes cause tau to detach from microtubules and stick to other tau molecules, forming threads that eventually join to form tangles inside neurons. These tangles block the neuron's transport system, which harms the synaptic communication between neurons. As a result, neurons fail to function normally and eventually die. The tangles are most commonly known as a primary marker of AD. Their presence is also found in numerous other diseases known as tauopathies, but little is known about their exact relationship to the different pathologies (see Figure 7.4).

Evidence is emerging that suggests that Alzheimer's-related brain changes may result from a complex interplay among abnormal tau and beta-amyloid proteins and several other factors. It appears that abnormal tau accumulates in specific brain regions involved in **memory**. Beta-amyloid clumps into plaques between neurons. As the level of beta-amyloid reaches a tipping point, there is a rapid spread of tau throughout the brain.

- ***Loss of connections between neurons responsible for memory and learning***: In AD, as neurons are injured and die throughout the brain, connections between networks of neurons may break down, and many brain regions begin to shrink. Neurons cannot survive when they lose their connections to other neurons. As neurons die throughout the brain, the affected regions begin to atrophy (or shrink). By the final stage of AD, this damaging process—called brain atrophy—is widespread and brain tissue has shrunk significantly, causing significant loss of brain volume.

Figure 7.4 – Showing how microtubules disintegrate in Alzheimer's disease

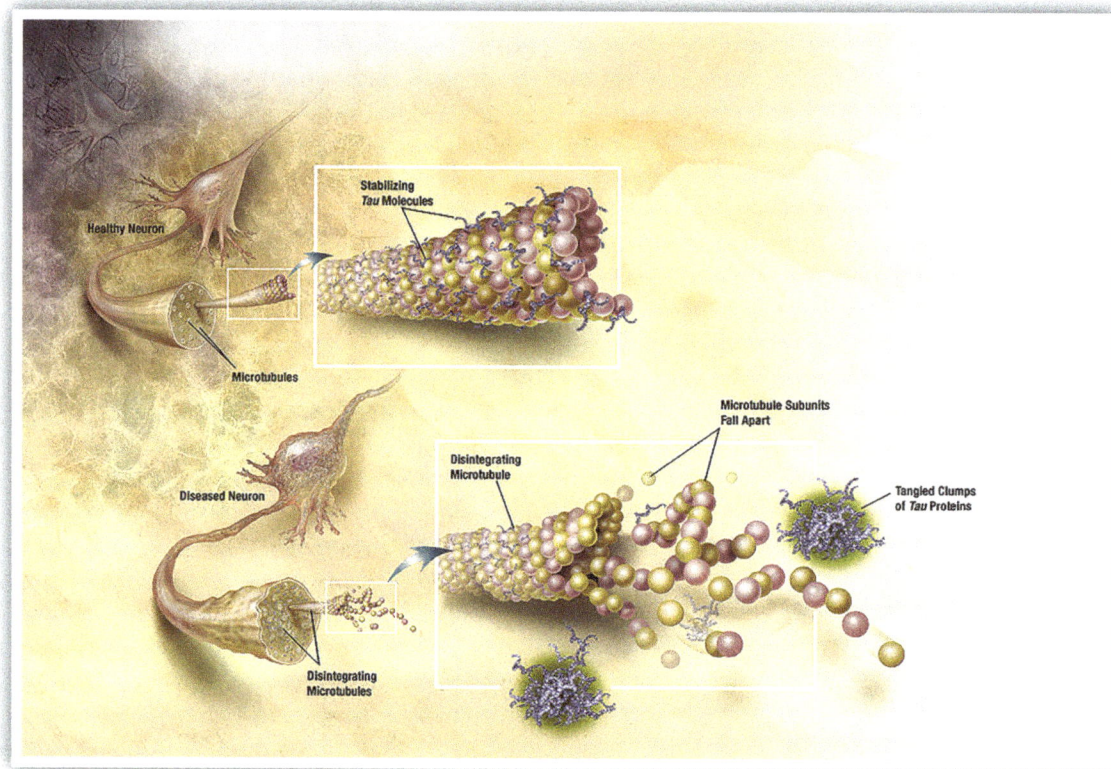

Source: National Institute on Aging, (U.S.) National Institutes of Health, Alzheimer's Disease Education and Referral Center **http:// www.nia.nih.gov/NR/rdonlyres/A01D12CE-17E3-4D3D-BCEF- 9ABC4FF91900/0/TANGLES_HIGH.JPG**

> *Chronic Inflammation:* Research suggests that chronic inflammation may be caused by the build-up of glial cells normally meant to help keep the brain free of debris. One type of glial cell, the "microglia", engulfs and destroys waste and toxins in a healthy brain. In AD, microglia fail to clear away waste, debris, and protein collections, including beta-amyloid plaques. Researchers are trying to find out why microglia fail to perform this vital function in AD. One focus of study is a gene called TREM2. Normally, TREM2 tells the microglial cells to clear beta-amyloid plaques from the brain and helps fight inflammation in the brain. In the brains of people where this gene does not function normally, plaques build up between neurons. "Astrocytes"—another type of glial cell—are signaled to help clear the buildup of plaques and

other cellular debris left behind. These microglia and astrocytes collect around the neurons but fail to perform their debris-clearing function. In addition, they release chemicals that cause chronic inflammation and further damage the neurons they are meant to protect.

As if beta amyloid plaques, neurofibrillary (tau) tangles, loss of neuronal connections and chronic inflammation are not sufficient, other complications essentially of a vascular nature arise.

On the presumed causes of AD

Based on identified risk factors, no less that **19** (yes,19!) **other theories** (or hypotheses) have been propounded for its cause(s), spanning genetics, the environment, and lifestyle. I discuss them in great detail in my 2017 book on AD (its Chapter 6). Such a wide array of hypotheses is by itself indicative of our lack of true understanding and knowledge of the disease and a sad testimonial to this shortcoming. Some of these hypotheses may not be completely independent of each other, some may occur in combination in whole or in part, and additional hypotheses may perhaps surface in the future. Unfortunately, except for two of them ('INT' and 'runaway autoimmune system'), all these hypotheses are merely risk (not causative) factors for AD.

It must be noted that whereas genetics is not a fundamental contributor to the disease, it still accounts for a not so small percentage (say, less than 10%) of all cases. **Gene mutations on chromosomes 1, 14, 19 and 21** are responsible for early onset AD but, unfortunately, we have not found a specific gene that directly causes late-onset AD.

Regarding the "beta-amyloid hypothesis", there are many subtle variations of it but, generally, the theory goes as follows: The beta-amyloid proteins accumulate in the brain then clump together and, somewhere in this process, nerve cells in the brain become damaged, which leads to **memory loss** and other symptoms. So, naively, the approach to treatment seemed rather straightforward: Stop the clumping and the disease will be arrested. Unfortunately, while treatment such as with *Aducanumab* (and the more recently FDA-approved drug *Leqembi* of the same family) cleared beta-amyloid in the brain, the disease continued unabated. In one clinical trial, it was even reported to worsen the symptoms. While perhaps helpful, reducing the amyloid-beta plaques is unlikely to lead to a cure. Should, then, the amyloid hypothesis for AD be abandoned? As a presumed root cause of AD, I think so! In reality, few neuroscientists still subscribe to the view that it is the beta-amyloid plaques themselves that cause the symptoms of AD.

The cause(s) of late-onset AD are not yet completely understood, but, as indicated earlier, they likely include a combination of **g**enetic, **e**nvironmental, and **l**ifestyle factors (acronym: **GEL**). Critical research findings about early-onset AD have helped identify key steps in the formation of brain abnormalities typical of the more common late-onset form of AD. Genetic studies have also helped explain why the disease develops in people at various ages. Research on the genetics of AD is continuing, particularly using genome wide association studies (GWAS) that have identified 33 regions of interest. Although an important genetic risk factor, ApoE ε4 does not necessarily lead to AD and its absence may not prevent AD, making a genetic intervention rather problematic.

Beyond genetics, research has shown that a number of other factors, indeed important factors, may play a role in the development and course of AD such as heart disease, stroke, and high blood pressure, as well as metabolic conditions such as diabetes and obesity. Ongoing research aims to understand whether and how reducing risk factors for these conditions may also reduce the risk of AD. Further, the emerging sciences of epigenetics and ecogenetics are also being co-opted in order to explain these and other risk factors. Although they may help reduce the severity of the symptoms and even help with certain behavioral problems, the 'treatment' approaches followed can only be effective for some, but not all people, and this for a limited time. AS indicated earlier, it is my conviction that AD is rather a **runaway autoimmune disease** so that any treatment should rather aim to rebalance the brain autoimmune system. In separate publications, I have even charted a path to a cure along this principle.

Diagnosis, staging, and treatment of AD

Diagnosis

AD is usually diagnosed based on three factors and two supportive factors with advanced neuroradiological imaging. These tests can also be used to help exclude other cerebral pathologies or subtypes of dementia. Chapter 7 of my book discusses the several tests employed for diagnosing 'possible' and 'probable' AD, including the so-called 'gold standard'. (I will not dwell at length on this topic here but again refer the interested reader to my book.) More recent tests are those of lipid and other molecules produced in the brain that are also found in the blood, and imaging of the retina which may turn out to be a mirror to the brain.

For each individual, it is possible to design a set of genetic, biochemical, and other tests that would provide a personalized risk profile for AD. These tests will identify those suboptimal conditions according to present health guidelines that would require attention and may aid in assessing the present risk status, charting a treatment path, and evaluating its results. Depending on that person's health condition, the number of suboptimal test results will vary.

Staging

The disease is staged either functionally or/and cognitively.

Functional staging: The Aging and Dementia Research Centers of New York University Medical Center have developed the Functional Assessment Staging Test (or FAST) for AD shown in Figure 7.5. It differs from the generally accepted functional and cognitive staging of the disease but is nonetheless helpful and easy to understand.

FAST includes seven stages that will help better understand how AD affects the hypothalamus and other regions of the brain. These are:

> **Stage 1:** Normal adult. No functional decline.
> **Stage 2:** Awareness of some functional decline.

- **Stage 3:** Early AD. Functions at about 12 years of age.
- **Stage 4:** Mild AD. Requires some assistance.
- **Stage 5:** Needs help getting dressed. Functions at 5-7 years of age;
- **Stage 6:** Needs 24/7 care. Functions at 2-4 years of age.
- **Stage 7:** Severe. Functions at the level of a newborn.

Figure 7.5 - The New York University Functional Assessment Staging Test (FAST) of Alzheimer's disease

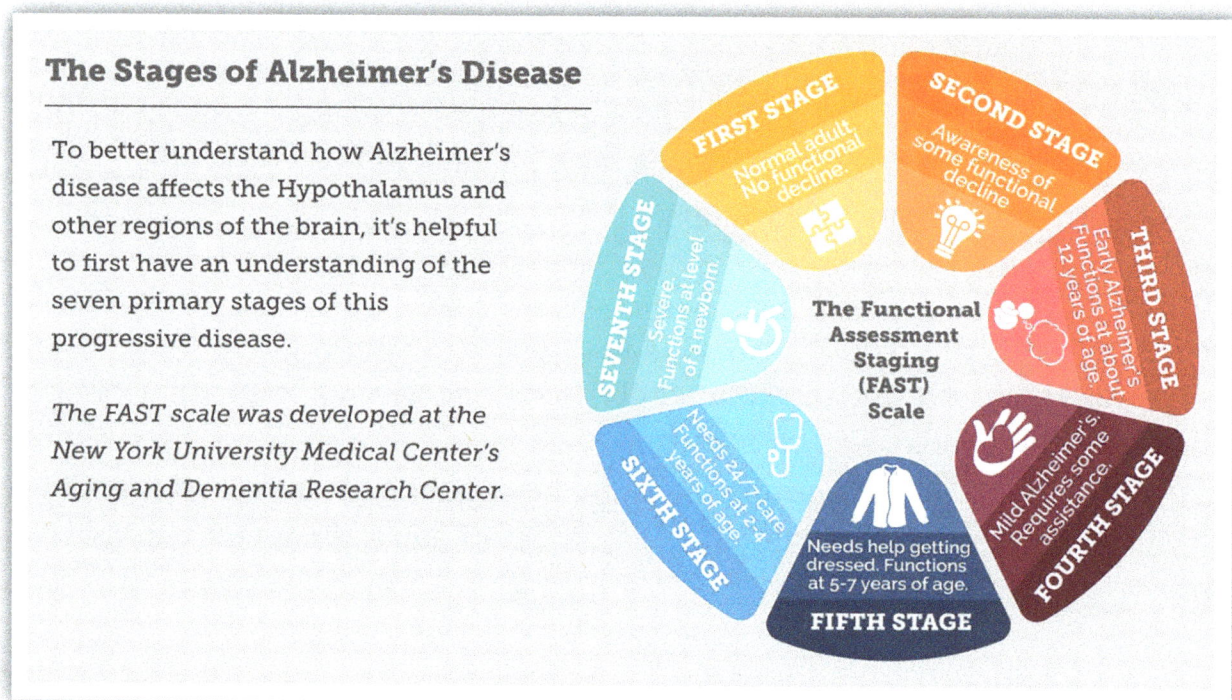

The Stages of Alzheimer's Disease

To better understand how Alzheimer's disease affects the Hypothalamus and other regions of the brain, it's helpful to first have an understanding of the seven primary stages of this progressive disease.

The FAST scale was developed at the New York University Medical Center's Aging and Dementia Research Center.

FIRST STAGE — Normal adult. No functional decline.

SECOND STAGE — Awareness of some functional decline.

THIRD STAGE — Early Alzheimer's. Functions at about 12 years of age.

FOURTH STAGE — Mild Alzheimer's. Requires some assistance.

FIFTH STAGE — Needs help getting dressed. Functions at 5-7 years of age.

SIXTH STAGE — Needs 24/7 care. Functions at 2-4 years of age.

SEVENTH STAGE — Severe. Functions at level of a newborn.

The Functional Assessment Staging (FAST) Scale

Functional and cognitive staging

The generally accepted staging follows a progressive pattern of cognitive and functional impairment whereas FAST is only concerned with the latter. There are the following six stages:

- **Stage 1: Subjective cognitive impairment (SCI).** It is a worsening condition that is noticeable to the individual but, in standard neuropsychological testing, still falls in the normal range. An MRI brain imaging scan may show some shrinkage. It may last a decade or two before the impairment progresses to the next stage.

- ➢ **Stage 2: Mild cognitive impairment (MCI).** MCI typically follows SCI. Neuropsychological tests show that **memory,** organizing, speaking, calculating, planning, or other cognitive abilities are abnormal (even though the individual may still be able to perform daily activities). MCI does not inevitably progress to AD but, in many people, especially those in whom there is memory loss, AD will follow within a few years. MCI is a preclinical transitional stage of the disease between normal aging and dementia. It can present with a variety of symptoms and, when **memory loss** is the predominant symptom, it is termed "amnestic MCI". It is frequently seen as a prodromal stage (that is, an early or premonitory symptom) of the disease.
- ➢ **Stage 3: Pre-dementia.** The first symptoms, often mistakenly attributed to aging or stress, are:
  - ○ Mild cognitive difficulties particularly **short term memory loss**. These are evidenced by detailed neuropsychological testing up to eight years before the clinical diagnostic criteria;
  - ○ Subtle problems with executive functions (attentiveness, planning, flexibility, abstract reasoning);
  - ○ Impairments in **semantic memory** (memory of meanings, concept relationships);
  - ○ Apathy (a most persistent neuropsychiatric symptom throughout the course of the disease); and
  - ○ Depressive symptoms, irritability and reduced awareness of subtle memory difficulties are also common.
- ➢ **Stage 4: Early disease.** This stage is characterized by the increasing impairment or difficulties of:
  - ○ Learning and **memory**;
  - ○ Language (shrinking vocabulary; decreased word fluency; impoverishment of oral and written language);
  - ○ Executive functions;
  - ○ Agnosia (lack perception);
  - ○ Apraxia (difficult execution of movements; difficulties in writing, drawing, dressing, coordination, planning) that may be more prominent than memory problems; and
  - ○ Various effects on **memory** capacities that may not be equally affected:

- It is important to note that AD does not affect all **memory** capacities equally among all those affected, particularly **episodic memory** (older memories of the person), **semantic memory** (facts learned), and **implicit memory** (how to do things, such as using a fork to eat or how to drink from a glass). Nonetheless, as the disease progresses, people with AD can often continue to perform many tasks independently, but may need assistance or supervision with the most cognitively demanding activities.

➢ **Stage 5: Moderate disease.** This stage is characterized by:
  - Progressive deterioration eventually hindering independence;
  - Inability to perform most common activities of daily living;
  - Paraphasia (speech difficulties due to an inability to recall vocabulary, incorrect word substitutions);
  - Reading and writing skills are progressively lost;
  - Complex motor sequences become less coordinated (so the risk of falling increases);
  - Worsened **memory** problems (failure to recognize close relatives);
  - Impaired long-term **memory**, which was previously intact; and
  - Behavioral and neuropsychiatric changes become more prevalent.

Common manifestations include some or all of the following:
  - Wandering;
  - Irritability;
  - Lability;
  - Crying, outbursts of unpremeditated aggression;
  - Resistance to caregiving;
  - Sundowning;
  - Illusionary misidentifications;
  - Delusions;
  - Anosognosia (lost insight of the disease process and limitations); and
  - Urinary incontinence possible development.

➢ **Stage 6: Advanced disease.** The final stages of the disease are characterized by:
  - Complete dependence of the patient upon caregivers;
  - Language reduction to simple phrases or even single words, eventually leading to complete loss of speech. However, despite

the loss of verbal language abilities, people can often understand and return emotional signals;

- ○ Although aggressiveness can still be present, extreme apathy and exhaustion are much more common;
- ○ Ultimately, inability to perform even the simplest tasks independently; and
- ○ Bedridden and inability to feed oneself.

The cause of death is usually an external factor (infection of pressure ulcers, pneumonia, etc.), not the disease itself.

Treatment

Although no particular preventive measure is effective against AD and AD-type dementia (ADD), many interventions can be helpful. They include: controlling certain medical conditions (including diabetes, depression, lipids and high blood pressure, cardiovascular risks), pharmaceutical products, cognitive training, mental and physical exercises, certain modifiable factors (physical activity, nutrition and diet, lipid-lowering, caloric restriction), stress management, sleep quality interventions; social engagement and integration.

Unfortunately, the approved drugs do not change the underlying disease process that goes on unabated. Tables 7.1 (a)-(c) summarize the treatments at a glance in term of changes in disease progression, treating cognitive symptoms (**memory** and thinking), and treating non-cognitive symptoms (behavioral and psychological), respectively.

There has recently been increased interest in the ketogenic diet (in one of several forms), especially as it has also been claimed to be preventive for those at risk of developing AD and other neurodegenerative diseases.

Table 7.1 (a) – Alzheimer's disease treatments claimed to change disease progression

Name (Generic/Brand)	Indicated for	Common side effects
Aducanumab/ Aduhelm®	AD: MCI or mild dementia	o ARIA o Headache o Fall
Lecanemab/ Leqembi®	AD: MCI or mild dementia	o ARIA o Headache o Infusion-related reactions

Table 7.1 (b) - Alzheimer's disease treatments of cognitive symptoms (memory and thinking)

Name (Generic/Brand)	Indicated for	Common side effects
Donepezil/ Aricept®	Mild to severe AD dementia	o Appetite loss o Bowel movements: Increased frequency o Muscle cramps o Nausea o Vomiting
Galantamine/ Razadyne®	Mild to moderate AD dementia	o Appetite loss o Bowel movements: Increased frequency o Nausea o Vomiting
Rivastigmine/ Exelon®	o Mild to moderate AD dementia or o PD dementia	o Appetite loss o Bowel movements: Increased frequency o Nausea o Vomiting
Memantine/ Namenda®	Moderate to severe AD dementia	o Confusion o Constipation o Dizziness o Headache

Memantine + Donepezil/ Namzaric®	Moderate to severe AD dementia	o Appetite loss o Bowel movements: Increased frequency o Headache o Nausea o Vomiting

Table 7.1(c) - Alzheimer's disease treatments of non-cognitive symptoms (behavioral and psychological)

Name (Generic/Brand)	Indicated for	Common side effects
Brexpiprazole/ Rexulti®	Agitation associated with AD dementia	o Common cold symptoms o Dizziness o Restlessness or feeling need to move o Sleepiness o Weight gain *Warning for serious side effects:* Increased risk of death in older adults with dementia-related psychosis. *Not approved for the treatment* of people with dementia-related psychosis without agitation that may happen with AD dementia
Suvorexant/ Belsomra®	Insomnia (has been shown to be effective in people living with mild to moderate AD)	o Alertness impaired o Depression worsening o Motor coordination impaired o Respiratory function compromised o Sleep behaviors complex o Sleep paralysis o Suicidal thinking compromised

ARIA= Amyloid-related imaging abnormalities

Achieving a deeper understanding of the molecular and cellular mechanisms—and how they may interact—is vital to the development of effective therapies. Much progress has been made in identifying various underlying factors. Additionally, advances in brain neuroimaging allow us to see the course of plaques and tangles in the living brain. Blood and fluid biomarkers are further providing insights about when the disease starts and how it progresses. More is also known about the genetic underpinnings of the disease and how they can affect particular biological pathways. These advances enable the development and testing of promising new therapies, including: Drugs that reduce or clear the increase of tau and amyloid proteins in the brain; therapies that target the vascular system, glucose metabolism, and inflammation; lifestyle interventions, like exercise or diet; and behavioral approaches like social engagement that may enhance brain health. Research is moving quickly, ever closer to the day when we can delay or even prevent the devastation of AD and dementia.

Lastly, a number of exciting out-of-the-box discoveries have recently been made. Thus, a new form of dementia (dubbed LATE) has been identified. It affects people older than 85 whose dementia did not arise from Alzheimer's but may have been erroneously so diagnosed. It may conceivably require a different treatment than heretofore offered:

➢ Reviving **working memory** in older adults with specialized electrical brain stimulations;
➢ Using the retina as a mirror of the brain and an early AD predictor;
➢ Utilizing blood tests to detect the risk of Alzheimer's;
➢ Employing biological fingerprints in the cerebrospinal fluid to improve the diagnosis of the different forms of dementia;
➢ Effecting visual and sound stimulations to reduce amyloid plaques and prevent neurodegeneration; and
➢ Applying virtual reality to vastly improve the quality of life with dementia.

Take-aways

- Over the past few decades, once considered a rare disorder, AD has emerged from obscurity to become a major public health problem impacting millions of people worldwide. Unless it can be effectively treated or prevented, the number of people with the disease will increase significantly if current population trends continue, posing considerable burdens on local economies.

- In ancient times, old age was associated with dementia, a broad term referring to a decline in cognitive function to the extent that it interferes with daily life and activities. In 2009, a new disease theory suggested that a close relative of the β-amyloid protein, and not necessarily the β -amyloid itself, may be a major culprit in the disease.

- Up till the present time, without the required biological understanding of the disease and its root cause(s), and like for other diseases (multiple sclerosis, diabetes, etc.), we had declared AD as incurable and been content to treat its symptoms, manage its risks, and consider its correlation(s) with other medical observations. I posited that AD is but a run-away autoimmune disease.

- Based on a lack of effective treatments, AD has been generally considered as an irreversible, progressive brain disease that slowly destroys **memory** and thinking skills, eventually even the ability to carry out the simplest tasks. It is a chronic neurodegenerative disorder of poorly (or not) understood cause(s).

- Toxic changes in the brain involve two proteins called beta-amyloid and tau. It appears that abnormal tau accumulates, eventually forming tangles inside neurons. Also, beta-amyloid clumps into plaques, which slowly build up between neurons. As the level of amyloid reaches a tipping point, there is a rapid spread of tau throughout the brain.

- Tau and beta-amyloid may not be the only factors involved in AD. Other changes that affect the brain may also play a role over time such as: a failing vascular system, a glucose-deprived brain, and chronic inflammation causing the deterioration and death of neurons.and brain shrinking. People may begin to experience **memory loss**, impaired decision-making, and language problems, gradual loss of the ability to think, remember, make decisions, and function independently.

- There are four major hallmarks (*not* causes of the disease) in the brain that are associated with the disease processes of AD: Amyloid (beta) plaques, neurofibrillary (tau) tangles, loss of connections between nerve cells (neurons), and chronic inflammation.

- Based on identified risk factors, no less that 19 theories (or hypotheses) have been propounded for the cause(s) of the disease, spanning genetics, the environment, and lifestyle. Some of these hypotheses may not be completely independent of each other, some may occur in combination in whole or in part, and additional hypotheses may perhaps surface in the future. Unfortunately, most (if not all) of these hypotheses are merely risk (not causative) factors for AD.

- AD is usually diagnosed based on three factors and two supportive factors with advanced neuroradiological imaging. These tests can also be used to help exclude other cerebral pathologies or subtypes of dementia. For each individual, it is possible to design a set of genetic, biochemical, and other tests that would provide a personalized risk profile for AD.

- The disease is staged either functionally (such as according to the New York University Functional Assessment Staging Test (FAST) or/ and cognitively.

- Although no particular preventive measure is effective against AD and AD-type dementia, many interventions can be helpful including: controlling certain medical conditions (diabetes, depression, lipids and high blood pressure, cardiovascular risks, etc.), pharmaceutical products, cognitive training, mental and physical exercises, certain modifiable factors (physical activity, nutrition and diet, lipid-lowering; caloric restriction), stress management, sleep quality interventions; and social engagement and integration. The approved drugs do not change the underlying disease process that goes on unabated.

- Achieving a deeper understanding of the molecular and cellular mechanisms—and how they may interact—is vital to the development of effective therapies. Additionally, advances in brain neuroimaging allow us to see the course of plaques and tangles in the living brain. Blood and fluid biomarkers are further providing insights about when the disease starts and how it progresses. More is also known about the genetic underpinnings of the disease and how they can affect particular biological pathways.

- Scientific advances are enabling the development and testing of promising new therapies, including: Drugs that reduce or clear the increase of tau and amyloid proteins in the brain; therapies that target the vascular system, glucose metabolism, and inflammation; lifestyle interventions, like exercise or diet; and behavioral approaches like social engagement that may enhance brain health.

8

Dementia- A primer

Contents

8

Dementia – A primer

*According to the definition provided by the World Health Organization (WHO, 2017), dementia is "...an umbrella term for several diseases affecting **memory**, other **cognitive abilities**, and behavior that interfere significantly with a person's ability to maintain their activities of daily living. Although age is the strongest known risk factor for dementia, it is not a normal part of aging".* It is a broad category of <u>brain diseases</u> that cause a long-term and often gradual decrease in the ability to <u>think</u> and remember that is great enough to affect a person's daily functioning. Other common <u>symptoms</u> include *"emotional problems, language difficulties, and decreased motivation"*. The definition provided by the U.S. National Institute of Neurological Disorders and Stroke (NINDS, 2018) is more detailed in that dementia is "... *a group of symptoms caused by disorders that affect the brain. It is not a specific disease"... and "...**memory loss** is a common symptom of dementia. However, **memory loss by itself does not mean having dementia**. People with dementia have serious problems with two or more brain functions, such as **memory** and language. Although dementia is common in very elderly people, it is not part of normal aging"*.

Many different diseases can cause dementia, including Alzheimer's disease (AD), frontotemporal dementia (FTD); Lewy body dementia (LBD), mixed dementia (MD), senility dementia (SD), syphilitic dementia (SD), vascular dementia (VD), or the combined effect of two or more types of dementia, and even stroke. About 10% of individuals present with MD, usually the combination of AD and another type of dementia such as FTD or VD.

However, not being a specific disease, the above potential contributors do not reach to the primary cause of the disease. There lies our greatest shortcoming: Unable to pinpoint the root cause of the disease, we are powerless in treating it. Sure, drugs are available to treat some of the symptoms of these contributing diseases but not the diseases themselves. Likewise, drugs available for dementia can also only alleviate its symptoms; they cannot cure it or repair brain damage. They may improve symptoms or at best slow down the disease. Indeed, there is no known cure for dementia. This is a sad observation on the state of the situation. It stems from our incomplete understanding of the deep biology of the contributing diseases and associated epigenetic/ecogenetic influences.

Epidemiology of the disease

With elongating lifespan in the developed world, dementia has emerged as an increasing public health concern. It was uncommon in pre-industrial times and relatively rare before the 20th century. As more people are living longer, and as risk factors are decreasing or better managed, dementia is becoming more common in the population as a whole. AD and other dementias are fifth among the top 10 global causes of mortality.

Worldwide, dementia affected 35.6 million (2010), 46 million (2015), and ~50 million people (2017). It is projected to reach 82 million (2030) and 152 million (2050), much of the increase located in low- and middle-income countries (nearly 60% of people affected). Table 8.1 shows the increasing percentage of dementia with age for low-to-middle income and developed countries.

Table 8.1 – Percentage of dementia cases as a function of age

Age* ==> % for different populations	65-74	75-84	Over 85
Low-to-middle income	3%	19%	~ 50%
Developed countries	5	%	20-40%

*Slightly higher in women than men at ages 65 and older

Causes of dementia depend on the age when symptoms begun. Thus, Table 8.2 illustrates the variations of dementia with age of occurrence:

Table 8.2 – Dementia variations with age of occurrence

Age	Contributor(s)	Treatment Effects
< 40	o Rare without other neurological disease o Genetic disorders can cause true neurodegenerative dementia (NDD): • AD • SCA 17 (dominant inheritance) • X-linked adenoleukodystrophy (ADL) • Gaucher's disease (GD) type 3 • Metachromatic leukodystrophy (MCLD) • Niemann-Pick disease (NPD) • Pantothenate kinase-associated neurodegeneration (PKAN) • Tay-Sachs disease (TSD) • Wilson's disease (WD)	o Treatment of underlying psychiatric illness, alcohol or drug abuse or metabolic disturbance o WD is particularly important since cognition can improve with treatment
< 65	o AD is most frequent o Inherited forms account for higher proportion o Frontotemporal lobar degeneration (FTLD) & Huntington's disease (HD) account for the rest o Vascular disease (VD) in cases of repeated brain traumas o Chronic traumatic encephalopathy (CTE)	
> 65	o AD, VD or both and DLB occurring alongside either AD or VD or both o Hypothyroidism o Normal pressure hydrocephalus (NPH)	o Fully reversible with treatment o Treatment may prevent progression and improve other symptoms

What is dementia?

Dementia is a major neurocognitive disorder that interferes with the patient's ability to perform everyday functions and activities. Its signs and symptoms result when once-healthy neurons (nerve cells) in the brain stop working, lose connections with other brain cells, and die. Everyone loses some neurons as they age, but people with dementia experience far greater loss, as illustrated in Figure 8.1.

Figure 8.1 – Illustrating healthy and damaged neurons

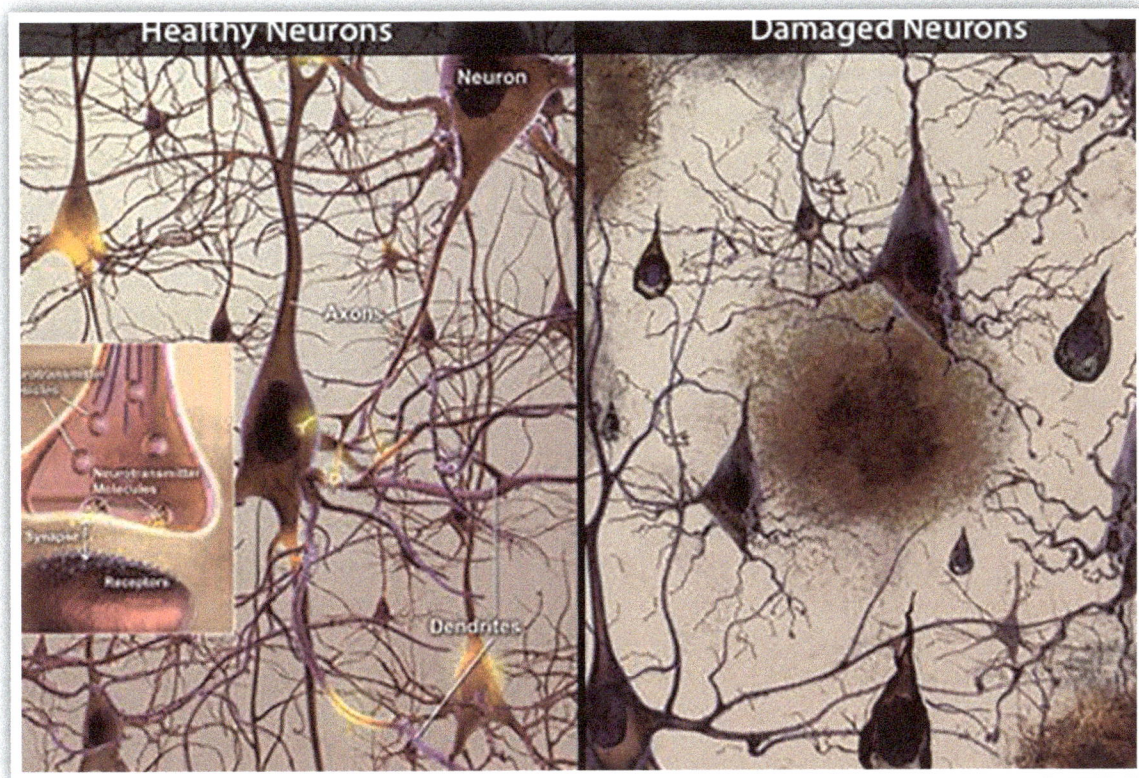

Figure 8.2 further contrasts the inside of a healthy and a diseased neuron.

While dementia is more common as people grow older (up to half of all people age 85 or older may have some form of dementia), it is **not** a normal part of aging. Many people live into their 90s and beyond without any signs of dementia. However, one type of dementia, frontotemporal disorders dementia (FTDD), is more common in middle-aged than older adults.

Figure 8.2 – Contrasting the inside of a healthy and a diseased neuron

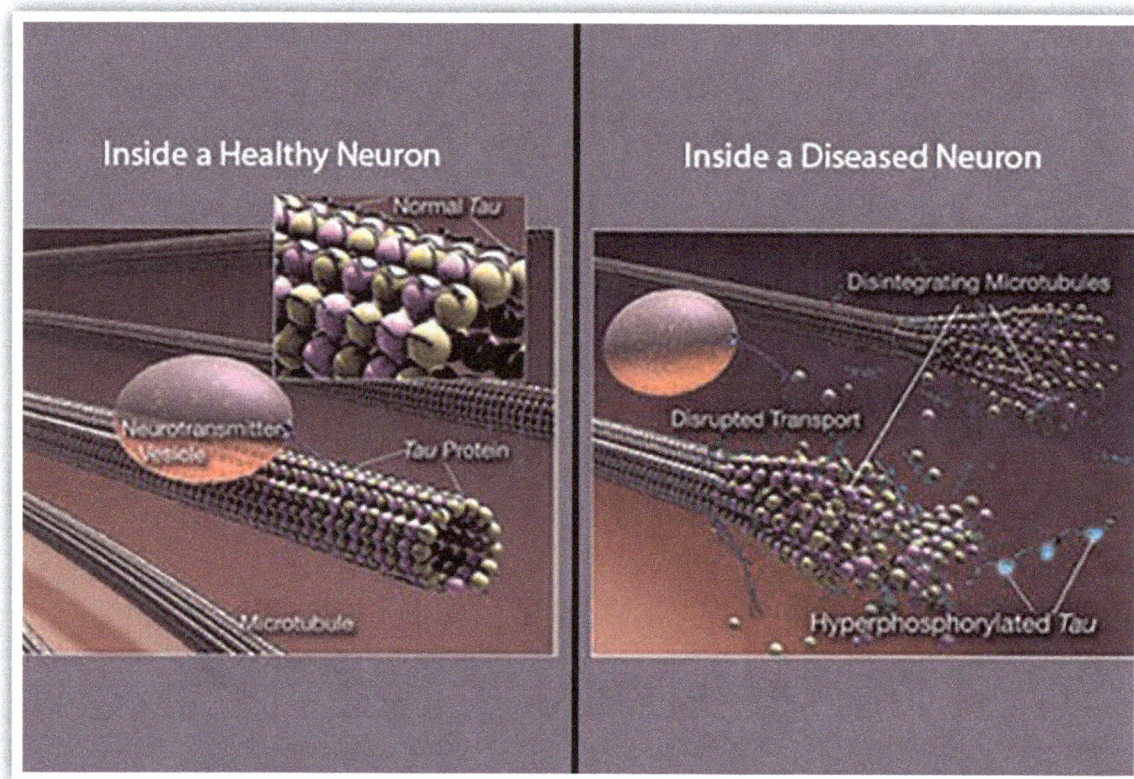

Considerably more details can be found in my book on this subject (Figure 8.3).

Signs and symptoms

Most dementia types are slow and progressive. In their early stages, the onset is gradual to the point of not being clearly noticeable. Symptoms vary across types and stages of the disease and vary with the individual. Signs and symptoms evolve along three phases (early, middle and late) that have been loosely categorized in Table 8.3 as psychological, **memory**, cognition, behavioral, and motor. Behavioral and psychological symptoms almost always occur in all types of dementia.

Figure 8.3 – Dementia – Fending-off the menacing and what you can do about it

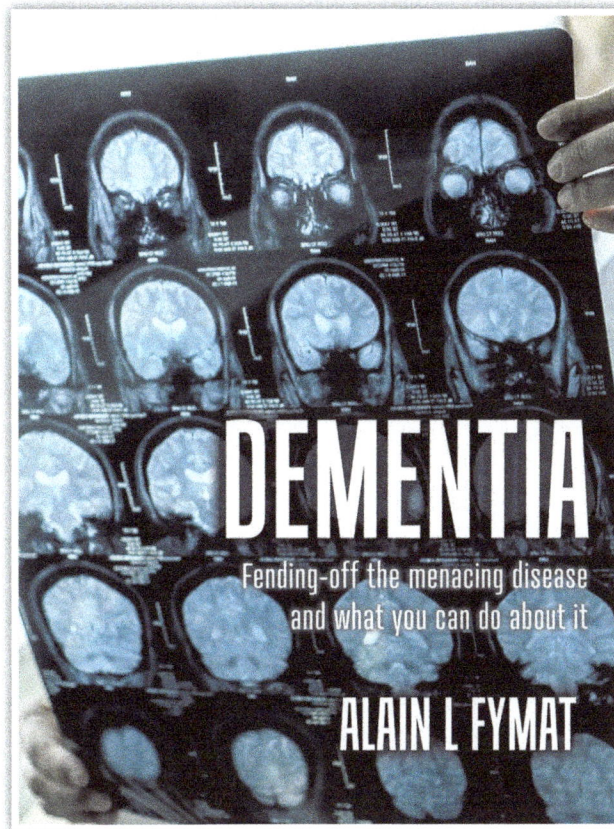

(Reference: Fymat A.L., Tellwell Talent Publishers, 2020)

Early and later signs and symptoms

Most dementia types are slow and progressive. Symptoms vary with the individual and across the types and stages of the disease. The signs and symptoms evolve in three phases (see also Table 8.3):

Early phase: The onset being gradual, this phase is often overlooked. Many patients are unaware that they have any problem. Common symptoms include: difficulty with learning new material (frequently one of the earliest signs of dementia), simple forgetfulness, losing track of the time, becoming lost in familiar places, losing items, and having problems performing tasks or activities that were previously done without effort.

Table 8.3 – Signs and symptoms of dementia

Phase	Psychological	Memory	Cognition	Behavioral	Motor
Early (gradual onset)	o Lost in time & space	o Forgetfulness	o Speech and language difficulties o Difficulties performing tasks or activities	o Lost in familiar places	
Middle (progressing disease)	o Communication difficulties o Attention deficit o Problem-solving difficulty o Having difficulty understanding what is occurring around	o **Memory distortions** o Lost at home o Forgetfulness o Confusion	o Increased speech and language difficulties (anomia)	o Wandering o Restlessness o Repeated questioning o Agitation o Anxiety o Apathy	o Requires help for personal care o Difficulty performing basic tasks o Balance problems o Tremors o Trouble eating & swallowing
Late (advanced disease)	o Unaware of time & space o Delusions o Hallucinations o Depression o Disinhibition o Impulsivity o Psychosis	o Serious **memory disturbances** o Difficulty recognizing relatives & friends		o Agitation o Aggression o Crying o Anger	o Total dependence & inactivity o Difficulty walking

Middle phase: As the disease progresses, the signs and symptoms become clearer and more restricting. These include: experiencing difficulty performing basic tasks such as getting dressed or using the bathroom; needing help with personal care; becoming lost at home; having balance problems; tremors; trouble eating and swallowing; speech and language difficulties; experiencing behavioral changes including wandering, restlessness and repeated questioning; becoming forgetful of recent events and people's names; forgetting pieces of information about oneself including one's address or telephone number, or even date of birth; having increasing difficulty with communication, attention, and problem-solving; **memory** distortions (believing that a **memory** has already happened when it has not, thinking an **old memory** is a new one, combining **two memories**, or confusing the people in a

memory); having difficulty understanding what is occurring around; and not remembering to eat and developing pronounced weight loss.

Late phase: This is a phase of near total dependence and inactivity, serious **memory** disturbances, and more obvious physical signs and symptoms. Symptoms include being no longer able to effectively care for oneself and requiring assistance for all activities of daily living; having an increasing need for assisted self-care; difficulty walking; experiencing behavioral changes that may escalate and include aggression, crying, anger (called a "catastrophic reaction"); having difficulty recognizing relatives and friends; ability to communicate effectively is markedly impaired; and becoming unaware of the time and place. Over time, patients can forget how to walk or even how to sit up.

Risk factors

While most dementias have several common risk factors, each dementia type has its own risk factors, but most forms have several risk factors. These are summarized in Table 8.4:

Table 8.4 – Principal risk factors for dementia

Age	Family History (ApoE ε4)	Other factors

- Biggest risk factor:
Age variation:
  < 60: rare
  >80: common:
    80-85: 1 in 6
    > 85: 1 in 3
    > 90: 1 in 2
	- Increased risk of AD if:
	o First degree relative with AD
	o Relative developed AD < 70
	- Decreased risk if:
	o Relative got AD late in life
	- Half of people with ApoE ε4 develop AD by age 90
		- Hypertension
		- Diabetes
		- Lifestyle factors (including lack of social connections, mental engagement)

Stages of dementia

The stages of dementia are loosely grouped into mild, moderate, and severe categories. Other stagings have also been adopted.

Utilizing scores in the Mini-Mental State Examination (MMSE), four progressive and subsequent stages are defined, as shown in Table 8.5 below. MMSE is a screening tool used to identify cognitive decline on a scale of 0 to 30. It also helps to assess the diagnosis stage to help the attending doctor create a treatment plan.

Table 8.5 – Mini-Mental State Examination (MMSE) and dementia stages

Dementia stage	Signs and symptoms	MMSE score
Mild cognitive impairment (MCI)	o Subtle (apparent in retrospect) o Not severe enough o 70% progress to dementia Mostly **memory** difficulties	27-30 (normal)
Early stage dementia (ESD)	o Interfere with daily activities o Difficulties: **memory**, anomia, executive functions, psychological, cognition, behavioral, and motor	20-25
Middle stage dementia (MSD)	o Worsen o Executive/ social judgment impaired o Assistance required (hygiene, care,...)	6-17
Late stage dementia (LSD)	o 24-hour assistance/ supervision o Changes in diet o Significant changes in sleeping habits	<< 6

- **Stage 1 - Mild cognitive impairment (MCI):** Here, the signs and symptoms of the disorder may be subtle and only become apparent in retrospect, including some **memory** problems and trouble finding words. They are not yet severe enough to affect the person's daily function, solving everyday problems, and handling one's own life affairs. Of those diagnosed with MCI, 70% progress to dementia at some point.

Around 70% of people with MCI go on to develop some form of dementia. MCI is generally divided into three categories:

  ➤ **Amnestic MCI:** Primarily **memory** loss. People with amnestic MCI may go on to develop a more advanced stage of dementia;

> *Non-amnestic MCI:* Not primarily memory difficulties. People with non-amnestic MCI may go on to develop other types of dementia; and

> *Fixed cognitive impairment (FCI):* In this advanced stage of MCI, long-term effects on cognition may result from:

Various types of brain injury: These may cause irreversible cognitive impairment that remains stable over time. Traumatic brain injury may cause generalized damage to the white matter of the brain (diffuse axonal injury), or more localized damage (as also may neurosurgery);

Temporary reduction in the brain's supply of blood or oxygen: May lead to hypoxic-ischemic injury. Strokes (ischemic stroke, or intracerebral, subarachnoid, subdural or extradural hemorrhage) or infections (meningitis or encephalitis) affecting the brain, prolonged epileptic seizures, and acute hydrocephalus may also have long-term effects on cognition; and

> *Excessive alcohol use:* May cause alcohol dementia (AD); Wernicke's encephalopathy (WE) or Korsakoff's psychosis (KP).

Diagnosis of MCI is often difficult, and requires *Petersen's criteria* that include: **memory** or other cognitive (thought-processing) complaint; **memory** or other cognitive problem. The problem must not be severe enough to affect the person's daily functioning and the person must not have dementia.

- **Stage 2 - Early stage dementia (ESD):** Here, symptoms begin to interfere with daily activities and become noticeable to people around. They depend on the type of dementia and usually include: **memory** difficulty; anomia (word-finding problems); executive function problems (planning and organizational skills); getting lost in new places; repeating things; personality changes; and social withdrawal and difficulties at work.

- **Stage 3 - Middle stage dementia (MSD):** Symptoms generally worsen. Solving problems and social judgement are impaired;

functioning outside of the home is precluded; and assistance is required for personal care and hygiene other than simple reminders.

- **Stage 4 - Late stage dementia (LSD):** Assistance is required with personal care and hygiene. 24-hour supervision is needed to ensure personal safety as well as to ensure that basic needs are being met. Lacking supervision, demented individuals wander or fall; may not recognize common dangers around them; and may become incontinent. Changes in diet and eating frequently occur, causing them to gain weight and risk choking. Some patients may not want to eat at all or get out of bed; may need complete assistance doing so; no longer recognize familiar people; and have significant changes in sleeping habits or have trouble sleeping at all.

However, other practitioners also use the following 7-stage system:

- ➤ Stage 1 - N**o impairment:** There are no obvious signs and people are able to function independently.
- ➤ Stage 2 - Very mild impairment: **Symptoms are slight and seem to appear as forgetfulness associated with aging.**
- ➤ Stage 3 – Mild impairment: **P**atients are still able to do daily routine and tasks. Symptoms include forgetfulness; **memory** lapses; losing objects daily; trouble managing finances; confusion while driving; **trouble managing medi**cations; and loss of concentration.
- ➤ Stage 4 - M**oderate impairment:** This is usually the longest stage of dementia. Patients typically have trouble performing daily routine and tasks. Symptoms include the following: trouble holding urine; increased **memory** loss and forgetfulness; forgetting personal details; inability to use or find the correct words; difficulty doing challenging mental mathematics; and increased social withdrawal.
- ➤ Stage 5 - Moderately severe **impairment:** Patients will need assistance in daily routine and tasks. Symptoms include the following: increased **memory** loss; confusion about location or previous events; trouble with less challenging mental mathematics; needing help with selecting appropriate wardrobe; increasing problems planning or organizing, disorientation; and may no longer be able to live alone;

- Stage 6 - Severe impairment: **P**atients will need more assistance in daily routine and tasks. Symptoms include the following: problems recognizing friends and family members; worsened **memory** loss; needing assistance when getting dressed; needing assistance when using the restroom; wandering and getting lost; unable to recall names of loved-ones or caregivers; sleep disturbances; and **changes in personality (paranoia or hallucinations).**
- Stage 7 – Very severe impairment: **Patients will need constant care. Symptoms include the following: b**ody systems decline; loss of language skills; loss of awareness of surroundings; assistance required when eating; unable to control urination; and l**oss of muscle control to smile, swallow, walk, or sit without support.**

Patients may seem to fall into two different stages at the same time, depending on what symptoms they are experiencing. The different stages of dementia cannot be used to predict how rapidly someone's condition might progress and patients may remain in one stage for many years or for only a few months. Every patient has a different disease progression.

Stage determination

Doctors will determine a patient's stage by asking a variety of questions to the patient and the caregiver. Defining the stages of disease progression for dementia is difficult such that management and duration of the disease vary greatly from person to person. To further complicate the stage assessment, the disease has a progressive but vacillating clinical course, one of its defining symptoms being fluctuating levels of cognitive abilities, alertness, and attention. Sudden decline is often caused by medications, infections or other compromises to the immune system. Usually the affected individual returns to his/her baseline upon resolution of the problem. But for some individuals, it may also be due to the natural course of the disease.

Mental disorders classification

The classification of mental disorders (also known as psychiatric nosology or taxonomy) is a key aspect of psychiatry and other mental health professions, and an important issue for people who may be diagnosed with a neurological disorder. The following classifications exist (Table 8.6):

Table 8.6 – Classification of mental disorders

International Classification of Diseases (ICD-10 or later)	Diagnostic & Statistical Manual of Mental Disorders (DSM-5)*	Others
-Similar categories than DSM-5: - 10 groups with subcategories - Includes personality disorders	Similar categories than ICD-10: - 5 dimensions (axes, domains) - Dementia is a neurocognitive disorder with various degrees of severity (axis 1, group 2)	- Chinese Classification of Mental Disorders (CCMD) - Psychodynamic Diagnostic Manual (PDM).

Reference: Produced by the American Psychiatric Association (APA)

Approaches to diagnosis

A diagnosis requires a change from a person's usual mental functioning and a greater decline than one would expect due to <u>aging</u>. Being very similar in all types of dementia, symptoms cannot by themselves help reach the correct diagnosis of demential type(s). Diagnosis usually proceeds along the following lines (Table 8.7). Screening the general population for dementia is not recommended.

Table 8.7 – Approaches to a dementia diagnosis

Type	Approach	Outcome/Characteristic
History	History of the illness	
Preliminary Tests	To rule out confounding diseases/disorders: o *Niacin, Folate or Vitamin B12 deficiency, statins* o *Delirium* (aka *acute confusional state*): deficits in **cognition**, perception, sleep-wake cycle, psychosis (hallucinations, delusions). May be caused by infection or drugs (anticholinergics, benzodiazepines, opioids) o *Mental illnesses (depression, psychosis)* o *Paralytic dementia* (aka *general paresis; general paralysis of the insane*): caused by chronic meningoencephalitis; leads to cerebral atrophy in late-stage syphilis. o *Infective conditions:* Cryptococcal meningitis; AIDS; Lyme disease, progressive <u>multifocal leukoencephalopathy</u> , <u>subacute sclerosing panencephalitis</u> , <u>syphilis</u> , and <u>Whipple disease</u>	o No solid evidence of benefit o Not a disease. Varies in severity over time. Sudden change in mentation. Not to be confused with depression, dementia, psychosis. May appear on background of mental illness or dementia o Use Neuropsychiatric Inventory (NPI) or Geriatric Depression Scale (GDS) tests o Severe neuropsychiatric disorders (classified as an organic mental disorder)
Cognitive Tests	Tests of **memory**, executive function, processing speed, attention, language skills, emotional, and psychological adjustment	o To rule out other etiologies o To determine relative cognitive decline over time: MMSE, AMTS, 3MS, TMT, CDT, MOCA, SAQ, IQCODE, ADCQ, GPAC
Laboratory tests	To rule out other treatable causes	Vitamin B12, Folic acid, TSH, CRP, full blood count (<u>electrolytes</u> , <u>calcium</u> , <u>renal function</u> , <u>liver enzymes</u>)
Imaging scans	o CT, MRI o Functional neuroimaging (SPECT, PET. PIB-PET)	o No evidence of diffuse metabolic changes. May suggest normal pressure hydrocephalus (NPH) (a potentially reversible cause of dementia). Can yield information on vascular dementia o For long-standing cognitive dysfunction. To differentiate vascular dementia from AD

Table 8.8 provides the sensitivity and specificity of common tests for dementia; MMSE; 3MS; and Abbreviated Mental Test Score (AMTS):

Table 8.8 – Sensitivity and specificity of common tests for dementia

Test	Sensitivity (%)	Specificity (%)
MMSE	71-92	56-96
3MS	83-93.5	85-90
AMTS	73-100	71-100

Reversible diseases

These are: Hypothyroidism; Vitamin B12 deficiency; Lyme disease; and Neurosyphilis. All people with **memory** difficulty should be checked for hypothyroidism and B12 deficiency. For Lyme and neurosyphilis, testing should only be done if there are risk factors for those diseases. Because risk factors are often difficult to determine, testing for neurosyphillis and Lyme disease, as well as other unmentioned factors, may be undertaken as a matter of course in cases where dementia is suspected.

Contributing diseases

The main contributors to dementia are summarized in Table 8.9 with other (unlisted) minor contributors, including senilitic dementia (SD) or senility, normal pressure hydrocephalus (NPH) and syphilis:

Table 8.9 – Contributors to dementia

Disease	Contribution (%)	Characteristics & symptoms
Alzheimer's disease (AD)	50-70	o Cause: death of nerve cells (neurons) in important parts of the brain o Symptoms: repetition, getting lost, difficulties keeping track of bills, forgetting to take medication, **short-term memory loss**, word-finding difficulties, trouble with visual-spatial areas, reasoning, judgement, insight o Signs: hippocampus, shrinkage of frontotemporal parts

Vascular dementia (VD)	25	o <u>Cause</u>: stroke(s); blood vessels diseases, hypertension, CVDs (particularly previous heart attack, angina), diabetes o <u>Symptoms</u>: minor strokes o <u>Signs</u>: lost or damaged ischemic brain areas
Lewy body dementia (LBD)	15	o <u>Cause</u>: abnormal protein structures within brain cells. Treatable with medication o <u>Symptoms</u>: PD (trembling, stiffness, slowness), visual hallucinations, difficulty with visual-spatial function, problems with attention, organization, executive functions, "Parkinsonism" (tremor, rigid muscles, stiffness, slowness, emotionless face,... o <u>Signs</u>: vivid, long-lasting hallucinations; "act out of dreams", occipital <u>hypoperfusion</u> hypometabolism
Parkinson's disease dementia (PDD)	)	o <u>Cause</u>: during the course of PD o <u>Symptoms</u>: very similar to DLB
Frontotemporal dementia (FTD)	)	o <u>Symptoms</u>: personality changes, abnormal social behavior, language difficulties (**memory** problems are not a main feature) o <u>Signs</u>: nerve cell loss in frontal and temporal lobes. Arises at earlier age than AD. 3 types: behavioral, temporal (or semantic), progressive nonfluent aphasia
Mixed dementia (MD)	)	o <u>Cause</u>: more than one (often AD and vascular) o <u>Signs</u>: over 80 years of age
Progressive supranuclear palsy (PSP)	)	o <u>Symptoms</u>: eye movement problems, falling backwards, balance problems, slow movements, rigid muscles, irritability, apathy, social withdrawal, depression, progressive difficulty eating and swallowing, eventually talking. Misdiagnosed as PD o <u>Signs</u>: atrophied midbrain
Corticobasal degeneration (CBD)	)	o Symptoms: many different types of neurological problems, get worse over time o Signs: affected frontotemporal lobes; difficulty using only one limb ("alien limb"), asymmetric symptoms (myoclonus or jerky movements of one or more limbs), strange repetitive movements (dystonia), speech difficulty (inability to move mouth muscles in coordinated way), numbness and tingling of limbs, neglect one side of vision or senses
Creutzfeldt-Jakob disease (CJD)	)	o Cause: Prions o Symptoms: slow (at times rapid) progression
Encephalopathy		o Causes: - Brain infection (viral or sclerosing encephalitis) and Whipple disease - Brain inflammation: limbic encephalitis <u>(LE);</u> <u>Hashimoto's encephalopathy (HE); cerebral vasculitis</u> <u>(CV);</u> tumors (lymphoma, glioma); drug toxicity (e.g., anticonvulsants) - Metabolic causes: liver or kidney failure, chronic subdural hematoma (CSH)

Immunologically mediated	)	o Causes: chronic inflammatory conditions, Behcet's disease (BD), multiple sclerosis (MS), sarcoidosis; Sjogren's syndrome (SS), systemic lupus errhythematosus (SLE), celiac disease (CD), and non-celiac gluten sensitivity o Signs: Can rapidly progress. Good response to early treatment (immuno-modulators, steroids)
Inherited conditions	)	o Causes: Alexander's disease (AD), cerebrotendinous xanthomatosis (CX), dentatorubal pallidoluysian atrophy (DPA), epilepsy, fatal familial insomnia (FFI), fragile X-associated tremor/ataxia syndome (FXTAS), glutaric aciduria type 1 (GA), Krabbe's disease (KD), maple syrup urine disease (MSUD), Niemann-Pick disease type C (NPD), neuronal ceroid lipofuscinosis (NCL), neuroacanthocytosis, organic acidemias, Pelizaeus-Merzbache disease (PMD), San Filippo syndrome type B (SFS), spinocerebellar ataxia type 2 (SCA), urea cycle disorders.
Other conditions	)	o Causes: cumulative damage in the brain (e.g., in chronic alcoholism, repeated head injuries, etc.)

Types of cognitive impairment

The following instances of cognitive impairment must be differentiated (Table 8.10):

Table 8.10 – Types of cognitive impairment

Cognitive Impairment Type	Subtypes	Characteristics	Diagnosis
Mild (MCI) MMSE=25-30	Amnestic	o **Memory** loss o Develop Alzheimer's disease	Difficult. Requires Petersen's criteria: - **Memory** or other cognitive problem not severe enough - Person must not have dementia
(70% of people with MCI develop some form of dementia)	Non-amnestic	o **Memory** loss not primary o Develop other dementias	
Fixed (FCI) Long-term effects	Various types of brain injury	o Irreversible cognitive impairment	- Diffuse axonal injury - Localized damage due to neurosurgery

	Temporary reduction in brain's blood or oxygen supply	o Hypoxic/ischemic injury o Strokes (ischemic stroke, intra-cerebral, subarachnoid, subdural or extradural hemorrhage) o Infections (meningitis, encephalitis) o Epileptic seizures o Acute hydrocephalus	- Long-term effects on cognition
	Excessive alcohol use	o Alcohol dementia (AD) o Wernicke's encephalopathy (WE) o Korsakoff's psychosis (KP)	

On neurodegenerative dementia

Dementia that begins gradually and worsens progressively over several years is usually caused by a neurodegenerative disease (NDD)—that is, by conditions that affect only or primarily the neurons of the brain and cause gradual but irreversible loss of function of these cells. Less commonly, a non-degenerative condition may have secondary effects on brain cells, which may or may not be reversible if the condition is treated.

Disease management

Except for the treatable types of dementia listed above, and in the absence of a thorough understanding of its deep biology, there is currently no cure for the disease. Medical interventions remain therefore palliative with aim to alleviate pain and suffering. They include:

- *Cognitive and behavioral interventions*;

- *Education and support for the patient and the patient's family and caregiver(s); and*
- *Activity and exercise program.*

Other management approaches include:

Psychological and reminiscence therapies

While benefits are small, these therapies can improve the quality of life, communication, and possibly mood in some circumstances. Areas covered include:

Quality of life, cognition, communication, mood, and cognitive reframing for caretakers;

- ➢ *Validation therapy;* and
- ➢ *Mental exercises:* such as cognitive stimulation programs (for people with mild to moderate cognitive impairment).

Care in adult centers, special units in nursing homes, and in the home

These institutions provide specialized care (supervision, recreation, meals, limited health care, music therapy,... as well as providing respite for caregivers). Home care can provide one-on-one support and allow for the more individualized attention that is needed as the disorder progresses.

Psychiatric nursing

Can make a distinctive contribution to patients' mental health.

Table 8.11 summarizes the psychotherapy for AD and other dementias:

Table 8.11 - Psychotherapy for Alzheimer's disease and other dementias

Pathology	Drugs	Precautions	Side Effects
Memory problems Monitored 8-week course	Provide no cure: o Cholinesterase inhibitors*: Donepezil (Aricept®), Galantamine (Razadyne®) Rivastigmine (Exelon®) o Memantine (Namenda®): Used in combination with anti-cholinesterase o N-Methyl D-Aspartate (NMDA) receptor blockers o Folate or Vitamin B12 o Statins o Blood pressure medications	o Symptoms may worsen if the treatment is stopped or after treatment o Periodic evaluation of the treatment required o May cause increase in cardiovascular-related events	o Nausea, vomiting, gastro-intestinal upset, diarrhea, weight loss, fainting spells, difficulty sleeping with very vivid dreams (when taken at bedtime), muscle cramping, slow heart rate and fainting in people with heart problem o Dizziness, aggression and hallucinations o No improved outcomes o No benefit o No clear link with dementia
Behavioral symptoms	o Environment change, physical exercise, avoiding triggers that cause sadness, socializing with others, engaging in pleasant activities o Antipsychotics:		o Agitation, anxiety, irritability o Not usually recommended due to little benefits, side effects, increased risk of death
Depression	o Behavioral therapy and/or medications o Selective serotonin re-uptake inhibitors (SSRI): Fluoxetine (Prozac®), Sertraline** (Zoloft®), Paroxetine (Paxil®), Citalopram** (Celexa®), Escitalopram (Lexapro®)		
Anxiety & Aggression	Medications		Can be caused by several factors: confusion, misunderstanding, disorientation, frightening, paranoid delusions, hallucinations, depression, sleep disorders, reduced sleep or altered sleep/wake cycles, medical conditions (such as difficulty urinating or severe constipation, other causes of physical pain or discomfort)

Sleep problems	o Medications or/and behavior changes o Benzodiazepines (diazepam) and non-benzodiazepine hypnotics: To be avoided: o Melatonin, Ramelteon, Trazodone		o Worsened confusion, increased risk of falls, increased cognitive impairment o Little evidence to improve sleep in dementia patients
Pain	Medications		Decreased ambulation, depressed mood, sleep disturbances, impaired appetite, falls, and exacerbation of cognitive impairment, profound functional, psychosocial, and quality of life implications
Eating difficulties	Assisted feeding, gastrostomy, feeding tube		Worsening pressure ulcers, fluid overload, diarrhea, abdominal pain, local complications,. risk of aspiration

* Precautions: Donepezil should be used with caution in people with: (a) cardiac problems: heart disease, cardiac conduction disturbances, chronic obstructive pulmonary disease (COPD), severe cardiac arrhythmias; (b) asthma; (c) sick sinus syndrome (SSD); (d) peptic ulcer disease (PUD) or taking non-steroidal anti-inflammatory drugs (NSAID); and (e) in case of predisposition to seizures.

** Sertraline and Citalopram do not reduce symptoms of agitation compared to placebo and do not affect outcomes.

Changes in medication management

The Medications Appropriateness Tool for Co-Morbid Health – Dementia (MATCH-D) criteria can help identify ways that a diagnosis of dementia changes medication management for other health conditions.

Alternative therapies

- ○ Aromatherapy and massage: U nclear benefits.
- ○ Cannabinoids: Can relieve behavioral and psychological symptoms of dementia.
- ○ Omega-3 fatty acid supplements from plants or fish sources: Do not appear to benefit or harm people with mild to moderate AD, or improve other types of dementia.

Dental hygiene

There is limited evidence linking poor oral health to cognitive decline. Poor oral hygiene can have an adverse effect on speech and nutrition, causing general and cognitive health decline. Oral bacteria (*P. gingivalis*, *F. Nucleatum; P. intermedia*, *T. Forsythia;* trepomena spirochetes) and oral viruses have been observed in the brains of Alzheimer's patients.

Note on spirochetes: These are neurotrophic in nature, meaning they act to destroy nerve tissue and create inflammation. Inflammatory pathogens are an indicator of AD. Bacteria related to gum disease have been found in the brains of AD individuals. They invade nerve tissue in the brain, increasing the permeability of the blood-brain barrier (BBB) and promoting the onset of AD among the elderly population (Fymat 2018b). (See also Sidebar 6.1.)

Note on Herpes simplex virus (HSV): Found in over 70% of the 50 and older population, it persists in the peripheral nervous system (PNS) and can be triggered by stress, illness or fatigue. High proportions of viral-associated proteins in amyloid-containing plaques or neurofibrillary tangles (NFTs) highly confirm the involvement of HSV-1 in AD pathology. HSV-1 produces the main components of NFTs, the primary marker of AD.

Palliative care

Recommended before the late stages of dementia. Given the progressive and terminal nature of the disease, palliative care can be helpful to patients and their caregivers by helping both people with the disorder and their caregivers understand what to expect, deal with loss of physical and mental abilities, plan out a patient's wishes and goals including surrogate decision-making, and discuss wishes for or against cardiopulmonary resuscitation (CPR) and life support.

Prevention

No medications or supplements have shown good preventative evidence, including blood pressure medications. Efforts to prevent dementia include:

- *Early education;*
- *Decrease of risk factors:* High blood pressure, smoking, diabetes and obesity, hearing loss, depression, social isolation;
- *Lifestyle changes:* Including physical exercise and social activities; and
- *Computerized cognitive training:* May improve memory.

Conclusions

While much is known about dementia and the underlying and contributing factors, and much has been published on the subject, we still do not understand the deep biology of the disease. Lacking this understanding, we have so far failed to find a cure and continue to be limited to symptomatic treatments that have limited or no effect. In the case of Alzheimer's dementia, the main contributor, there is a ray of hope in the recent suggestion (Fymat, 2018) that the root cause of Alzheimer's may be an autoimmune disease gone rogue, and that deposits (or plaques) of beta-amyloid (a protein) and the neurofibrillary tangles (disorganized masses of protein fibers within the brain cells) may only be the signs of a brain homeostasis that had broken down under an avalanche of brain insults. Similar innovative ideas and suggestions should be pursued for the other contributors to dementia.

Take-aways

- Dementia describes symptoms of a major neurocognitive disorder that interferes with the patient's ability to perform everyday functions and activities. Its signs and symptoms result when once-healthy neurons (nerve cells) in the brain stop working, lose connections with other brain cells, and die. While everyone loses some neurons as they age, people with dementia experience far greater loss.
- While dementia is more common as people grow older (up to half of all people age 85 or older may have some form of dementia), it is not a normal part of aging and it varies with the age of occurrence. The several contributors and associated symptoms have been described for ages over 65, under 65, and up to 40 years.
- Early and later signs of the disease have been described. Most dementia types are slow and progressive. The onset is gradual to the point of not

being clearly noticeable. Symptoms vary across types and stages of the disease and vary with the individual. Signs and symptoms evolve along three phases (early, middle and late) that have been loosely categorized in terms of psychological, **memory**, cognition, behavioral, and motor. Behavioral and psychological symptoms almost always occur in all types of dementia.

- While most dementias have several common risk factors, each dementia type has its own risk factors, and most forms of dementia have several risk factors

- Several disease staging approaches have been developed, including the Mini-Mental State Examination (MMSE), which is a screening tool used to identify cognitive decline on a scale of 0 to 30. It also helps to assess the diagnosis stage. It involves seven stages that range from no impairment to very severe impairment. Patients may fall into two different stages at the same time, depending on what symptoms they are experiencing.

- The different stages of dementia cannot be used to predict how rapidly someone's condition might progress and patients may remain in one stage for many years or for only a few months. Every patient has a different disease progression. Stage diagnosis can help create a personalized treatment plan.

- The classification of mental disorders (also known as psychiatric nosology or taxonomy) is a key aspect of psychiatry and other mental health professions, and an important issue for people who may be diagnosed with a neurological disorder.

- A diagnosis requires a change from a person's usual mental functioning and a greater decline than one would expect due to aging. Being very similar in all types of dementia, symptoms cannot by themselves help reach the correct diagnosis of demential type(s).

- Screening the general population for dementia is not recommended. However, all people with memory difficulty should be checked for hypothyroidism and B12 deficiency. For Lyme and neurosyphilis, testing should only be done if there are risk factors for those diseases.

- The main contributors to dementia include: Alzheimer's, vascular, Lewy body, Parkinson's, frontotemporal, mixed, progressive supranuclear palsy, corticobasal degeneration, Creutzfeldt-Jakob disease, encephalopathy, immunologically-mediated, inherited, and other conditions. Other minor contributors include senilitic dementia or senility, normal pressure hydrocephalus, and syphilis.

- Mild and fixed cognitive impairments must be differentiated.
- Except for the treatable types of dementia, and in the absence of a thorough understanding of its deep biology, there is currently no cure for the disease. Medical interventions remain therefore palliative with aim to alleviate pain and suffering. They include: Cognitive and behavioral interventions; education and support for the patient and the patient's family and caregiver(s); and activity and exercise program.
- Other management approaches include: Psychological and reminiscence therapies which, while of small benefit, can nonetheless improve the quality of life, communication, and possibly mood in some circumstances. They include: Quality of life (**cognition**, communication, mood, cognitive reframing for caretakers, validation therapy, and mental exercises); care in adult centers and in the home; and psychiatric nursing.
- The psychotherapy for Alzheimer's disease and other dementias has been described, including for **memory** problems, behavioral symptoms, depression, anxiety and aggression, sleep problems, pain and eating difficulties.
- Pharmacotherapy for dementia, and its changes during the course of the disease, have been briefly discussed.
- Alternative therapies (aromatherapy and massage cannabinoids, omega-3 fatty acid supplements), dental hygiene, and palliative care have also been briefly discussed.
- No medications or supplements have shown good preventative evidence, including blood pressure medications, early education, decrease of risk factors (such as high blood pressure, smoking, diabetes, obesity, hearing loss, depression, social isolation), and lifestyle changes (including physical exercise and social activities). Computerized **cognitive** training may, however, improve memory.
- In sum, while much is known about dementia and the underlying and contributing factors, and much has been published on the subject, we still do not understand the deep biology of the disease. Lacking this understanding, we have so far failed to find a cure and continue to be limited to symptomatic treatments that have limited or no effect.

9

Other neurodegenerative diseases-A primer

Contents

9

Other neurodegenerative diseases- A primer

A neurodegenerative disease (NDD) is caused by the progressive loss of structure or function of neurons in the process known as neurodegeneration. Such neuronal damage may ultimately involve cell death. NDDs include Alzheimer's disease (AD), amyotrophic lateral sclerosis (ALS), Huntington's disease (HD), multiple sclerosis (MS), multiple system atrophy (MSA), Parkinson's disease (PD), and prion diseases. Neurodegeneration can be found in the brain at many different levels of neuronal circuitry, ranging from molecular to systemic. Because there is no known way to reverse the progressive degeneration of neurons, these diseases are considered to be incurable; however, research has shown that the two major contributing factors to neurodegeneration are oxidative stress and inflammation. Biomedical research has also revealed many similarities between these diseases at the subcellular level, including atypical protein assemblies (like proteinopathy) and induced cell death. These similarities suggest that therapeutic advances against one NDD might ameliorate other diseases as well.

Some brain diseases and corresponding effects on the blood-brain barrier

There are approximately 400 known neurological disorders (NDDs), some of which having been classified as mental disorders). A number of these are due to a disruption or failure of the blood-brain barrier (BBB) such as, for example: Alzheimer's disease (AD - a disease in which amyloid beta contained in blood plasma enters the brain and adheres to the surface of astrocytes); epilepsy (chronic or acute seizures caused by inflammation); meningitis (an inflammation of the meninges or membranes surrounding the brain and spinal cord); multiple sclerosis (MS - a disease of either the immune system or/and the breaking down of the BBB in a section of the brain or spinal cord); possibly prion and prion-like diseases such as Parkinson's disease (PD) and AD; HIV encephalitis (HIVE - a precursor of HIV-associated dementia - HIVAD in which latent HIV can cross the BBB inside circulating monocytes in the blood stream); and systemic inflammation (sterile or infectious) that may lead to effects on the brain, cause sickness behavior, and induce or/and accelerate brain diseases such as MS and PD.

Table 9.1 summarizes for each disease the corresponding BBB factor.

Table 9.1: Some brain diseases and their corresponding effects on the blood-brain barrier

Disease	BBB Factor	Disease	BBB Factor
Alzheimer's	Disruption/ Breakdown	**Multiple sclerosis** (Immune system deficiency)	Breakdown
Brain abscess	*Unknown mechanism*	**Neuromyelitis optica** (Devic's disease)	Breakdown
Cerebral edema	Opening (due to hypoxia)	**Prion and prion-like diseases** (Parkinson's; Alzheimer's)	*Unknown penetration mechanism*
De Vivo	*Unknown mechanism*	**Progressive multi-focal leukoencephalopathy**	Disruption
Epilepsy	Disruption/ Failure	**Rabies**	Increased permeability

HIV Encephalitis	Damage (inflammatory) Latent HIV crosses	**Systemic inflammation** (Sterile infectious)	Disruption?
Meningitis	Disruption	**Tripanosomasis** (Sleep thickness)	Disruption

Reference: Fymat (2017).

Some other specific disorders

Chapter 6 has already listed and briefly discussed the multiple possible contributors to memory impairments that would theoretically need to be considered, as appropriate, for a correct diagnosis and treatment. Thus:

Among the central nervous system (CNS) diseases due to inflammation, only encephalitis is of interest. Its severity can be variable with symptoms including reduction or alteration in consciousness and memory problems.

Among the CNS diseases due to encephalopathies, one must distinguish between:

> **Degenerative diseases:** They include:
>   ○ *Extrapyramidal & movement disorders:* Particularly Huntington's disease; myoclonus; Alzheimer's disease; Creutzfeldt-Jakob disease; Parkinson's disease and parkinsonism; panthotenate kinase-associated neurodegeneration; and progressive supranuclear palsy.
>   ○ *Dementia:* Including Alzheimer's; primary progressive aphasia; posterior cortical atrophy; frontotemporal lobar degeneration; and the various dementias (early onset; frontotemporal; HIV; juvenile; Lewy bodies; late onset; pugilistica; and vascular); Parkinson's synucleinopathies; and tauopathy.
>   ○ Seizures/epilepsy: Dravet's syndrome; Lennox-Gastaut syndrome.
> **Demyelinating diseases:** They include:
>   ○ Multiple sclerosis; and
>   ○ Canavan's disease.
> **Episodic paroxysmal diseases:** They include:
>   ○ Seizures;

- Cerebrovascular diseases (acute aphasia; stroke; transcranial global and anteretrograde amnesia)
- Sleep disorders, especially sleep apnea.
- **Other related diseases:** They include the encephalopathies of:
  - Wernicke's;
  - Anti-mild dementia stage receptor; and
  - HIV.

Among the CNS neurodegenerative diseases:
- **Motor neuron diseases:** They include particularly:
  - Amyotrophic lateral sclerosis.

Chapters 7 and 8 have already covered at some length Alzheimer's disease (AD) and Parkinson's disease (PD), respectively. They will not be further considered here. I will only provide brief remarks on a few of the other NDDs.

Huntington's disease (HD)

HD is a rare autosomal dominant NDD caused by mutations in the huntingtin gene (HTT). It is characterized by the loss of medium spiny neurons and astrogliosis. The first brain region to be substantially affected is the striatum, followed by degeneration of the frontal and temporal cortices. The striatum's subthalamic nuclei sends control signals to the globus pallidus, which initiates and modulates motion. The weaker signals from subthalamic nuclei thus cause reduced initiation and modulation of movement, resulting in the characteristic movements of the disorder, notably chorea. Huntington's disease presents itself later in life even though the proteins that cause the disease work towards manifestation from their early stages in the humans affected by the proteins. Along with being a NDD, HD has links to problems with neurodevelopment.

HD is caused by polyglutamine tract expansion in the huntingtin gene, resulting in the mutant HTT. Aggregates of mutant huntingtin form as inclusion bodies in neurons, and may be directly toxic. Additionally, they may damage molecular motors and microtubules to interfere with normal axonal transport, leading to impaired transport of important cargoes such as BDNF. HD currently has no effective treatments that would modify the disease.

Multiple sclerosis (MS)

MS is a chronic debilitating demyelinating disease of the CNS, caused by an autoimmune attack resulting in the progressive loss of myelin sheath on neuronal axons. The resultant decrease in the speed of signal transduction leads to a loss of functionality that includes both **cognitive** and motor impairment depending on the location of the lesion. The progression of MS occurs due to episodes of increasing inflammation, which is proposed to be due to the release of antigens such as myelin oligodendrocyte glycoprotein, myelin basic protein, and proteolipid protein, causing an autoimmune response. This sets off a cascade of signaling molecules that result in T-cells, B-cells, and macrophages to cross the BBB and attack myelin on neuronal axons leading to inflammation. Further release of antigens drives subsequent degeneration causing increased inflammation.

MS presents itself as a spectrum based on the degree of inflammation. A majority of patients experience early relapsing and remitting episodes of neuronal deterioration following a period of recovery. Some of these individuals may transition to a more linear progression of the disease, while about 15% of others begin with a progressive course on the onset of MS. The inflammatory response contributes to the loss of the grey matter and, as a result, current literature devotes itself to combatting the auto-inflammatory aspect of the disease. While there are several proposed causal links between the Epstein-Barr virus (EBV) and the HLA-DRB1*15:01 allele to the onset of MS – they may contribute to the degree of autoimmune attack and the resultant inflammation – they do not determine the onset of MS.

Amyotrophic lateral sclerosis (ALS)

ALS (or Lou Gehrig's disease) is a disease in which motor neurons are selectively targeted for degeneration. It is a NDD that negatively impacts the upper motor neurons (UMNs) and lower motor neurons (LMNs). A mutation in chromosome 9 (C9orf72) is thought to be the most common known cause of sporadic ALS. It is diagnosed by skeletal muscle weakness that progresses gradually. Early diagnosis of ALS is harder than with other NDDs as there are no highly effective means of determining its early onset. Currently, there is research being done regarding the diagnosis of ALS through UMN tests.

The Penn Upper Motor Neuron Score (PUMNS) consists of 28 criteria with a score range of 0–32. A higher score indicates a higher level of burden present on the upper motor neurons. The PUMNS has proven quite effective in determining the burden that exists on upper motor neurons in affected patients. The specific mechanism of toxicity still needs to be investigated, but the findings are significant because they implicate cells other than neuron cells in neurodegeneration.

Creutzfeldt–Jakob disease (CJD)

CJD is a prion disease that is characterized by rapidly progressive **dementia**. Misfolded proteins called prions aggregate in brain tissue leading to nerve cell death. Variant Creutzfeldt–Jakob disease (vCJD) is the infectious form that comes from the meat of a cow that was infected with bovine spongiform encephalopathy (BSE), also called 'mad cow disease'.

Risk factors

The greatest risk factor for NDDs is aging. Both mitochondrial DNA (mDNA) mutations as well as oxidative stress (OS) contribute to aging. Many of these diseases are late-onset, meaning there is some factor that changes as a person ages for each disease. One constant factor is that, in each disease, neurons gradually lose function as the disease progresses with age. It has been proposed that DNA damage accumulation provides the underlying causative link between aging and NDD. About 20%–40% of healthy people between 60 and 78 years old experience discernible decrements in cognitive performance in several domains including **working, spatial, and episodic memory**, and processing speed.

Mechanisms

There are five recognized mechanisms underlying the formation of NDDs: Genetics (including, epigenetics, and ecogenetics), protein misfolding, intracellular mechanisms, programmed cell death, and transglutaminase. Only a brief presentation of these mechanisms is given below.

Genetics

Many NDDs are caused by genetic mutations, most of which are located in completely unrelated genes. In many of the different diseases, the mutated gene has a common feature: A repeat of the CAG nucleotide triplet (CAG codes for the amino acid glutamine), which results in a polyglutamine (polyQ) tract. Diseases associated with such mutations are known as trinucleotide repeat disorders (TNRD). Polyglutamine repeats typically cause dominant pathogenesis. Extra glutamine residues can acquire toxic properties through a variety of ways, including irregular protein folding and degradation pathways, altered subcellular localization, and abnormal interactions with other cellular proteins. Nine inherited NDDs are caused by the expansion of the CAG trinucleotide and polyQ tract, including Huntington's disease and the spinocerebellar ataxias (SCA).

> **Epigenetics**

The presence of epigenetic modifications for certain genes has been demonstrated in this type of pathology. An example is FKBP5 gene, which progressively increases its expression with age and has been related to Braak staging and increased tau pathology both *in vitro* and in mouse models of AD.

Protein misfolding

Several NDDs are classified as proteopathies because they are associated with the aggregation of misfolded proteins. Protein toxicity is one of the key mechanisms of many NDDs:

- **Alpha-synuclein:** Can aggregate to form insoluble fibrils in pathological conditions characterized by Lewy bodies, such as PD, DLB, and MSA. Alpha-synuclein is the primary structural component of Lewy body fibrils. In addition, an alpha-synuclein fragment, known as the non-Abeta component (NAC), is found in amyloid plaques in AG.
- **Tau:** Hyperphosphorylated tau protein is the main component of neurofibrillary tangles in AD. Tau fibrils are the main component of Pick bodies found in behavioral variant frontotemporal dementia (FTD).

- **Amyloid beta:** The major component of amyloid plaques in AD.
- **Prion:** Main component of prion diseases and transmissible spongiform encephalopathy.

Intracellular mechanisms

They include:

- ➤ **Protein degradation pathways;**
- ➤ **Membrane damage;**
- ➤ **Mitochondrial dysfunction:** Together with oxidative stress, it plays a causal role in NDD pathogenesis, including four of the more well known diseases (AD, PD, HD, and ALS).
- ➤ **DNA damage:** Reactive oxygen species produced by oxidative metabolism (the brain metabolizes as much as a fifth of consumed oxygen) are a major source of DNA damage in the brain. This is associated with AD and PD. Defective DNA repair has been linked to AD, PD, ALS, telangiectasia, Cockayne's syndrome (CS), and xeroderma pigmentosum.
- ➤ **Axonal transport:** It can be disrupted by a variety of mechanisms including damage and disruption of degenerative pathways.

Programmed cell death (PCD)

PCD is death of a cell in any form mediated by an intracellular program. This process can be activated in NDDs including AD, PD, HD, and ALS. It may be directly pathogenic or, alternatively, occur in response to other injury or disease processes. It includes:

Figure 9.1 – Parkinson's: Elucidating the disease and what you can do about it

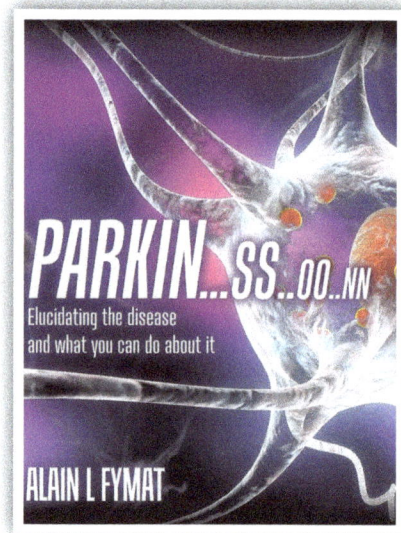

(Reference: Fymat A.L., Tellwell Talent Publishers, April 2020)

- **Apoptosis (type I):** One of the main types of PCD in multicellular organisms. It involves a series of biochemical events leading to a characteristic cell morphology and death. It may involve extrinsic as well as intrinsic pathways.

Figure 9.2 – Epilepsy: The electrical storm in the brain

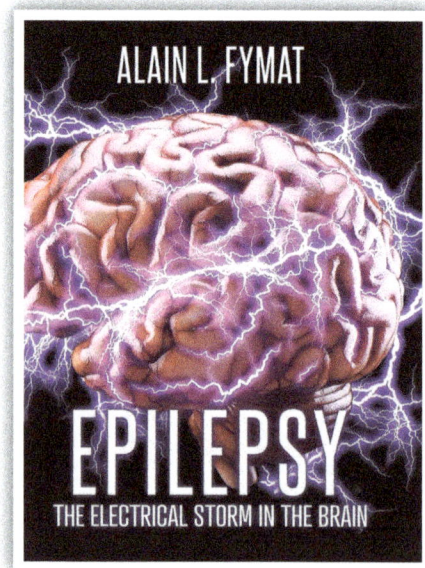

(Reference: Fymat A.L., Tellwell Talent Publishers, September 2022)

- **Caspases (cysteine-aspartic acid proteases):** They cleave at very specific amino acid residues. Initiator caspases cleave inactive forms of effector caspases. This activates the effector caspases that, in turn, cleave other proteins resulting in apoptotic initiation.

Figure 9.3 – Multiple sclerosis: The progressive demyelinating autoimmune disease

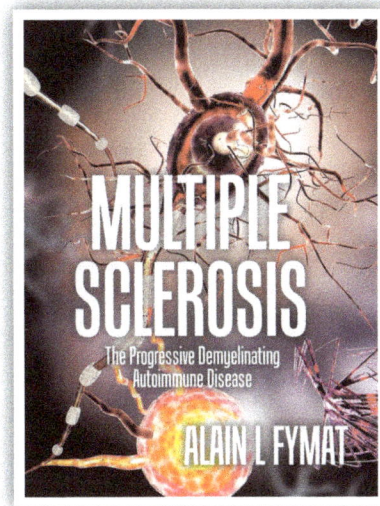

(Reference: Fymat A.L., Tellwell Talent Publishers, March 2022)

Figure 9.4 – Multiple system atrophy: The chronic, progressive, neurodegenerative synucleopathic disease

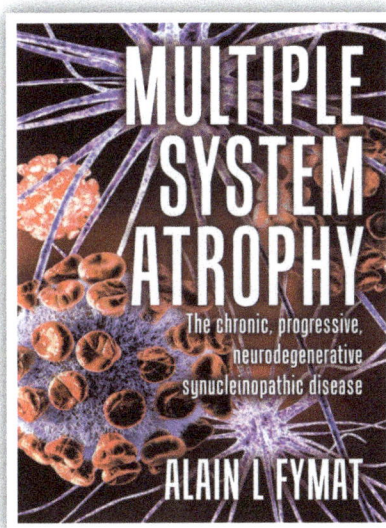

(Reference: Fymat A.L., Tellwell Talent Publishers, May 2023

- **Autophagic (type II):** Autophagy is a form of intracellular phagocytosis in which a cell actively consumes damaged organelles or misfolded proteins by encapsulating them into an autophagosome, which fuses with a lysosome to destroy the contents of the autophagosome. Because many NDDs show unusual protein aggregates, it is hypothesized that defects in autophagy could be a common mechanism of neurodegeneration.
- **Cytoplasmic (type III):** PCD can also occur via non-apoptotic processes, also known as Type III or cytoplasmic cell death.

Transglutaminases

Transglutaminases are human enzymes ubiquitously present in the human body and in the brain in particular. Their main function is to bind proteins and peptides, intra- and inter-molecularly, by a type of covalent bonds termed isopeptide bonds, in a reaction termed transamidation or cross-linking. This makes them clump together, the resulting structures being extremely resistant to chemical and mechanical disruption. Most relevant human NDDs share the property of having abnormal structures made up of proteins and peptides. Each of these NDDs has one (or several) specific main protein or peptide. In AD, these are amyloid-beta and tau; in PD, it is alpha-synuclein; in HD, it is huntingtin. In these NDDs, the expression of the transglutaminase enzyme is increased.

Disease management

The process of neurodegeneration is not well understood, so the diseases that stem from it have, as yet, no cures. For a detailed run-down of disease management in many of these NDDs, I refer the reader the reader to my books on these several subjects (Figures 9.1 to 9.4, and Figures 7.1 and 8.3).

Take-aways

> **There are approximately 400 known neurological disorders, some of which having been classified as mental disorders). A**

number of these are due to a disruption or failure of the blood-brain barrier.

- **A neurodegenerative disease is caused by the progressive loss of structure or function of neurons, in the process known as neurodegeneration. Such neuronal damage may ultimately involve cell death. Neurodegenerative diseases include Alzheimer's disease, amyotrophic lateral sclerosis, Huntington's disease, multiple sclerosis, multiple system atrophy, Parkinson's disease, and prion diseases. Neurodegeneration can be found in the brain at many different levels of neuronal circuitry, ranging from molecular to systemic.**

- Among the central nervous system diseases due to inflammation, only encephalitis is of interest. Among those due to encephalopathies, one must distinguish between degenerative diseases (extrapyramidal & movement disorders, dementias, and seizures/epilepsy).

- Demyelinating diseases include multiple sclerosis and Canavan's disease.

- Episodic paroxysmal diseases include seizures, cerebrovascular diseases, and sleep disorders, especially sleep apnea.

- Among the CNS neurodegenerative diseases, we find motor neuron diseases that include particularly amyotrophic lateral sclerosis.

- The greatest risk factor for neurodegenerative diseases is aging. Both mitochondrial DNA mutations as well as oxidative stress contribute to aging. Many of these diseases are late-onset. One constant factor is that in each disease, neurons gradually lose function as the disease progresses with age, and discernible decrements in cognitive performance in several domains including working, spatial, and episodic memory, and processing speed.

- There are five recognized mechanisms underlying the formation of neurodegenerative diseases: Genetics (including epigenetics and ecogenetics), protein misfolding, intracellular mechanisms, programmed cell death, and transglutaminase.

PART D
THE AGING BRAIN

10

The aging brain

Contents

Sidebar

10

The aging brain

Aging of the brain is a process of transformation of the brain in older age. It encompasses changes experienced by all healthy individuals as well as those changes caused by illnesses (including unrecognized illnesses). It is a major risk factor for most common neurodegenerative diseases (NDDs) such as mild cognitive impairment (MCI) and dementias of various types, including: Alzheimer's disease dementia (ADD); cerebrovascular disease dementia (CVDD); Parkinson's disease dementia (PDD); and amyotrophic lateral sclerosis (or Lou Gehrig's disease) dementia (ALSD). The brain is very complex and composed of many different areas and types of tissue or matter. The brain matter can be broadly classified as either 'grey matter' or 'white matter'. Grey matter consists of cell bodies in the cortex and subcortical nuclei. On the other hand, white matter consists of tightly packed myelinated axons connecting the neurons to each other and with the periphery. The different functions of the various brain tissues may be more or less susceptible to age-induced changes. Figure 10.1 is a pictorial representation of the human brain in the sagittal plane. (For other images, see Chapters 3-5.) Figure 10.2 is a lateral view of the brain showing the principal fissures and lobes of the cerebrum.

While much research has focused on diseases of aging, there are few informative studies on the molecular biology of the aging brain in the absence of neurodegenerative disease and likewise for the neuropsychological profile of healthy older adults. However, research suggests that **the aging process is associated with several structural, chemical, and functional changes in the brain as well as a host of neurocognitive changes**. In addition, recent reports on model organisms suggest that, as organisms age, there are distinct changes in the expression of genes at the single neuron level. These various changes are discussed below.

Structural changes

Aging entails many physical, biological, chemical, and psychological changes. The brain is no exception to this phenomenon. In 2009, scientists have attempted to map these various changes utilizing conceptual models like the 'scaffolding theory of aging and cognition' (STAC). The STAC model looks at factors like: (a) neural changes to the white matter, (b) cortical thinning, (c) shrinkage, and (d) dopamine depletion.

CT scans have found that the cerebral ventricles expand as a function of age. More recent MRI studies have reported age-related regional decreases in cerebral volume. This regional volume reduction (RVR) is not uniform in that some brain regions shrink at a rate of up to 1% per year, whereas others remain relatively stable until the end of the life-span.

Figure 10.1 - The human brain in the sagittal plane

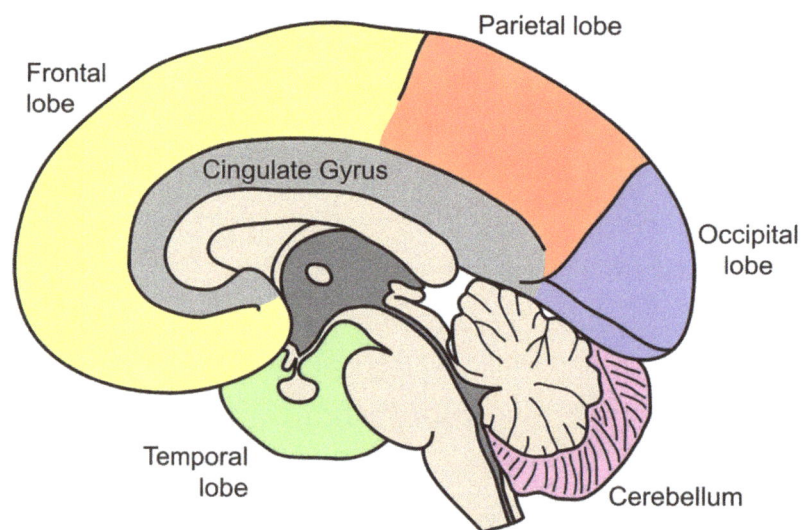

Source: NEUROTiker

Loss of neural circuits and brain plasticity

Brain plasticity refers to the brain's ability to change structure and function. In animals, one proposed mechanism for the observed deficits in age-related plasticity is the result of age-induced alterations in calcium regulation. Here, the changes in the organism's abilities to handle calcium will ultimately influence neuronal firing and the ability to propagate action potentials, which, in turn, would affect the ability of the brain to alter its structure or function (i.e. its plastic nature). Due to the complexity of the brain, with all of its structures and functions, it is logical to assume that some areas would be more vulnerable to aging than others. Two circuits worth mentioning here are the hippocampal and neocortical circuits. It has been suggested that **age-related cognitive decline is due in part not to neuronal death but to synaptic alterations**. Evidence in support of this idea from animal work has also suggested that this cognitive deficit is due to functional and biochemical factors such as changes in enzymatic activity, chemical messengers, or gene expression in cortical circuits.

**Figure 10.2 - Principal fissures and lobes
of the cerebrum (lateral view)**

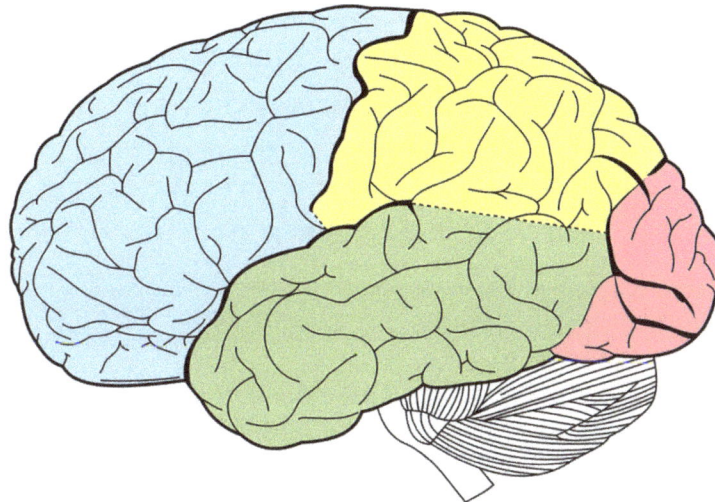

*Source: Henry Vandyke Carter et al. - Henry Gray
(1918) "Anatomy of the Human Body"*

Thinning of the cortex

Advances in MRI technology have provided the ability to see *in vivo* the brain structure in great detail in an easy, non-invasive manner. For example, Bartzokis *et al.*, have noted that there is a decrease in grey matter volume between adulthood and old age, whereas white matter volume was found to increase from age 19 to 40, and decline after this age.

Studies using voxel-based morphometry have identified areas such as the insula and superior parietal gyri as being especially vulnerable to age-related losses in grey matter of older adults. Sowell *et al.*(2003) reported that the first six decades of an individual's life were correlated with the most rapid decreases in grey matter density, and this occurred over dorsal, frontal, and parietal lobes on both inter-hemispheric and lateral brain surfaces. It is also worth noting that areas such as the cingulate gyrus, and occipital cortex surrounding the calcarine sulcus appear exempt from this decrease in grey matter density over time. Age effects on grey matter density in the posterior temporal cortex appear more predominantly in the left versus right hemisphere, and were confined to posterior language cortices. Certain language functions such as word retrieval and production were found to be located to more anterior language cortices, and deteriorate as a function of age. Sowell *et al.*, also reported that these anterior language cortices were found to mature and decline earlier than the more posterior language cortices. It has also been found that the width of sulcus not only increases with age, but also with cognitive decline in the elderly.

Table 10.1 – Age-thinning of the cortex

	Adulthood	Older age
Grey matter Insula; superior parietal gyri	Age 0-60: o Most rapid density decrease: Dorsal, frontal, parietal lobe on both inter-hemispheric and lateral brain surfaces *Note:* Cingulate gyrus and occipital cortex surrounding the calcarine sulcus are exempt from this decrease o More predominant in left vs. right hemisphere and confined to language cortices	o Decrease from adulthood
White matter	o Age 19-40: Increase	o Age > 40: Decrease

Morphology and microstructure

Age-related decrease in grey matter volume was the largest contribution to changes in brain volume. Moreover, neuronal density appears to decrease, white matter microstructure gets altered, and energy metabolism in the cerebellum gets altered. General cortical atrophy (shrinkage) occurs in aging; for example, the caudate nucleus volume appears to decrease.

Age-related neuronal morphology

There is converging evidence from cognitive neuroscientists around the world that age-induced **cognitive deficits** may not be due to neuronal loss or cell death, but rather may be the result of small region-specific changes to the morphology of neurons. Studies by Duan *et al.* (2003), have shown that dendritic arbors and dendritic spines of cortical pyramidal neurons decrease in size and/or number in specific regions and layers of human and non-human primate cortex as a result of age. A 46% decrease in spine number and spine density has been reported in humans older than 50 compared with younger individuals. An electron microscopy study in monkeys reported a 50% loss in spines on the apical dendritic tufts of pyramidal cells in prefrontal cortex of old animals (27–32 years old) compared with young ones (6–9 years old).

Neurofibrillary tangles

Age-related neuropathologies such as AD, PD, diabetes, hypertension, and arteriosclerosis make it difficult to distinguish the normal patterns of aging. One of the important differences between normal aging and pathological aging is the location of neurofibrillary tangles (NFT). NFT are composed of paired helical filaments (PHF). In normal, non-demented aging, the number of tangles in each affected cell body is relatively low and restricted to the olfactory nucleus, parahippocampal gyrus, amygdala and entorhinal cortex. As the non-demented individual ages, there is a general increase in the density of tangles, but no significant difference in where tangles are found. Tau-protein disorders cause microtubule destruction and formation of neurofibrillary tangles.

The other main neurodegenerative contributor commonly found in the brain of patients with AD is amyloid plaques. However, unlike tangles, plaques have not been found to be a consistent feature of normal aging.

DNA damage

At least 25 studies have demonstrated that DNA damage accumulates with age in the mammalian brain. This DNA damage includes: (a) the oxidized nucleoside 8-hydroxydeoxyguanosine (8-OHdG), (b) single- strand breaks, (c) double-strand breaks, (d) DNA-protein cross-links, and (d) malondialdehyde adducts (as reviewed in Bernstein *et al.*).

Increasing DNA damage with age has been reported in the brains of mice, rats, gerbils, rabbits, dogs, and humans. Young 4-day-old rats have about 3,000 single-strand breaks and 156 double-strand breaks per neuron whereas, in rats older than 2 years, the level of damage increases to about 7,400 single-strand breaks and 600 double-strand breaks per neuron.

Lu *et al.* studied the transcriptional profiles of the human frontal cortex of individuals ranging from 26 to 106 years of age. This led to the identification of a set of genes whose expression was altered after age 40. They further found that the promoter sequences of these particular genes accumulated oxidative DNA damage, including 8-OHdG, with age (see DNA damage theory of aging). They concluded that DNA damage may reduce the expression of selectively vulnerable genes involved in learning and memory and neuronal survival, initiating a pattern of brain aging that starts early in life.

Immune system and fluids

Blood-brain barrier (BBB) permeability, neuroinflammation, neurodegeneration, and gut microbiota-induced systemic chronic inflammation appear to be linked and interact with aging, e.g. as gut microbiota homeostasis could be disturbed by increasing age. Neuroinflammatory changes, including microglial activation and production of inflammatory cytokines, occur with normal aging.

Figure 10.3 - Diagram of how microtubules disintegrate with Alzheimer's disease

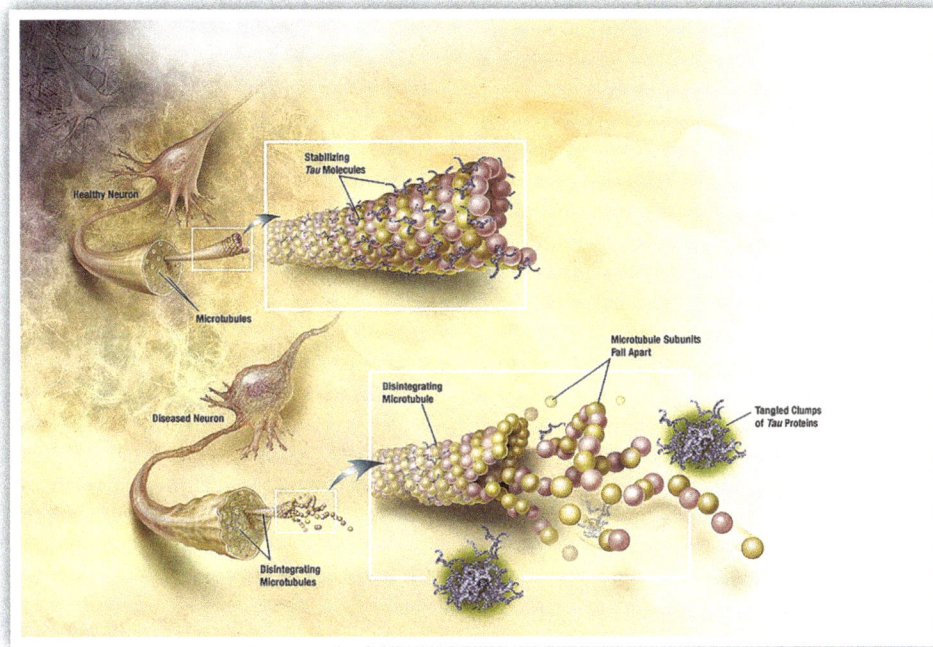

Source: Alzheimer's Disease Education and Referral Center (ADEAR)
A service of the (U.S.) "National Institute on Aging (NIA).
http://www.nia.nih.gov/NR/rdonlyres/A01D12CE-17E3-4D3D-BCEF-
9ABC4FF91900/0/TANGLES_HIGH.JPG

Cerebral blood flow was shown to decrease 0.3-0.5% per year in healthy aging. An efficiently functioning glymphatic system, involved in waste clearance, may be important for maintaining brain health and its transport efficiency appears to be declining with aging. Factors in the circulation have been shown to modulate aging and to rejuvenate the brain. Figure 10.4 shows the circulation of the cerebrospinal fluid in the subarachnoid space around the brain and spinal cord, and in the ventricles of the brain

Role of oxidative stress

Cognitive impairment has been attributed to oxidative stress (OS), inflammatory reactions, and changes in the cerebral microvasculature. The exact impact of each of these mechanisms in affecting cognitive aging is unknown. OS is the most controllable risk factor and is the best understood;

it is that physiological stress on the body that is caused by the cumulative damage done by free radicals inadequately neutralized by antioxidants and that is held to be associated with aging. Hence, OS is the damage done to the cells by free radicals that have been released from the oxidation process.

Figure 10.4 - Circulation of the cerebrospinal fluid

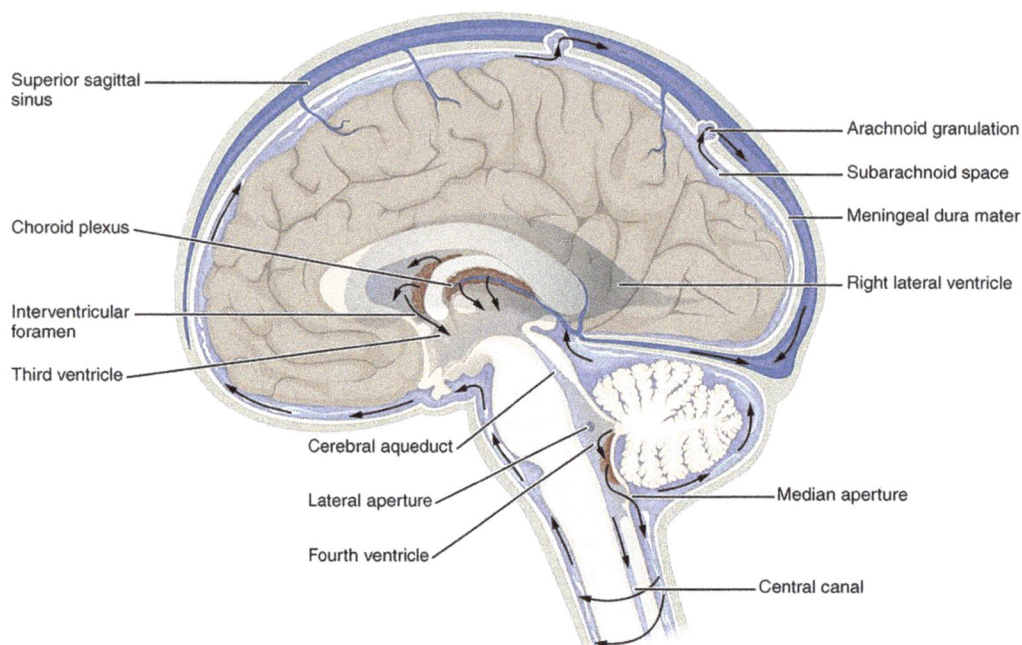

Reference: OpenStax "Anatomy and Physiology", 2016.- https://cnx.org/contents/FPtK1zmh@8.25:fEI3C8Ot@10/Preface

Compared to other tissues in the body, the brain is deemed unusually sensitive to oxidative damage. Increased oxidative damage has been associated with NDDs, MCI, and individual differences in cognition in healthy elderly people. In 'normal aging', the brain is undergoing OS in a multitude of ways. The main contributors to OS include: (a) protein oxidation, (b) lipid peroxidation, (c) oxidative modifications in nuclear DNA, and (d) oxidative modifications in mitochondrial DNA. OS can damage DNA replication and inhibit repair through many complex processes, including telomere shortening in DNA components. Each time a somatic cell replicates, the telomeric DNA component shortens. As telomere length is partly inheritable, there are individual differences in the age of onset of **cognitive decline**.

Biochemical changes

In addition to the structural changes that the brain incurs with age, the aging process also entails a broad range of biochemical changes. More specifically, neurons communicate with each other via specialized chemical messengers called neurotransmitters. Several studies have identified a number of these neurotransmitters, as well as their receptors, that exhibit a marked alteration in different regions of the brain as part of the normal aging process. These neurotransmitters include:

Figure 10.5 – Dopamine and serotonine functions and pathways

Reference: Original: NIDA / Derivative work: Quasihuman - Dopamine Pathways.png

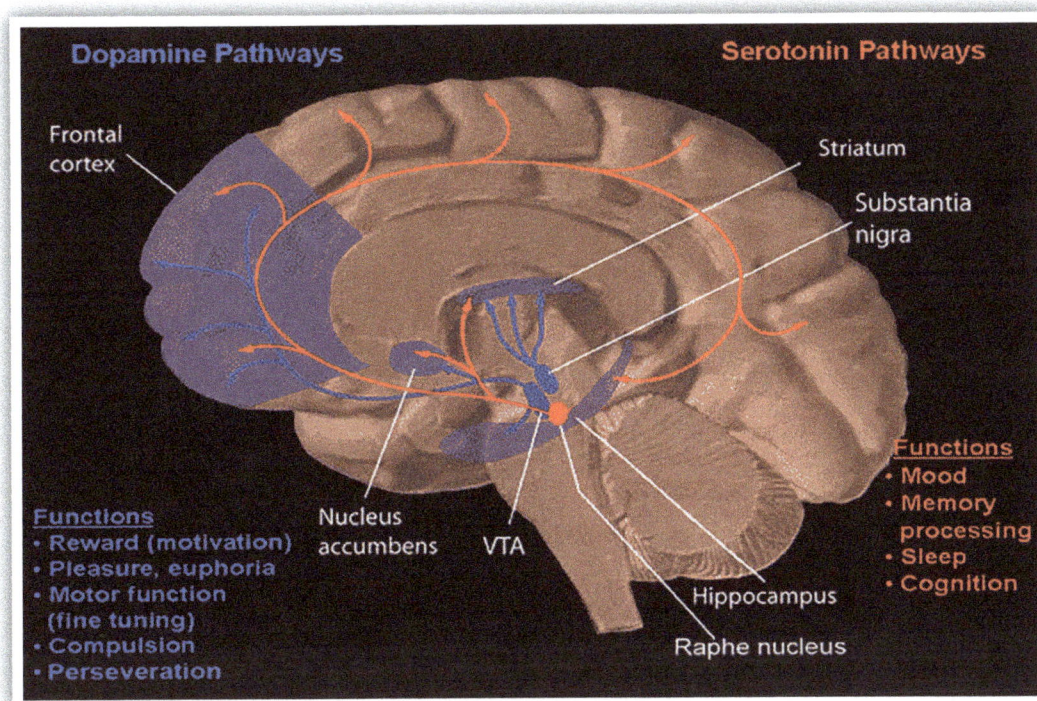

NIH - http://www.drugabuse.gov/pubs/teaching/largegifs/slide-2.gif

> **Dopamine:** In the brain, dopamine plays an important role in the regulation of reward and movement. An overwhelming number of studies have reported age-related changes in dopamine synthesis, binding sites, and number of receptors. Positron emission tomography (PET) in living human subjects have shown a significant age-related

decline in dopamine synthesis, notably in the striatum and extrastriatal regions (excluding the midbrain). Significant age-related decreases in dopamine receptors D1, D2, and D3 have been highly reported. A general decrease in D1 and D2 receptors has been shown, and more specifically a decrease of D1 and D2 receptor binding in the caudate nucleus and putamen. A general decrease in D1 receptor density has also been shown to occur with age. Significant age-related declines in D2 and D3 dopamine receptors were detected in the anterior cingulate cortex, frontal cortex, lateral temporal cortex, hippocampus, medial temporal cortex, amygdala, medial thalamus, and lateral thalamus. One study also indicated a significant inverse correlation between dopamine binding in the occipital cortex and age. *Post-mortem* studies also show that the number of D1 and D2 receptors decline with age in both the caudate nucleus and the putamen, although the ratio of these receptors did not show age-related changes.The loss of dopamine with age is thought to be responsible for many neurological symptoms that increase in frequency with age, such as decreased arm swing and increased rigidity. Changes in dopamine levels may also cause age-related changes in cognitive flexibility (Tables 10.2 and 10.3).

Table 10.2 – Age-related decreases in dopamine receptors

Dopamine receptor	Brain regions affected	Effects
D1	o Striatum & extrastriatal regions (excluding midbrain) o Caudate nucleus; putamen	o Significant decline in synthesis o Significant and general decrease in receptors o General decrease in receptor density
D2	o Striatum & extrastriatal regions (excluding midbrain) o Caudate nucleus; putamen; cortex (anterior cingulate; frontal; lateral temporal; medial temporal); hippocampus; amygdala; thalamus (medial; lateral)	o Significant decline in synthesis o Significant and general decrease in receptors

D3	o Striatum & extrastriatal regions (excluding midbrain) o Caudate nucleus; putamen; cortex (anterior cingulate; frontal; lateral temporal; medial temporal); hippocampus; amygdala; thalamus (medial; lateral)	o Significant decline in synthesis o Significant decrease in receptors

Shown in Figure 10.5 are the dopamine pathways, offering the following functions: Reward (motivation); pleasure – euphoria, motor functions (fine tuning); compulsion; and perseveration. As part of the reward pathway, dopamine is manufactured in nerve cell bodies located within the ventral tegmental area (VTA) and is released in the nucleus acumbens and the prefrontal cortex. Its motor functions are linked to a separate pathway, with cell bodies in the substantia nigra that manufacture and release dopamine into the striatum. By contrast, the functions offered by serotonin are: Mood, **memory processing**; sleep; and **cognition**.

- **Serotonin:** Decreasing levels of different serotonin receptors and the serotonin transporter (5-HTT), have also been shown to occur with age. *In vivo* studies conducted using PET methods on humans show that levels of the 5-HT2 receptor in the caudate nucleus, putamen, and frontal cerebral cortex, decline with age. A decreased binding capacity of the 5-HT2 receptor in the frontal cortex was also found, as well as a decreased binding capacity of the serotonin transporter (5-HHT) in the thalamus and the midbrain. *Post-mortem* studies on humans have indicated decreased binding capacities of serotonin and a decrease in the number of S1 receptors in the frontal cortex and hippocampus as well as a decrease in affinity in the putamen.

Table 10.3 – Age-related decreases in serotonin receptors and transporters

Serotonin	Brain regions affected	Effects
Receptors (5-HT2)	o Caudate nucleus; putamen; and frontal cerebral cortex	o Decline
S1-receptor	o Frontal cortex; hippocampus	o Decreased binding capacity
Transporters (5-HTT)	o Thalamus; midbrain	o Decline o Decreased binding capacity

> **Glutamate:** Glutamate is another neurotransmitter that tends to decrease with age. Studies have shown older subjects to have lower glutamate concentration in the motor cortex compared to younger subjects. A significant age-related decline especially in the parietal gray matter, basal ganglia, and to a lesser degree, the frontal white matter, has also been noted. Although these levels were studied in the normal human brain, the parietal and basal ganglia regions are often affected in degenerative brain diseases associated with aging and it has therefore been suggested that brain glutamate may be useful as a **marker of aging brain diseases** (Table 10.4 and Figure 10.6).

Table 10.4 - Age-related decreases in glutamate concentration

Glutamate	Brain regions affected	Effects
Concentration	o Motor cortex o Parietal grey matter; basal ganglia; and.. to a lesser degree, frontal white matter	o Decrease o Significant decline

The image in Figure 10.6 shows the tissue distribution of excitatory amino acid transporter 2 (EAAT2), a.k.a. glutamate transporter 1 (GLT1), in the brain. The expression of glutamate transporter 1 in glial cell facilitates reuptake of glutamate and decreases extracellular glutamate concentration.

Figure 10.6 - Expression of glutamate transporter 1 in glial cells

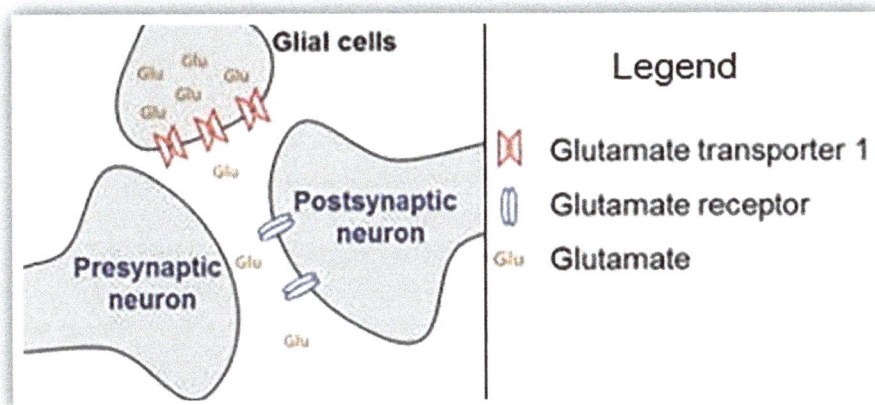

Reference: PSS Rao et al. (2015)

Neuropsychological changes

Neuropsychological changes include changes in orientation, attention, **memory**, and language, as discussed below:

Changes in orientation

Deficits in orientation are one of the most common symptoms of brain disease, hence tests of orientation are included in almost all medical and neuropsychological evaluations. Research studies have been inconclusive as to whether there is a normal decline in orientation among healthy aging adults. Results have been somewhat inconclusive. However, some studies have suggested that mild changes in orientation may be a normal part of aging and not necessarily a sign of a particular pathology.

Changes in attention

Attention is a broad construct that refers to *"the cognitive ability that allows a person to deal with the inherent processing limitations of the human brain by selecting information for further processing"*. Since the human brain has limited resources, people use their attention to zone-in on specific stimuli and block out others.

Many older adults notice a decline in their attentional abilities. If older adults have fewer attentional resources than younger adults, we would expect that when two tasks must be carried out at the same time, older adults' performance will decline more than that of younger adults. However, this hypothesis has not been wholly supported. While some studies have found that older adults have a more difficult time encoding and retrieving information when their attention is divided, other studies have not found meaningful differences from younger adults. Similarly, sustained attention shows no decline with age.

There are factors other than true attentional abilities that might relate to difficulty paying attention such as, for example, sensory deficits (impaired hearing or vision) may impact older adults' attentional abilities.

Changes in memory

Many different types of **memory** have been identified in humans (see Chapter 12). Memory functions, more specifically those associated with the medial temporal lobe, are especially vulnerable to age-related decline. A multitude of studies utilizing a variety of methods (histological, structural imaging, functional imaging, and receptor binding) have supplied converging evidence that the frontal lobes and frontal-striatal dopaminergic pathways are especially affected by age-related processes resulting in memory changes.

Changes in language

Behavioral changes associated with age include compromised performance on tasks related to word retrieval, comprehension of sentences with high syntactic and/or **working memory** demands, and production of such sentences.

Changes in behavioral flexibility

The rapid neurotransmitter GABA (gamma aminobutyric acid)-boosting may be a major potential explanation-component for why learning is often more efficient in children and takes longer or is more difficult with age. Late-stage aging and/or late-life dementias decrease behavioral flexibility and impair deliberation about courses of action.

Qualitative changes

Most research on **memory** and aging has focused on how older adults perform worse at a particular memory task. However, researchers have also discovered that simply saying that older adults are doing the same thing, only less of it, is not always accurate. In some cases, older adults seem to be using different strategies than younger adults. For example, brain imaging studies have revealed that **older adults are more likely to use both hemispheres when completing memory tasks than younger adults**. In addition, older adults sometimes show a positivity effect when remembering information, which seems to be a result of the increased focus on regulating emotion seen with age. For instance, eye tracking reveals that older adults showed preferential looking toward happy faces and away from sad faces.

Genetic changes

Variations in the effects of aging among individuals can be attributed to genetic, health, lifestyle, and environmental factors. The search for genetic factors has always been an important aspect in trying to understand neuropathological processes. Here, research has focused on discovering the genetic component in developing "autosomal dominant" (AD) – the pattern of inheritance characteristic of some genetic disorders where "autosomal" means that the gene in question is located on one of the numbered, or non-sex, chromosomes and "dominant" means that a single copy of the mutated gene (from one parent) is enough to cause the disorder. The search for AD has greatly contributed to understanding the genetics behind normal or "non-pathological" aging.

The human brain shows a decline in function and a change in gene expression. This modulation in gene expression may be due to oxidative DNA damage at promoter regions in the genome. Genes that are down-regulated over the age of 40 include:

- ➤ GluR1 AMPA receptor subunit;
- ➤ NMDA R2A receptor subunit (involved in learning);
- ➤ Subunits of the GABA-A receptor;
- ➤ Genes involved in long-term potentiation e.g. calmodulin 1 and CaM Kinase II alpha;
- ➤ Calcium signaling genes;
- ➤ Synaptic plasticity genes; and
- ➤ Synaptic vesicle release and recycling genes;

Genes that are upregulated include:

- ➤ Genes associated with stress response and DNA repair; and
- ➤ Antioxidant defense.

Measurements

Epigenetic age-analysis of brain regions

According to an epigenetic biomarker of tissue age known as 'epigenetic clock', the cerebellum is the youngest brain region (and probably body part) in centenarians: it is about 15 years younger than expected in a centenarian. By contrast, all brain regions and brain cells appear to have roughly the same epigenetic age in subjects who are younger than 80. These findings suggest that the **cerebellum is better protected from aging effects**, which in turn could explain why the cerebellum exhibits fewer neuropathological hallmarks of age-related dementias compared to other brain regions.

Other biomarkers of aging

There is research and development of biomarkers of aging, and detection and software systems to measure the biological age of the brain. For example, a deep-learning software using anatomic MRI estimated brain age with relatively high accuracy, including detecting early signs of Alzheimer's disease and varying neuroanatomical patterns of neurological aging.

Delaying the effects of aging

The current state of biomedical technology does not allow to stop and reverse aging. However, one may potentially delay the effects and severity of the symptoms of aging. While there is no consensus of efficacy, the following (unprioritized) factors are reported as delaying **cognitive decline**:

- High level of education.
- Staying intellectually engaged, i.e. reading and mental activities (such as crossword puzzles).
- Brain protection.
- Treating cardiovascular risk factors and other chronic conditions.
- Avoiding anticholinergic medications.
- A number of pharmacological strategies are under investigation, including nicotinamide riboside.
- Maintaining a healthy diet, including omega-3 fatty acids, protective antioxidants (e.g., flavonols-containing foods) as well as potentially anthocyanins- and flavanones-containing ones as in, more generally, Mediterranean diet patterns.
- Caloric restriction and intermittent fasting.
- The microbiome also plays a role. Scientists have shown that transplantation of fecal microbiota from young donor mice into aged recipient mice substantially rejuvenates brain biomarkers of the latter, complementing similar results of a 2020 study. Diet and other factors influence the microbiome. Probiotics such as of *L. plantarum* may also have relevant effects.
- Physical exercise.
- Limiting stress, having adequate sleep, managing sensory impairments, ceasing smoking, limiting alcohol use.
- Maintaining social and friendship networks.

Cognitive reserve

The ability of an individual to demonstrate no cognitive signs of aging despite an aging brain is called 'cognitive reserve'. This hypothesis suggests that two patients might have the same brain pathology, with one person experiencing noticeable clinical symptoms, while the other continues to function relatively normally. Studies of cognitive reserve explore the specific biological, genetic, and environmental differences which make some people more resistant to cognitive decline than others.

Sidebar 10.1 reports on the results of longitudinal studies of aging conducted in the U.S.A.

Take-aways

- Aging of the brain is a process of transformation of the brain in older age. It encompasses changes experienced by all healthy individuals as well as those changes caused by illnesses (including unrecognized illnesses). It is a major risk factor for most common neurodegenerative diseases such as mild cognitive impairment and the various types of dementia.
- While much research has focused on diseases of aging, there are few informative studies on the molecular biology of the aging brain in the absence of neurodegenerative disease and likewise for the neuropsychological profile of healthy older adults.
- The aging process is associated with several structural, chemical, and functional changes in the brain as well as a host of neurocognitive changes. In addition, there are distinct changes in the expression of genes at the single neuron level.
- Aging entails many physical, biological, chemical, and psychological changes. The brain is no exception to this phenomenon.
- Structural changes include: Loss of neural circuits and alterations in brain plasticity, thinning of the cortex, decrease in neuronal density, alteration in white matter microstructure, and alteration in energy metabolism in the cerebellum. General cortical atrophy (shrinkage) occurs in the caudate nucleus; general increase in the density of neurofibrillary tangles but no significant difference in where tangles are found, and tau-protein disorders causing microtubule destruction, accumulation of DNA damage, and decrease in the central blood flow without forgetting the role of oxidative stress.

- The aging process additionally entails a broad range of biochemical changes relating to the specialized chemical messengers called neurotransmitters (dopamine, serotonin, and glutamate).
- Neuropsychological changes include changes in orientation, attention, **memory**, language, and behavioral flexibility.
- The search for genetic factors has always been an important aspect in trying to understand neuropathological processes. The human brain shows a decline in function and a change in gene expression, which may be due to oxidative DNA damage at promoter regions in the genome.
- Measurements of brain changes due to aging include epigenetic age-analysis of brain regions, which suggested that the cerebellum is better protected from aging effects. This, in turn, explains why the cerebellum exhibits fewer neuropathological hallmarks of age-related dementias compared to other brain regions. Other biomarkers of aging are still under development such as detection and software systems to measure the biological age of the brain.
- The current state of biomedical technology does not allow to stop and reverse aging. However, one may potentially delay the effects and severity of the symptoms of aging. While there is no consensus of efficacy, several factors have been reported as delaying cognitive decline.
- Studies of cognitive reserve have explored the specific biological, genetic, and environmental differences which make some people more resistant to cognitive decline than others.

Sidebar 10.1 – Longitudinal studies of aging

1. The Nun Study (1986 -)

Purpose of the study: "To investigate whether activities, academics, past experiences, and disposition are correlated to continued cognitive, neurological, and physical ability as individuals got older, as well as overall longevity".

Cohort of participants: A group of 678 volunteer American Roman Catholic Sisters who were members of the School Sisters of Notre Dame - a relatively homogeneous group (no drug use, little or no alcohol, similar housing and reproductive histories) to minimize the extraneous variables that may confound other similar research studies.

Inclusion criteria: Be cognitively intact, at least 75 years of age, and participate in the study until time of death, give permission for researchers to have access to their autobiographies and personal documented information, and participate in regular physical and mental examinations.

After-death permission: Permission to donate one's brain for research purposes after death so that it could be neuropathologically evaluated for changes related to Alzheimer's disease (AD) and other dementias.

Consent form: The form agreeing to the terms of the study was willingly signed.

Documents reviewed:

- **Personal documents:** Autobiographical essays written by the nuns upon joining the sisterhood.
- **Convent archives:** Researchers accessed the convent archive to review documents amassed throughout the lives of the nuns in the study.

Examinations:

- **Annual cognitive and physical function examinations:** They were conducted throughout the remainder of the participants' lives. They were designed to test the subject's proficiency with object identification, **memory**, orientation, and language. These categories were tested through a series of mental state examinations with the data being recorded with each passing test.
- **Neuropathology evaluations:** They were performed by creating microscope slides from brain autopsy samples and carefully evaluated for AD changes by neuropathologists.

Findings:

- **Education:**
  - Participants who had an education level of a bachelor's degree or higher were less likely to develop Alzheimer's later in life. They also lived longer than their colleagues who did not have higher education.
  - An essay's lack of linguistic density (e.g., complexity, vivacity, fluency) functioned as a significant predictor of its author's risk for developing AD in old age. Roughly 80% of nuns whose writing was measured as lacking in linguistic density went on to develop AD; meanwhile, of those whose writing was not lacking, only 10% later developed the disease.
  - Participants' word choice and vocabulary were also correlated to the development of AD.
  - Participants writing positively in their personal journals were more likely to live longer than their counterparts.

- **Cognition:** Three indicators of longer life were found: Amount of positive sentences, positive words, and variety of positive emotions used. Less positivity used was associated with greater mortality.

- **Other variables not considered:** Long term hopefulness or bleakness in one's personality, optimism, pessimism, ambition, and others.

- **Lifestyle:** Exercise was inversely correlated with the development of AD, conducing to retaining cognitive abilities during aging. Participants who started exercising later in life were more likely to retain cognitive abilities, even if not having exercised before.

- **Neuropathology:**
  - **Tau neurofibrillary tangles** located in regions of the brain outside the neocortex and hippocampus: May have less of an effect than amyloid beta plaques located within those same areas.
  - **Brain weight:** Brains weighing under 1000 grams were seen as higher risk than those in a higher weight class.

- **Age and disease:** Do not always guarantee impaired cognitive ability and "that traits in early, mid, and late life have strong relationships with the risk of AD, as well as the mental and cognitive disabilities of old age".

> **Influence on studies by others:**

  ○ If a person has a stroke, there is a smaller requirement of Alzheimer's brain lesions necessary to diagnose a person with dementia.

  ○ *Post-mortem* MRI scans of the hippocampus can help distinguish that some non-demented individuals fit the criteria for AD.

  ○ There is a relationship between the number of teeth an individual has at death with how likely they were to have had dementia; those with fewer teeth were more likely to have dementia while living.

  ○ Higher idea density is correlated with better cognition during aging, even if the individual had brain lesions resembling those of AD.

  ○ Vocation and lifestyle of nuns correlated with higher potential for developing dementia.

  ○ Correlation between longevity and autonomy. Subjects were shown to have a longer lifespan based on the amount of purposeful and reflective behavior shown in their writing.

2. The Religious Orders Study (1994 -)

The Religious Orders Study follows the earlier Nun Study.

Purpose of the study: "To explore the effects of aging on the brain".

Cohort of participants: More than 1,000 nuns, priests, and other religious professionals across the United States.

Findings:

> Cognitive exercise including social activities and learning new skills has a protective effect on brain health and the onset of dementia, while negative psychological factors like anxiety and clinical depression are correlated with cognitive decline.

11

Aging and superaging

Contents

11

Aging and superaging

The mechanisms of superaging are a growing area of scientific research interest. In the absence of a formal definition, for the purpose of this chapter, "superagers" are people ages 80 and older with the memory function of people decades younger than them. **O**ctogenarians with sharp memory **retention also perform better on movement tests (they "move quicker") and have lower rates of anxiety and depression compared to older adults with cognitive decline. The question immediately arises as to why superagers are resistant to neurodegenerative diseases and associated age-related progressive** memory **decline and loss. The purpose of this chapter is to look into some fundamental questions such as the superagers' resistance to age-related** memory **loss, genetic predisposition to longevity, role of inflammation, influence of aging disparities among certain demographics, influence of gender and socio-economic factors, and influence of nutrition.**

Why are superagers resistant to age-related memory loss?

A new research study conducted at the Technical University of Madrid, Spain aimed to answer this question, continuing the tradition of the founder of modern neuroscience (Dr. Santiago Ramón y Cajal) in his own home country and *alma mater* University (see Chapter 2). The study comprised

64 superagers who had been previously identified through a memory test taken in an earlier study on Alzheimer's disease (AD) together with 55 typical control older adults. All study participants (subjects and controls) were aged 79.5 years or older. The findings of that study are as follows:

> Superagers performed better on both the timed "up-and-go" test, which gauges mobility and a "finger tapping" test that measures fine motor function. These results held even when they reported no significant difference in exercise levels than the control group of older adults.

> Though reporting similar activity levels to typical older people, superagers may possibly do more physically demanding activities than the control group.

> Superagers exhibited no significant difference in biomarkers or genetic risk factors for neurodegenerative diseases (NDDs) compared to other adults of a similar age, suggesting that some other protective factor could be at work.

> Superagers and typical older adult groups exhibited similar concentrations of dementia blood biomarkers, suggesting that group differences reflect inherent superager resistance to typical age-related memory loss.

> Confirming past research results, superagers have a greater volume of grey matter associated with **memory** in parts of the brain. This finding primarily focused on the medial temporal lobe of the brain, consistent with previous research.

> Superagers appear to live longer and are cognitively healthier and resistant to age-related **memory** decline because they have better brain and physical health and are aging at a different rate than the rest of the population.

> Superagers may either be truly resistant to age-related **memory** decline, as suggested by the research, or/and have coping mechanisms that help them overcome this decline better than their peers.

> The "greater performance of superagers relative to typical older adults might not only be a result of better memory function but could also reflect differences in motivation, executive function, and persistence in the face of difficulty", which suggests that superagers have a higher

level of tenacity than typical older adults. This may result from the activity of **the anterior mid-cingulate cortex, which is involved in a variety of functions that, include attention, memory, executive function, and motivation.**

Are superagers genetically predisposed to longevity?

The better movement performance by superagers that was noted in the Spanish study may support the hypothesis of a genetic basis for the "biological time clock ticking at a slower rate" for some people. In other words, the time clock of superagers may differ from their biological time clock …. and there may be "no secret to longevity"! As the noted aging scientist Dr. Olshansky stated: "… *it's absurd to ask superagers their secret to longevity; they have no clue. They've just won the genetic lottery at birth*".

Longitudinal research studies have recently conducted genetic analyses of centenarians and their offspring to identify protective factors against the negative effects of aging. In particular, they found that:

> ➢ The **CETP gene is linked to prevention of cognitive decline and Alzheimer's disease.** Specifically, CETP homozygotes but not heterozygotes experienced a relative 51% less decline in memory compared to a reference group after adjusting for demographic factors and APOE status.

[Remark: Actually, most diseases, including the subject of this chapter, could be succinctly (mathematically) described by the weighted linear algebraic equation: $g\mathbf{G} + e\mathbf{E} + l\mathbf{L} = \mathbf{O}$, where G, E, and L stand respectively for genetics, environment, and lifestyle; g, e, and l are the corresponding weights in the combination such that $g + e + l = 1.0$; and O is the disease outcome.]

Extraordinary memory abilities

Memory capacity can be far more immense than it is for most of most people on even their most lucid days.

Hyperthymesia and memory champions

What is at is hyperthymesia?

Hyperthymesia, also known as hyperthymestic syndrome or highly superior **autobiographical memory** (HSAM) is the ability to remember far more about one's own life than is typical, including details of personal experiences and when they occurred. However, people with HSAM do not show such unusual memory for all kinds of information, their autobiographical memory is not perfect, and they may not stand out on other cognitive characteristics. Two defining characteristics of hyperthymesia have been advanced: Spending an excessive amount of time thinking about one's past and displaying an extraordinary ability to recall specific events from that past.

Hyperthymesia is an extraordinarily rare condition (as of 2021, only 62 people in the world have been so diagnosed). These awe-inspiring individuals have developed highly unusual abilities to remember particular kinds of information, even in the absence of extensive training. The cause is often unclear.

Memory athletes and champions

A memory athlete is someone who participates in memory competitions, which can involve a variety of tests of memory ability. Competitors train their ability to recall information with the aid of mental techniques called mnemonics. Some people accomplish impressive feats of memory, not because of a radical difference in cognitive functioning relative to other people, but through training and the use of techniques for enhancing memory. The examples of these memory champions suggest that even relatively ordinary minds can take memory to extraordinary levels.

Some of the feats performed by memory champions include memorizing long strings of digits, series of random words, sequences of cards in decks, and names and faces.

Role of inflammation

A study found that myeloid cells are drivers of a maladaptive inflammation element of brain-aging in mice and that this can be reversed or prevented via inhibition of their EP2 signaling. In particular, the subarachnoidal lymphatic-like membrane is a "host for a large population of myeloid cells", the number of which increases in response to inflammation and aging.

Cerebrospinal fluid

Another study showed that infusing the nourishing cerebrospinal fluid (CSF) from around brain cells of young mice into aged brains rejuvenates certain aspects of the brain, proving that CSF plays a role in brain aging. A key target for potential therapeutics, including for anti-aging, was the FGF17 protein.

The subarachnoidal lymphatic-like membrane likely plays a role in CSF functions as both a protective barrier and a host of immune cells that monitor the brain for infection and inflammation. It appears to be substantially involved in major brain diseases and brain aging.

Hypothalamus inflammation and the GnRH hormone

In a 2013 study, it was suggested that the inflammation of the hypothalamus may be connected to our overall aging bodies. The researchers focused on the activation of the protein complex NF-κB in mice test subjects, which showed increased activation as the mice aged. This activation not only affects aging, but affects a hormone known as GnRH. It has shown new anti-aging properties when injected into mice outside the hypothalamus while causing the opposite effect when injected into the hypothalamus. However, the mechanism of GnRH's anti-aging properties is not understood, foreclosing for the time being the potential application of this finding to humans in any meaningful way.

Influence of ethnic aging disparities

For certain demographics lacking access to or having reduced medical care, the effects of normal cognitive aging may be especially pronounced. As the global population grows, diversifies, and ages, there is an increasing need to understand these inequities. The following are brief observations regarding certain ethnic groups.

African-Americans

In the U.S., Black and African-American demographics disproportionately experience metabolic dysfunction with age with a toll on cardiovascular health. Metabolite profiles of the healthy aging index (HAI) - a score that assesses neurocognitive function among other correlates of health through the years - are associated with cardiovascular disease. Healthy cardiovascular function is critical for maintaining neurocognitive efficiency into old age. Attention, verbal learning, and cognitive set ability are related to diastolic blood pressure, triglyceride levels, and high density lipoprotein (HDL) cholesterol levels, respectively.

Latinos

In the U.S., the Latino demographic is most likely to develop metabolic syndrome (the combination of high blood pressure, high blood sugar, elevated triglyceride levels, and abdominal obesity), which not only increases the risk of cardiac events and type II diabetes but also is associated with lower neurocognitive function during midlife. This takes place even though life expectancy for Latinos in the U.S. is higher than for whites and blacks.

Table 11.1 summarizes the percent frequency of the dementia-predisposing alleles (ε2, ε3, and ε4) among different Latin heritages: Caribbean Latinos (Cubans, Dominicans, Puerto Ricans) and mainland Latinos (Mexicans, Central Americans, and South Americans).

Table 11.1 – Percent frequency of dementia-predisposing alleles among Latinos

Allele of ApoE	Caribbean	Mainland
ε2	5.2 – 8.6	2.9 – 3.9
ε3	73.9 – 81.5	85.2 – 86.2
ε4	12.6 – 17.5	11.0 – 11.2

However, one genetic risk factor, having one form of the apolipoprotein E (ApoE ε4) gene on chromosome 19, does increase a person's risk. ApoE comes in several different forms, or alleles:

- **ApoE ε2:** It is relatively rare and may provide some protection against AD. If AD occurs in a person with this allele, it usually develops later in life than it would in someone with the ε4 gene.
- **ApoE ε3:** This is the most common allele. It is believed to play a neutral role in the disease - neither decreasing nor increasing risk.
- **ApoE ε4:** It increases risk for AD and is also associated with an earlier age of disease onset. A person has zero, one, or two ApoE ε4 alleles. Having more ApoE ε4 alleles increases the risk of developing AD and is also associated with an earlier age of disease onset. However, inheriting it does not mean that a person will definitely develop AD. Some people with an ApoE ε4 allele never get the disease, and others who develop AD do not have any ApoE ε4 alleles. Also, some persons with no ApoE ε4 may nonetheless develop the disease.

Indigenous peoples

Indigenous populations are often understudied in research. Reviews of current literature studying natives in Australia, Brazil, Canada, and the United States from participants aged 45 to 94 years old reveal varied prevalence rates for cognitive impairment not related to dementia, from 4.4% to 17.7%. These results can be interpreted in the context of culturally biased neurocognitive tests, preexisting health conditions, poor access to healthcare, lower educational attainment, and/or old age.

Influence of gender and socioeconomic factors

Gender

Compared to their male counterparts, women's scores on the Mini Mental State Exam (MMSE) tend to decline at slightly faster rates with age. Males with mild cognitive impairment (MCI) tend to show more microstructural damage than females with MCI, but seem to have a greater cognitive reserve due to larger absolute brain size and neuronal density. As a result, women tend to manifest symptoms of cognitive decline at lower thresholds than men do. This effect seems to be moderated by educational attainment - higher education is associated with later MCI diagnosis as neuropathological load increases. Currently, there are no known studies to identify a characteristic pattern of cognitive decline with age in transgender people.

Socioeconomic factors

Socioeconomic status (SES) is the interaction between social and economic factors. It has been demonstrated that sociodemographic factors can be used to predict cognitive profiles within older individuals to some extent. This may be because families of higher SES are equipped to early on provide their children with resources to facilitate cognitive development. For these children, small changes in parental income were associated with small changes in surface area within these regions. By contrast, for children in families of low SES, relatively small changes in parental income were associated with large changes in brain surface area, which are associated with language, reading, executive functions, and spatial skills.

With respect to global cortical thickness, low SES children showed a curvilinear decrease in thickness with age while those of high SES demonstrated a steeper linear decline, suggesting that synaptic pruning is more efficient in the latter group. This trend was especially evident in the critical language and literacy supporting areas (left fusiform and left superior temporal gyri).

A study showed that 50+ aged users of the dietary program SNAP "had about 2 fewer years of cognitive aging over a 10-year period compared with non-users" despite it having nearly no conditions for the sustainability and healthiness of the food products purchased with the coupons (or coupon-credits).

Influence of food types and elements

Influence of nutrition is summarized in Table 11.2 for several food types and elements:

Table 11.2 – Influence of various food types and elements on health and aging

Food type	Effects	Consequences
1. Spices	o Make blood vessels swell and even break o Raise body temperature o Increase sweating to cool body back down, adding to purple marks on the face	o When mixed with bacteria on the skin, can cause breakouts and blotches
2. Margarine	o Raises 'bad' blood cholesterol o Reduces "good" cholesterol	o Creates **inflammation** linked to heart disease and stroke that can give an **aged appearance**
3. Sodas & energy drinks	o Have more calories and added sugar than any other beverage	o The more drinks, the quicker cells age o Combined with bacteria in the mouth, sugar forms acid that wears down tooth enamel and causes decay o Leads to weight gain and **higher risk of stroke and dementia**
4. Alcohol	o Dehydrates the skin	o Additional water will hydrate other organs before the skin, causing dry skin and wrinkles
5. Frozen dinners	o One can pack half the sodium of a healthy diet	o Too much salt causes more drinking than normal, flooding the kidneys o Any extra water moves to body places that have less salt, causing puffiness
6. Processed meats	o Sodium and chemical preservatives in them cause inflammation	o Too much inflammation can cause **heart disease, stroke, and diabetes**
7. Fried foods	o Frying promotes the formation of free radicals	o These unstable molecules damage other molecules in the body's cells
8. Baked goods	o High in fat and sugar	o Can cause **diabetes, high blood pressure, tooth decay**, etc. o Inflammation increases chances of **arthritis, depression, Alzheimer's, and some cancers**
9. Charred meats	o Creates advanced glycation end-products (AGE)	o High amounts cause inflammation that "inflammages" the body and triggers **heart disease and diabetes**
10. High-fructose corn syrup	o Interferes with body's ability to use copper o Full of calories	o Interferes with collagen and elastin formation (that keep skin healthy) o Risk of **diabetes and heart disease**
11. Caffeine	o A diuretic	o Stimulates the brain and need to urinate o Can cause dehydration, stop skin from releasing toxins o May cause dry skin, wrinkles, and **psoriasis**
12. Agave	o Is 90% fructose (type of sugar that can only be broken in the liver)	o An overworked liver turns fructose into fat, makes more radicals

13. Strawberries	o Packed with essential nutrients: Vitamins A, B-9 (folate), and C; magnesium; potassium, and folate o Polyphenols (anti-oxidants) o Phytosterols (anti-oxidants)	o Daily consumption can **enhance cognitive function, reduce blood pressure, bolster anti-oxidant capacity** o Anti-inflammatory properties o Aid in cholesterol reduction o May improve **cognitive function and cardiovascular health**
14. Selenium and selenoproteins	o Essential trace mineral o Anti-oxidant	o **Anti-aging properties** o **Anti-age-related diseases (type 2 diabetes, Alzheimer's disease)** o May prevent **age-related health issues** (tumors, cardiovascular disease, and neuropsychiatric disorders) o May reduce **chronic inflammation** o Protects the skin against **ultraviolet (UV) oxidative stress** o May play a role in cancer prevention by protecting cells against DNA damage and mutations

Take-aways

- Superagers are people aged 80 and older with the memory function of people decades younger than them. **Octogenarians with sharp memory retention also perform better on movement tests and have lower rates of anxiety and depression compared to older adults with cognitive decline.**

- Superagers are resistant to age-related memory loss. They perform better on both the timed "up-and-go" test, which gauges mobility and a "finger tapping" test that measures fine motor function.

- Compared to other adults of a similar age, superagers may possibly do more physically demanding activities, and exhibit no significant difference in biomarkers or genetic risk factors for neurodegenerative diseases, and exhibit similar concentrations of dementia blood biomarkers.

- Superagers appear to live longer and are cognitively healthier and resistant to age-related memory decline because they have better brain and physical health and are aging at a different rate than the rest of the population.

- Superagers may either be truly resistant to age-related memory decline or/and have coping mechanisms that help them overcome this decline better than their peers.
- **The "greater performance of superagers relative to typical older adults might not only be a result of better memory function but could also reflect differences in motivation, executive function, and persistence in the face of difficulty", which suggests that superagers have a higher level of tenacity than typical older adults.**
- **Superagers may be predisposed to longevity. A genetic basis has been hypothesized in that the time clock of superagers may differ from their biological time clock …. and there may be "no secret to longevity"!**
- **The CETP gene was found to be linked to the prevention of cognitive decline and Alzheimer's disease.**
- Memory capacity can be far more immense than it is for most people on even their most lucid days.
- Hyperthymesia, also known as hyperthymestic syndrome or highly superior autobiographical memory (HSAM) is an extremely rare condition. It is the ability to remember far more about one's own life than is typical, including details of personal experiences and when they occurred. However, people with HSAM do not show such unusual memory for all kinds of information.
- Two defining characteristics of hyperthymesia have been advanced: Spending an excessive amount of time thinking about one's past and displaying an extraordinary ability to recall specific events from that past.
- Hyperthymesia is an extraordinarily rare condition (as of 2021, only 62 people in the world have been so diagnosed). These awe-inspiring individuals have developed highly unusual abilities to remember particular kinds of information, even in the absence of extensive training. The cause is often unclear.
- **Inflammation plays a role in aging.**
- Ethnic aging disparities, gender and socioeconomic factors, as well as various food types and elements play a role in health and aging.

PART E
MEMORY

On memory and its particulars

Contents

Sidebars:

12

On memory and its particulars

Memory refers to the **psychological processes** of **acquiring, retaining, storing,** and later **retrieving information**. There are four major processes involved: encoding, preservation, storage, and retrieval. However, this is not a flawless process and errors may occur in one or more of these processes. Sometimes people forget or misremember things. Other times, information is not properly encoded in memory in the first place. While often minor, memory problems can also be a sign of serious conditions such as Alzheimer's disease (AD), other kinds of dementia (see Part C of this book), and other neurodegenerative diseases. These conditions affect the quality of life and the ability to function. I will begin this chapter by presenting the different memory processes from memory creation to how memory works, to various forms of memory. This will be continued by a brief presentation on using and organizing memory. I will then discuss in some detail the several types of memory (sensory, short-term, long-term, episodic, prospective, procedural, and others). I will follow by suggesting ways gleaned from the published research literature on how to protect and effectively improve memory as well as palliating memory loss.

Memory processes

Various processes characterize memory, but first why are memories created?

Why are memories created?

We all have a strong intuitive sense of what the different types of memory are. One of the fundamental roles of memory is to make our behavior appropriate for our current situation and, based on past experiences, to allow us to rapidly change and adapt our behavior when our environment changes. Memories serve many purposes, from allowing us to revisit and learn from past experiences to storing knowledge about the world and how things work. Memory helps us survive! However, when memory becomes dysfunctional, resulting in memories that are too strong or in memory loss, problematic changes in our behavior and our emotions devolve and potentially contribute to a variety of mental health disorders including addiction, anxiety, dementias, post-traumatic stress disorder (PTSD), etc. Memory contributes to mental health states and, conversely, both mental and physical states can dramatically impact it, what memories we store, and what memories we recall at any given time.

The creation of a memory is a conversion process

The creation of memory is a conversion process in which a select amount of perceived information is converted into a more permanent form. A subset of that memory will be secured in long-term storage, accessible for future use. Many factors during and after the creation of a memory influence what (and how much) gets preserved.

Researchers have long believed that memories form due to changes in brain neurons (nerve cells). Our understanding today is that memories are created through the connections that exist between these neurons—either by strengthening these connections or through the growth of new connections. Changes in the connections between nerve cells (known as synapses) are associated with the learning and retention of new information. Strengthening these connections helps commit information to memory. This is why reviewing and rehearsing information improves the ability to remember it. Practice strengthens the connections between the synapses that store that memory.

Figure 12.1 – Brain regions involved in memory formation

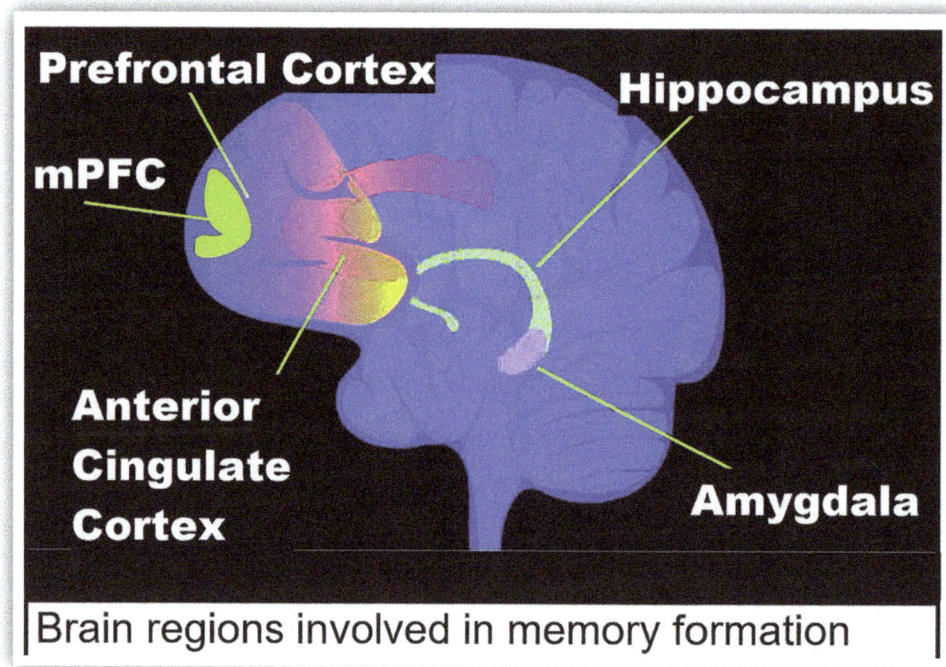

Brain regions involved in memory formation

How memory works? A theoretical construct

Memory is a continually unfolding process. Initial details of an experience take shape in memory; the brain's representation of that information then changes over time. With subsequent reactivations, the memory grows stronger or fainter and takes on different characteristics. Memories reflect real-world experience, but with varying levels of fidelity to that original experience. The degree to which the memories formed is accurate or easily recalled depends on a variety of factors, from the psychological conditions in which information is first translated into memory to the manner in which we seek—or are unwittingly prompted—to conjure details from the past. The working process of the memory is encapsulated by the following theoretical model. (It is important to note that this is only a theoretical model devised to help understand how memory works, and not a true description of reality.)

- **Encoding:** This is the first stage. It is the process by which the details of a person's experience are converted into a form that can be stored in the brain. People are more likely to encode details of what they are paying attention to and details that are personally significant.

- **Retention and consolidation:** While memories are usually described in terms of mental concepts, such as single packages of personal experience or specific facts, they are ultimately reducible to the workings and characteristics of the ever-firing cells of the brain. Scientists have narrowed down regions of the brain that are key to memory and developed an increasingly detailed understanding of the material form of these mental phenomena. The *hippocampus* and other parts of the *medial temporal lobe* are critical for many forms of memory. However, various other parts of the brain play roles as well, including: the more recently evolved *cerebral cortex* (the outermost layer of the brain); the deep-seated structures such as the *basal ganglia;* and the *amygdala.* Other processes are also important for memory as well, including the integration of emotional responses into memory. The extent to which different brain regions are involved in memory depends on the type of memory (see Figure 12.1).
- **Storage:** Memory involves changes to the brain's neural networks. Neurons in the brain are connected by synapses, which are bound together by chemical messengers (the neurotransmitters) to form larger networks. Memory storage is thought to involve changes in the strength of these connections in the areas of the brain that have been linked to memory.
- **Retrieval:** Much of our stored memory lies outside of our awareness most of the time, except when we actually need to use it. The memory retrieval process allows us to bring stored memories into conscious awareness. After memories are stored in the brain, they must be retrieved in order to be useful. While we may or may not be consciously aware that information is being summoned from storage at any given moment, this stage of memory is constantly unfolding—and the very act of remembering changes how memories are subsequently filed away. Retrieval follows the stages of encoding and storage. It is the stage in which the information saved in memory is recalled, whether consciously or unconsciously. Retrieval includes both 'intentional remembering' (as when one thinks back to a previous experience or tries to put a name to a face) and more 'passive recall' (as when the meanings of well-known words or the notes of a song come effortlessly to mind). There are retrieval cues in the above process (different types

of stimulus that initiate remembering). Cues can be external (such as an image, a text, a scent, or some other stimulus that relates to the memory) or internal (such as a thought or sensation that is relevant to the memory). They can be encountered inadvertently or deliberately sought in the process of deliberately trying to remember something.

Figure 12.2 is a working model of memory, showing the mutual relationships between the central executive, the phonological loop, and the visuo-spatial sketchpad.

Figure 12.2 – Working model of memory

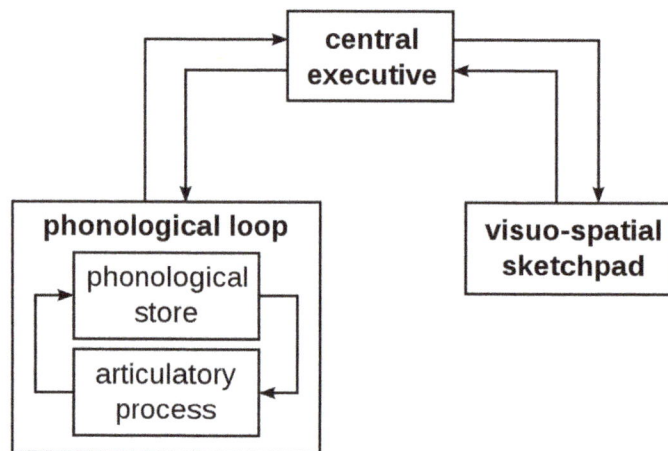

Figure 12.3 shows an engineer wearing a helmet of sensors, part of a brain scanner, at the Martinos Center for Biomedical Imaging, Massachusetts General Hospital. Scanners such as this one are employed to study the brain and its processes.

What do we remember?

Most people do not remember everything, so **how do their brains sort out what information to remember and what not to remember? Time**, **emotion**, and **repetition** (acronym: TER) all seem to contribute to whether information or an event is remembered. The basic rule is that events and information with significance are remembered. In particular, remembering recent events is likely to be more relevant for functioning than most things from long ago. But, w**hy is this selectivity in memory important? Why**

not just remember everything? Is it simply a question of capacity (not enough synapses in the brain to store all the information from every day)? We do not know. Even if we do have the storage capacity, storing all memories is inefficient.

Figure 12.3 – The Massachusetts General Hospital's brain scanner

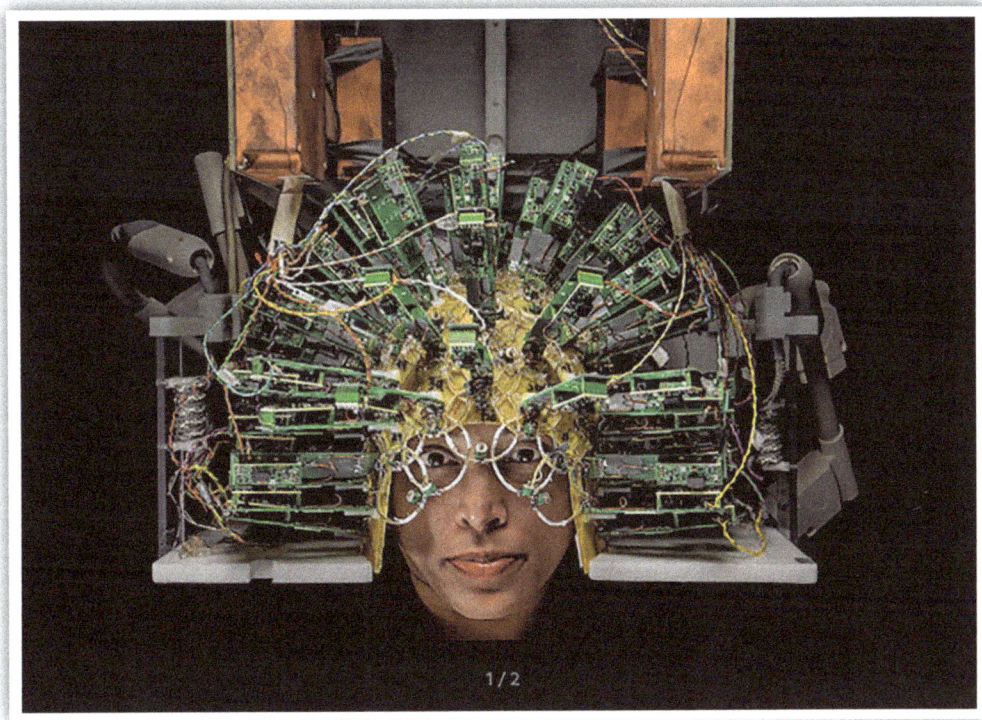

Photograph by Robert Clark

If the purpose of memory is to guide behavior and allow survival, then, a lot of every day experience will be largely irrelevant to the ability to function in the future. But, some events will be critical for survival. **Recency**, **emotion,** and **repetition** (acronym: RER), all indicate how important this information is likely to be in the current environment. So emotion contributes to not only the content of the memory but also whether something is remembered at all.

Individuals with "highly superior autobiographical memory" (HSAM) remember almost everything about events from their lives—yet they lead normal lives, exhibit normal IQ, and are indistinguishable from others across a range of other cognitive functions. Why? This may be because HSAM individuals do not show the same kinds of extreme memory for all kinds of memory (autobiographical, semantic, unconscious, associative conditioning, etc.). It may also be that HSAM individuals are less likely to have interference between these different types of memories.

What if the brain gets it wrong? Of course, if the brain *can* do something, it can also go wrong, and this is no exception: How the brain codes for "important" information can be hacked or disrupted by one's own experiences. For example, drugs are widely thought to hijack the brain's system for pleasure and reward, cause stronger memories for people, places, and things associated with them, which in turn contributes to drug-taking and relapse to drug-taking in addiction. And strong emotions during trauma contribute to strong, long-lasting, and intrusive memories that are one component of post-traumatic stress disorder (PTSD).

Memory strength

Modality is important in determining the strength of the memory. For instance, auditory creates stronger memory abilities than visual. This is shown by the higher recency and primacy effects of an auditory recall test compared to that of a visual test. Research has shown that auditory training can help preserve memory abilities as one ages and increases the life span on cognition abilities in one's advanced years.

False and distorted memories

The memory system has been built to craft a useful account of past experiences, not a perfect one. Memories have to be reconstructed in order to be used, and the piecing-together of details may at times be inaccurate or even false, contaminating the record. Memories may be distorted or rendered less accurate based on conditions when they were first formed, such as how much attention was paid during the experience. False memories can be simple (such as erroneously concluding having been shown a word that actually was not) or believing having experienced a dramatic event that did not take place. People may produce such false recollections by unwittingly drawing on the details of actual, related experiences, or in some cases, as a response to another person's detailed suggestions (perhaps involving some true details) about an imaginary event that is purported to be real.

The malleability of memories over time means internal and external factors can introduce errors. These may include a person's knowledge and expectations about the world (used to fill in the blanks of a memory) and misleading suggestions by other people about what occurred.

How long do memories last?

Some memories are very brief, just seconds long, and allow people to take in sensory information about the world. Short-term memories are a bit longer and last about 20 to 30 seconds. These memories mostly consist of the information people are currently focusing on and thinking about. Some memories are capable of enduring much longer—lasting days, weeks, months, or even decades. Most of these long-term memories lie outside of one's immediate awareness but can be drawn into consciousness when needed.

Why do we remember painful memories?

Many times, painful memories tend to hang on for long periods of time? Research suggests that this is because of increased biological arousal during the negative experience, which increases the longevity of that memory.

Memory failure

Forgetting is a surprisingly common event. There are four basic underlying explanations:

- ➢ Failure to store a memory;
- ➢ Interference;
- ➢ Motivated forgetting; and
- ➢ Retrieval failure.

Research has shown that one of the critical factors that influence memory failure is time. Information is often quickly forgotten, particularly if not actively reviewed and rehearsed. It can be simply lost from memory or it was never stored correctly in the first place. Further, some memories compete with one another, making it difficult to remember certain information. In other instances, people actively try to forget things that they simply do not want to remember.

How we remember things – The types of amnesia

To understand how we remember things, it is incredibly helpful to study how we forget them - which is why neuroscientists study amnesia (the loss of memories or the ability to learn). Amnesia is usually the result of some kind of trauma to the brain, such as a head injury, a stroke, a brain tumor, or chronic alcoholism.

There are two main types of amnesia:

> **Retrograde amnesia:** It occurs when things known before the brain trauma are forgotten after it.
> **Anterograde amnesia:** It occurs when brain trauma curtails or stops someone's ability to form new memories.

It seems that short-term and long-term memories do not form in exactly the same way, nor do declarative and procedural memories. There is no one place within the brain that holds all of the memories. Different areas of the brain form and store different kinds of memories, and different processes may be at play for each. For instance, emotional responses such as fear reside in the amygdala; memories of skills learned are associated with the striatum. The hippocampus is crucial for forming, retaining, and recalling declarative memories. The temporal lobes play a crucial role in forming and recalling memories.

Using memory

To use the information that has been encoded into memory, it first has to be retrieved. There are many factors that can influence this process, including the type of information being used and the retrieval cues that are present.

An example of a perplexing memory retrieval issue is known as 'ethological' or the 'tip-of-the-tongue' phenomenon.

Organizing Memory

The ability to access and retrieve information from long-term memory allows us to actually use these memories to make decisions, interact with others, and solve problems. But, in order to be retrievable, memories have to be organized in some way. When areas of the brain connected to memory are damaged, the ability to identify persons, events,... is impaired.

One way of thinking about memory organization is the 'semantic network model'. This model suggests that certain triggers activate associated memories, for example, seeing or remembering a specific place might activate memories that have occurred in that location.

Certain stimuli can also sometimes act as powerful triggers that draw memories into conscious awareness. Scent is one example, which can help trigger autobiographical memories in people who have Alzheimer's disease (AD), underscoring just how powerful memories can be.

Types of Memory

A person's memory is a sea of images and other sensory impressions, facts and meanings, echoes of past feelings, and ingrained codes for how to behave—a diverse well of information. Naturally, there are many ways (some experts suggest there are hundreds) to describe the varieties of what people remember and how. While the different brands of memory are not always described in exactly the same way by memory researchers, some key concepts have emerged.

The flow chart diagram of Figure 12.4 is a representation of the multi-store model of memory. It shows the transformation process from sensory to short-term memory through attention, to long-term memory through transfer and retrieval, and rehearsal within short-term memory.

These forms of memory, which can overlap in daily life, have also been arranged into broad categories. Memory that lingers for a moment (or even less than a second) could be described as **short-term memory**, while any kind of information that is preserved for remembering at a later point can be called **long-term memory**. Memory experts have also distinguished **explicit memory**, in which information is consciously recalled, from **implicit memory**, the use of saved information without conscious awareness that it is being recalled.

Characteristic details of these various types of memory are briefly described below (Table 12.1).

Figure 12.4 – The multi-store model of the memory processes

MULTI-STORE MODEL

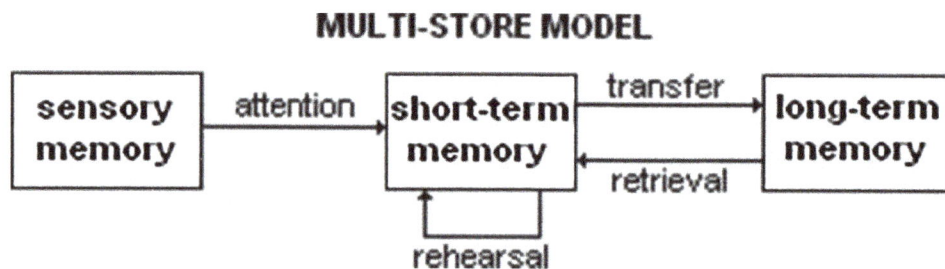

Sensory memories

Sensory memories are what psychologists call "the short-term memories of just-experienced sensory stimuli such as sights and sounds".

Sensory memory is the earliest stage of memory. During this stage, sensory information from the environment is stored for a very brief period of time, generally for no longer than a half-second for visual information and three or four seconds for auditory information. Attending to sensory memory allows some of this information to pass into the next stage: short-term memory. Sense-related memories, of course, can also be preserved long-term.

The several sensory memories corresponding to the various sensory triggers include: **Visual-spatial** *(or* **iconic***)* **memory** *refers to memory of how objects are organized in space; it lasts for less than a half.-second.* **Auditory** *(or* **echoic***)* **memory** *is the brief memory of something just heard; it can* *last for 3-4 seconds.* **Olfactory memory** and **haptic memory** are terms for stored sensory impressions of smells, and skin sensations, respectively.

Short-term memory

Short-term memory (also known as **active memory** or **working memory**) refers to the processes that are used to temporarily store, organize, and manipulate information. It corresponds to the information we are currently aware of or thinking about. The terms *short-term memory* and *working memory* are sometimes used interchangeably, and both refer to storage of information for a brief amount of time. However, working memory can be distinguished from general short-term memory in that working memory specifically involves the temporary storage of information that is being mentally manipulated and held in mind so that it can be used in the moment. In Freudian psychology, this memory would be referred to as the **conscious mind.** As indicated previously, information in short-term memory is generated from sensory memories.

While many short-term memories are quickly forgotten, attending to this information allows it to continue to the next stage: long-term memory. Most of the information stored in active memory will be kept for approximately 20 to 30 seconds. This capacity can be stretched somewhat by using memory strategies such as 'chunking', which involves grouping related information into smaller chunks.

Additional forms of short-term sensory memory are thought to exist for the other senses as well.

Long-term memory

Long-term (or **semantic**) memory refers to the continuing storage of information. It is the ability to recall concepts and general facts that are not related to specific experiences. It is composed of pieces of information such as facts, meanings, concepts, and definitions. The details that make up semantic memory can correspond to other forms of memory. In Freudian psychology, this memory would be called the **preconscious and unconscious mind**. This information is largely outside of our awareness, but can be called into working memory to be used when needed. Some memories are fairly easy to recall, while others are much more difficult to access.

While most people do not remember much from their first years of childhood, the memories that remain can be vivid and personally meaningful. These earliest long-term memories, which often date back to the preschool years, help make up the beginning of the individual's autobiographical memory. Yet well before these lasting memories are formed, babies' brains retain information learned from the world around them. The youngest age one can remember is the fourth year of life (specifically ages 3 to 3-and-a-half) although people tend to misdate these memories and that they may actually be formed somewhat earlier. There is also variation in the age of these early memories between individuals:

The various types of memory

For convenience, these are listed below in alphabetical order:

> **Associative learning:** Another type of **episodic memory** (see below).
> **Autobiographical:** Autobiographical memory is a broad category of conscious memories about one's own experiences. It encompasses facts and other non-episodic forms of information.related to a person's own life. This complex body of information can range from basic details about one's past to vivid impressions of significant personal experiences. Together, they form a person's internal life story. It is important because it allows for the development and refinement of a sense of self, including who one is, how one has changed, and what one might be like in the future. It allows a person to identify connections between personally relevant events across time (and between those events and one's sense of self), but also significant changes—all of which can be sources of meaning. The life stories people develop based on autobiographical memory also become a way to communicate who they are to others.
> **Declarative** (see **explicit**): The acquisition or encoding, storage and consolidation, and retrieval of representations of facts and events. It provides the critical substrate for relational representations, i.e.,

for spatial, temporal, and other contextual relations among items, contributing to representations of events (episodic memory) and the integration and organization of factual knowledge (semantic memory). These representations facilitate the inferential and flexible extraction of new information from these relationships.

➤ **Emotional and nostalgia:** Emotion is a powerful force for sealing experiences into memory, and some of the most important parts of our life stories are memories of emotionally-intense experiences (e.g., moments of ecstasy, awe, or tranquility). Numerous studies have shown that the most vivid autobiographical memories tend to be of emotional events, which are likely to be recalled more often and with more clarity and detail than neutral events. The activity of emotionally-enhanced memory retention can be linked to human evolution; during early development, responsive behavior to environmental events would have progressed as a process of trial and error. Artificially inducing this instinct through traumatic physical or emotional stimuli essentially creates the same physiological condition that heightens memory retention by exciting neuro-chemical activity affecting areas of the brain responsible for encoding and recalling memory. This memory-enhancing effect of emotion has been demonstrated in many laboratory studies, using stimuli ranging from words to pictures to narrated slide shows, as well as autobiographical memory studies. However, emotion does not always enhance memory. Nostalgia is a longing for the past, an experience often described as bittersweet. The "emotional enhancement" of memory may have evolved in part because it helps to preserve information that is useful for future behavior.

➤ **Episodic:** It captures the "what," "where," and "when" of daily lives. It refers to the recall of a particular event (or "episode") experienced in the past. The experiences conjured by episodic memory can be very recent or decades-old. A related concept is **autobiographical memory**, which is the memory of information that forms part of a person's life story. However, while autobiographical memory includes memories of events in one's life, it can also encompass facts and other non-episodic forms of information.

- ➤ **Explicit::** Consists of the sorts of memories experienced consciously. Some are facts or "common knowledge", others consist of past events experienced. (See **declarative**.)
- ➤ **Implicit:** Unconscious build-up of memories (includes **procedural memory).**
- ➤ **Intrusive:** Sensory memories of a traumatic event(s) that spring to mind involuntarily, and can evoke strong emotions and disrupt functioning in daily life. They are their debilitating core features and are triggered by certain clinical symptoms (PTSD, anxiety, depression, and insomnia).
- ➤ K*inesthetic (see implicit):* Refers specifically to memory for physical behaviors. (A related
- ➤ **Long term** (or semantic): The memory which refers to the continuing storage of information; the ability to recall concepts and general facts that are not related to specific experiences. It is composed of pieces of information such as facts, meanings, concepts, and definitions.
- ➤ **Motor:** Required by motor skills without which behavior is only reflexes and stereotypes.
- ➤ **Non-declarative** (see implicit): Can shape the body's unthinking responses.
- ➤ **Objective:** The objective recollection of places, events, dates, people, persons. (See also subjective memory.)
- ➤ **Photographic memory:** The memory of things seen only once (photographs, objects, written documents, etc.).
- ➤ **Procedural** (see implicit): The long-term memory of how to do things (both physical and mental) *such as, for example, how to tell time by reading the numbers on a clock) typically stays the same.*(both physical and mental). It is involved in the process of learning skills (from the basic ones people take for granted to those that require considerable practice). A related term is ***kinesthetic memory***, which refers specifically to memory for physical behaviors.
- ➤ **Prospective memory:** The forward-thinking memory - recalling an intention from the past in order to do something in the future. It is essential for daily functioning in that memories of previous intentions, including very recent ones, ensure that people execute their plans and

meet their obligations when the intended behaviors cannot be carried out right away, or have to be carried out routinely.

➤ **Semantic** (see long-term memory): The ability to recall concepts and general facts that are not related to specific experiences. For example, understanding the concept that clocks are used to tell time. This type of memory also includes vocabulary and knowledge of language.

➤ **Sensory:** The earliest stage of memory *corresponding to the various sensory triggers. It includes:*

Verbal: Used in cognitive psychology, it *refers to memory of words and other abstractions involving language.*

*Visual-spatial (or **iconic**) **memory:** It* refers to memory of how objects are organized in space; it lasts for less than a half.-second.

*Auditory (or **echoic**) **memory** is the brief memory of something just heard. It can last for 3-4 seconds.*

*Olfactory **memory:** The memory of stored sensory impressions of smells.*

*Haptic **memory:** The memory for stored sensory impressions of skin sensations.*

➤ **Short-term** (also known as **active memory**): The storage of information for a brief amount of time. It is generated from sensory memories. To be distinguished from working memory (see below).

➤ **Spatial:** In cognitive psychology and neuroscience, it is a form of memory responsible for the recording and recovery of information needed to plan a course to a location and to recall the location of an object or the occurrence of an event. It is necessary for orientation in space. IT can also be divided into 'egocentric' and 'allocentric 'spatial memory. Spatial memory has representations within working, short-term memory and long-term memory. Research indicates that there are specific areas of the brain associated with spatial memory. Many methods are used for measuring spatial memory in children and adults.

➤ **Subjective:** The subjective recollection of places, events, dates, people, persons. (See also objective memory.)

➤ **Working: The active maintenance and flexible updating of goal/ task relevant information (items, goals, strategies, etc.) in a form that has limited capacity and resists interference. It** involves the manipulation of information that is being obtained and, then, using this information to complete a task. Working memory can be distinguished from general short-term memory in that it specifically involves the temporary storage of information that is being mentally manipulated and held in mind so that it can be used in the moment. In Freudian psychology, this memory would be referred to as the conscious mind.

Table 12.1 lists certain types of memory in Freudian psychology. It is not comprehensive.

Table 12. 1 – Certain types of memory in Freudian psychology

Type	In Freudian psychology	Features
Autobiographical	Broad category of memories related to a person's own life	Earliest memories (from childhood) to adult ones
Emotional	Powerful force for sealing memories	Emotional memory enhancement that may have evolved in part because it helps to preserve useful information for future behavior.
Sensory	The short-term memories of just-experienced sensory stimuli	o **Visual-spatial** (or **iconic**) o **Auditory** (or **echoic**) o **Olfactory** o **Haptic**
Short-term (or **active** or **working) memory**	The **conscious mind (explicit memory)**	o Generated from sensory memories o Kept ~ 20-30 sec o Can be stretched using memory strategies
Long-term (or **semantic**)	**Preconscious and unconscious mind** (**implicit memory**)	o Can be recalled into short-term memory
Episodic (related: **autobiographical**)		o Can be very recent or very old

Prospective		o Forward thinking recalling from the past
Procedural (includes **kinesthetic** for physical behaviors)		o How to do things (physical, mental)

How to protect memory?

While AD and other age-related memory problems affect many older adults, the loss of memory during later adulthood might not be inevitable. While certain abilities do tend to decline with age, researchers have found that individuals in their 70s often perform just as well on many cognitive tests as those in their 20s. By the time people reach their 80s, it is common to experience some decline in cognitive function. But some types of memory even increase with age.

The following lifestyle strategies may help protect the brain of the aging person:

> **Avoiding stress:** Stress can have detrimental effects on areas of the brain associated with memory, including the hippocampus.
> **Avoiding drugs, alcohol, and other neurotoxins:** Drug use and excessive alcohol consumption have been linked to the deterioration of synapses (the connections between neurons). Exposure to dangerous chemicals such as heavy metals and pesticides can also have detrimental effects on the brain.
> **Getting enough exercise:** Regular physical activity helps improve oxygenation of the brain, which is vital for synaptic formation and growth.
> **Stimulating the brain:** People who have more mentally stimulating jobs are less likely to develop dementia.
> **Maintaining a sense of self-efficacy:** Self-efficacy refers to the sense of control that people have over their own lives and destiny. Having a strong sense of self-efficacy has been associated with maintaining good memory abilities during old age and has also been linked to lowered stress levels.

How to improve memory effectively?

Human memory is a complex process that researchers are still trying to better understand. Our memories make us who we are, yet the process is not perfect. While we are capable of remembering an astonishing amount of information, we are also susceptible to memory-related mistakes and errors. Fortunately, there are plenty of things that can be done to increase memory power. While simply revisiting a newly learned fact, the definition of a word, or some other information can help reinforce someone's memory for it and additional tools and processes can help make the effort to retain those details more powerful. The following research-proven strategies can effectively improve memory, enhance recall, and increase retention of information. As few or as many such strategies are differently needed by different people.

1. Focusing attention

Attention is one of the major components of memory. Actively attending to it (such as, away from distractions and diversions, setting aside a short period of time to be alone, getting some space to focus on one's work, etc.) is needed for information to move from short-term memory into long-term memory.

2. Avoiding cramming

"Cramming"—studying in one long, continuous period—can be an unhelpful study habit. Studying materials over a number of sessions gives the time needed to adequately process information.

3. Structuring and organizing

Researchers have found that information is organized in memory in related clusters. To help group related concepts, one can structure and organize materials, group similar concepts and terms together, or make an outline of notes and textbook readings.

4. Utilizing mnemonic devices

Mnemonic devices are ways of enhancing memory that can involve elaboration—connecting what one is trying to remember to other information in memory—organizing to-be-remembered details more efficiently in memory, and making use of mental visualization. Examples of mnemonics include: Forming a series of words into an acronym; grouping to-be-remembered items together into categories; creating a 'memory palace' by visualizing a series of objects, events, or other things appearing in a familiar physical space.

5. Chunking the information

'Chunking' is the combination of to-be-remembered pieces of information, such as numbers or letters, into a smaller number of units (or "chunks"), making them easier to remember. A simple example is the reduction of a phone number into three parts (which one might repeat to oneself in three bursts), though more complex forms of chunking are thought to help account for experts' superior memory for certain kinds of information (such as chess positions).

6. Elaborating and rehearsing

In order to recall information, one needs to encode it into long-term memory. One of the most effective encoding techniques is known as 'elaborative rehearsal'.

7. Testing memory of learned material

Testing memory of learned material, such as a passage of text, can enhance memory for that material - above and beyond re-reading it. Self-testing can help with learning, whether responding to self-generated questions or flashcards related to that information or questions provided by others. Explaining a newly learned concept to oneself or someone else may also help reinforce memory for it.

8. Visualizing concepts

Many people benefit greatly from visualizing information (for example, photographs, charts, and other graphics). Personal cues (such as charts, figures, notes on margins, color highlighting, making flashcards of various terms etc.) can be created if visual ones are not available.

9. Relating new information to things already known

When studying unfamiliar material, relate this information to what is already known. By establishing relationships between new ideas and previously existing memories, one can dramatically increase the likelihood of recalling the recently learned information.

10. Reading out-loud

Reading materials out loud significantly improves memory of the material. Teaching new concepts to others enhances understanding and recall.

11. Paying closer attention to details

Paying closer attention to details in the moment can make it easier to remember them later. People can learn to focus better. Mindfulness techniques may help. Minimizing distractions and avoiding multitasking while learning information could also help with remembering.

12. Paying extra attention to difficult information

The order of information can play a role in recall (this is known as 'serial position effect'). The beginning and the ending of a text may be easier to recall. While recalling middle information can be difficult, it can be overcome by spending extra time rehearsing this information. Another strategy is to try restructuring it.

13. Varying the study routine

Another way to increase information recall is to occasionally change the study routine. By adding an element of novelty to the study sessions such as change of place or/and time, spacing apart the time spent studying, rather than massing it together, etc.) one can increase the effectiveness of efforts and significantly improve long-term recall.

14. Securing enough sleep

Sleep is important for memory and learning. It has been linked to memory loss. It is thought to play an important role in the consolidation of memories. So has restless sleep and sleep that gets disturbed often. Getting enough healthy sleep is a priority. Taking a nap after learning something new can actually help learn faster and remember better. Sleeping after learning something new actually leads to physical changes in the brain. Mice experiments have shown that sleep-deprived mice experienced less dendritic growth following a learning task than well-rested mice.

Procedural memories (memory for physical skills, for example) as well as memories for experiences and for new knowledge, seem to benefit from sleep. Consequently, failing to prioritize sleep (or struggling with sleep for other reasons) is detrimental to optimal memory consolidation.

15. Maintaining healthy behavior

In addition to the above strategies, striving to live a healthy and active lifestyle can help enhance short term memory and preserve memory ability over time.

Why we forget?

Forgetting can be frustrating but much of what people forget escapes memory quietly. Experts say "it is a feature, not a bug, of the way memory works". Forgetting may actually be ... helpful for remembering ... in the sense that the forgotten less-useful details will not interfere with the retrieval of useful ones. And forgetting unpleasant or painful memories can make one feel better about past experiences and reduce the burden of negative ones.

What conditions can cause memory loss?

Information may be forgotten because one was not paying close enough attention initially or has not reinforced the memory of the information by retrieving it. A more recently acquired memory may interfere with the retrieval of an earlier one. Several health-related conditions can cause memory loss, some of which such as stress, lack of sleep, and certain behaviors (e.g., excessive alcohol consumption) can also temporarily impair memory (causing a "blackout," in the case of drinking). Often, these causes may occur individually or together and usually resolve after treatment. These include:

> **Aging:** Aging can change the structures and chemistry of the brain, affecting a person's ability to learn new information and retrieve previously known information. The symptoms of age-related memory loss are usually mild and temporary.

> **Alcohol use disorder (AUD):** Heavy alcohol consumption or alcohol use disorder (AUD) can lead to the loss of brain cells (neurons) and cause cognitive decline.

> **Alzheimer's disease (AD):** Memory loss is one of the most common symptoms of AD. A person with this condition may have difficulty remembering important information and completing daily tasks.

> **Depression:** People with one or more symptoms of depression can have memory complaints. Some antidepressants can cause memory loss.

> **Head trauma:** Moderate to severe traumatic brain injury (TBI) from sports or accidents can affect the retention of short- and long-term memory.

> **Medications:** Certain medications can interfere with the brain's chemistry and lead to short- and long-term memory loss. However, this often resolves with medication changes. Examples of medications that may cause memory loss include psychoactive and nonpsychoactive drugs, antidepressants, anticonvulsants, and others. Older adults are also more likely to develop drug-induced cognitive impairment than

young adults. This may be due to drug toxicity from impaired liver and kidney functions.

- ➤ **Sleep deprivation:** People who lack quality sleep can have memory issues, which can directly affect their daytime activities.
- ➤ **Stress:** Stress affects memory in a time-dependent fashion. It can affect the formation of short- and long-term memory, the type of memories a person forms, and the ability to recall vital information.
- ➤ **Vitamin B-12 deficiency:** People with a vitamin B-12 deficiency have a greater likelihood of memory loss and other cognitive issues. This may be due to poor myelination — a condition that damages the myelin sheath that covers the nerve fibers in the brain.
- ➤ **Other causes:** People with certain conditions, such as COVID-19, herpes, HIV, gum disease, Lyme disease (LD), syphilis, urinary tract infection, and lung infections, may have a higher risk of neurological complications, including memory loss. Other causes may include diabetes, chronic obstructive pulmonary disease (COPD), renal dysfunction, endocrine disorders, cardiovascular diseases (CVD), and other neurodegenerative conditions. In many instances, treating the underlying infection can resolve the memory loss.

How to palliate memory loss?

For most people, it would be hard to imagine a life in which the mind did not routinely discard once-remembered details. A normal degree of forgetting is a core element of memory, allowing people to dispense with information for which they no longer have much use. Of course, forgetting causes problems, too. Minor failures to remember can be inconvenient at any age, and they may become more frequent and troublesome later in life. As indicated above, declines in certain types of memory ability are a typical part of aging and do not necessarily reflect the development of a medical condition such as AD. Although there are no guarantees when it comes to preventing memory loss or dementia, some activities might help. Experts have proposed a variety of tactics for staving off memory decline and managing typical levels of memory loss, including the following simple ways to sharpen memory advocated by the Mayo Clinic:

1. Being physically active every day

Physical activity raises blood flow to the whole body, including the brain. This might help keep memory sharp. For most healthy adults, the (U.S.) Department of Health & Human Services (DHHS) recommends "at least 150 minutes a week of moderate aerobic activity, such as brisk walking, or 75 minutes a week of vigorous aerobic activity, such as jogging". It is best if this activity is spread throughout the week".

2. Staying mentally active

Just as physical activity keeps the body in shape, mind activities (for example, reading, solving cross-word puzzles, playing games, learning to play a musical instrument, trying a new hobby, volunteering at a local school or with a community group.etc.) help keep the brain in shape and prevent some memory loss.

3. Spending time with others

Social interaction helps ward off depression and stress can contribute to memory loss, especially if living alone.

4. Staying organized

Staying organized can be accomplished by some or all of the following measures: uncluttering one's own environment; keeping track of tasks, appointments, and other events in a notebook, calendar or electronic planner; repeating each entry out-loud as as it is being written down; keeping to-do lists up to date; checking off finished items; keeping one's wallet, keys, glasses, and other essential items in a set place in the home so they are easy to find.

5. Eating a healthy diet

A healthy diet is good for your brain. It includes: Eating fruits, vegetables, and whole grains; choosing low-fat protein sources, such as fish, beans and skinless poultry; not abusing alcohol that can lead to confusion and memory loss.

6. Managing chronic health problems

These chronic conditions include: High blood pressure, diabetes, obesity, depression, and hearing loss. The better one takes care of oneself, the better memory is likely to be. Medicines taken should be regularly reviewed as some can affect memory.

Sidebar 12.1 discusses how emotional significance enhances memories.

Take-aways

> Memory refers to the psychological processes of acquiring, retaining, storing, and later retrieving information. There are four major processes involved: encoding, preservation, storage, and retrieval. However, this is not a flawless process.

> Memories are created to help ensure that our behavior fits the present situation and we can adjust them based on experience. They serve many purposes, from allowing us to revisit and learn from past experiences to storing knowledge about the world and how things work.

> When memory becomes dysfunctional, resulting in memories that are too strong or in memory loss, problematic changes in our behavior and our emotions devolve and potentially contribute to a variety of mental health disorders.

> The creation of memory is a transformation process in which a select amount of perceived information is converted into a more permanent form. A subset of that memory will be secured in long-term storage, accessible for future use. Many factors during and after the creation of a memory influence what (and how much) gets preserved.

> Memories are created through the connections that exist between neurons—either by strengthening these connections or through the growth of new connections. Changes in the connections between nerve cells (known as synapses) are associated with the learning and

retention of new information. Strengthening these connections helps commit information to memory.

➤ Memory is a continually unfolding process, reflecting real-world experience with varying levels of fidelity and accuracy. The working process includes: Encoding, retention and consolidation, storage, and retrieval.

➤ The memory system has been built to craft a useful account of past experiences, not a perfect one. Memories may be distorted or rendered less accurate based on conditions when they were first formed. False memories can be simple or complex. The malleability of memories over time means internal and external factors can introduce errors.

➤ Memories last for different times, some are very brief lasting just seconds. Short-term memories last about 20-30 seconds. Others are capable of enduring much longer, lasting days, weeks, months, or even decades. Most of these long-term memories lie outside of immediate awareness but can be drawn into consciousness when needed. Many times, painful memories tend to hang on for long periods of time.

➤ To use the information that has been encoded into memory, it first has to be retrieved. Many factors that can influence this process, including the type of information being used and the retrieval cues that are present.

➤ The ability to access and retrieve information from long-term memory allows us to actually use these memories to make decisions, interact with others, and solve problems. But, in order to be retrievable, memories have to be organized in some way. One way of thinking about memory organization is the 'semantic network model'.

➤ Certain stimuli can sometimes act as powerful triggers that draw memories into conscious awareness.

➤ A person's memory is a sea of images and other sensory impressions, facts and meanings, echoes of past feelings, and ingrained codes for how to behave—a diverse well of information. These forms of memory, which can overlap in daily life, have been arranged into broad categories: Sensory memories corresponding to the various sensory triggers (visual-spatial or iconic), auditory (or echoic), short-term memory (or active, working, or the conscious mind), long-term memory (or pre-conscious and unconscious mind). Memory experts have also distinguished *explicit and implicit memory.* Characteristic details of these various types of memory have been described.

➤ While Alzheimer's disease, other neurodegenerative disorders, and other age-related memory problems affect many older adults, the loss of memory during later adulthood might not be inevitable. It is common to experience some decline in cognitive function, but some types of memory even increase with age. Simple lifestyle strategies have been suggested to help protect the brain of the aging person.

➤ Human memory is a complex process that researchers are still trying to better understand. Research-proven strategies have been presented to effectively improve memory, enhance recall, and increase retention of information. As few or as many such strategies are differently needed by different people. Although there are no guarantees when it comes to preventing memory loss or dementia, some simple ways exist to sharpen memory.

Sidebar 12.1 - Emotional significance enhances memories

A normal function of emotion is to enhance memory in order to improve recall of experiences that have importance or relevance for our survival. Emotion emphasizes certain aspects of experiences to make them more memorable. It affects all the phases of memory formation: registering information, processing and storage, and retrieval.

Emotional learning to strengthen memory

➤ **Attention:** Attention guides the focus to select what is most relevant for our lives; it is normally associated with novelty. Nothing focuses the mind like surprise. Emotional intensity acts to narrow the scope of attention so that a few objects are emphasized at the expense of many others. Focusing upon a very narrow area allows for an optimal use of our limited attentional capacity.

➤ **Memory consolidation:** Most of the information we acquire is forgotten and never makes it into long-term memory. When we learn a complex problem, the short-term memory is freed up and the action becomes automatic. Emotionally charged events are remembered better than those of neutral events. The stress hormones epinephrine and cortisol enhance and consolidate memory. Dangerous situations are imprinted with extra clarity so that they may be avoided in the future.

> **Memory recall:** Memories of painful emotional experiences linger far longer than those involving physical pain.

> **Priming:** Past memories are often triggered or primed by one's environment. Priming refers to activating behavior through the power of unconscious suggestion. The goal stored in long-term memory is retrieved and placed in short-term memory.

> **Mood memory:** Current emotional state facilitates recall of experiences that had a similar emotional tone. Moods bring different associations to mind.

> **Blanking out:** Stress can lead to memory deficits, such as the common experience of mentally blanking during a high-pressure exam or interview. In general, anxiety influences cognitive performance in a curvilinear manner (this is the 'Yerkes–Dodson law'). When levels of arousal are either too low or too high, performance is likely to suffer. The optimal situation is moderate arousal.

> **Duration neglect ('peak-end rule'):** The way we remember events is not necessarily made up of a total of every individual moment. Instead, we tend to remember and overemphasize the peak (best or worst) moment and the last moment, and we neglect the duration of an experience.

In sum: Much of learning takes place in the form of emotional learning, and to make our memory stronger, it helps to attach emotional significance.

Impact of post-stroke memory loss and emotional responses

Coping with memory loss after a stroke can be a daunting and emotionally overwhelming journey. Approximately one-third of patients are affected by memory loss and profound cognitive changes within the first year after their stroke, leading to confusion, frustration, and despair. However, understanding the emotional impact of memory loss is an important factor in dealing with its challenges.

Stroke and memory loss

Memory loss following a stroke often occurs because the areas of the brain responsible for memory encoding and retrieval, primarily the **hippocampus and the adjacent structures in the medial temporal lobe**, get damaged. Depending on the severity and location of the stroke, memory loss can range from mild forgetfulness to severe anterograde amnesia, where the person cannot form new memories. For instance, a stroke affecting the left side of the brain may lead to difficulties in remembering verbal information. In contrast, a stroke affecting the right side may affect the recall of visual or spatial information.

Emotional impact

Memory loss after a stroke is a complex, multifaceted issue that often provokes a profound emotional response. The sudden inability to recall familiar faces, cherished memories, or daily routines presents emotional challenges. Specifically, it can cause fear, confusion, and frustration for stroke survivors and their loved ones.

Emotional response

Recognizing the emotional response to memory loss is critical because it lays the foundation for effective coping strategies.

- **Sadness:** It ranges from mild unhappiness to deep, clinical depression. The inability to remember valued memories or even simple, everyday tasks can trigger feelings of loss and grief.

- **Anger:** It can be directed toward oneself for perceived failings or others for their inability to understand the depth of the struggle. It is a natural response to a complex and unexpected situation. While anger might be perceived as a negative emotion, it can be channeled positively, using it as a motivation for change rather than a source of self-destruction.

- **Fear:** This debilitating emotion can lead to worsened anxiety and depression. The fear of losing oneself, and the fear of the unknown future, can be paralyzing, preventing the individual from progressing in their recovery journey.

Coping Strategies

Despite the difficulties posed by memory loss after a stroke, various coping methods and techniques can help manage the symptoms. These strategies are intended to compensate for memory deficits and enhance memory performance:

- **Routines and checklists:** They can provide structure and predictability, reducing the demand for memory.
- **Memory aids:** Calendars, diaries, note-taking, and electronic reminders can help with remembering appointments, tasks, or important information.
- **Associating new information with something familiar** (or elaborative **encoding**): This technique can make it easier to remember.
- **Lifestyle changes:** Regular physical exercise, a balanced diet, adequate sleep, and stress management have all been shown to benefit cognitive health and support memory function.

For many, memory loss following a stroke becomes a silent thief, quietly stealing precious moments and personal histories. However, through compassion, understanding, and knowledge, stroke survivors and their loved ones can navigate the emotional challenges of post-stroke memory loss, turning obstacles into opportunities for growth and resilience. Remember, emotional reactions to memory loss are normal and part of the recovery journey. They are not a sign of weakness but rather a testament to the strength and adaptability of stroke survivors.

In sum: Post-stroke memory loss impacts about a third of patients. Memory loss and other cognitive impairments often depend on stroke severity and location. Sadness, anger, and fear are common emotional responses to post-stroke memory loss.

Sidebar 12.2 - Respiration modulates cognitive function and memory

Breathing, an involuntary reflex, may shape cognitive function and memory. During off-line brain states such as sleep, respiration is known to coordinate hippocampal activity, acting as a memory modulator and playing a role in memory consolidation. Mice experiments have shown that certain components of central respiratory activity (such as frequency) during on-line encoding contribute substantially to shaping hippocampal ensemble cell dynamics and memory performance.

Thus, breathing could potentially be actively recruited during on-line memory encoding. The correlation between breathing patterns and memory encoding may yield innovative approaches in the treatment of memory-related disorders, such as Alzheimer's disease and other forms of dementia. Customized respiration exercises might be developed as part of therapeutic regimens to enhance cognitive function.

Sidebar 12.3 – Vision and the brain

Eyes tell much more than just where one is looking. They provide valuable insights into thoughts and underlying brain health. Basic eye movements such as, for example, following a dot across a screen, can inform of the current status of brain health. The ability to process and perceive visual motion can be read-out in eye movements, which can also inform how brain circuits are performing. Similar to a muscle, the brain circuitry can strengthen over time.

Vision loss is associated with cognitive impairment

Visual impairment increases the risk of cognitive decline and dementia for older adults. One study concluded that poor vision may have led to up to 100,000 cases of dementia in the U.S. In addition:

> **Worse vision is associated with more rapid cognitive decline:** Specifically, worse visual acuity and impaired depth perception are associated with greater declines in language and memory, whereas worse contrast sensitivity is associated with declines in language, memory, attention, and visuospatial ability.
> **Vision loss is associated with cognitive decline patterns:** Patterns of cognitive decline in older adults may differ by the type of vision loss they may experience.

> **Impaired contrast sensitivity is associated with a wider range of cognitive decrement.**

There are several possible reasons why visual impairment is associated with cognitive decline. There are essentially two possible causal pathways or, possibly, their combination:

> **The common causal pathway:** Having a shared pathology underlying both vision and cognitive impairments, such as nerve or vascular disease, is a possibility.

> **The sensory loss consequence pathway:** Here, vision loss may be associated with cognitive decline through conditions known to affect cognition, such as depression, social isolation, decreased engagement in cognitively stimulating activities, and increased cognitive load due to the greater dedication of cognitive resources to visual processing.

> **The combined pathway:** A combination of the above two mechanisms may likely contribute to the greater cognitive decline noted in older adults with vision loss.

Tips for eye and associated brain health

The following recommendations have been provided by the National Eye Institute (NEI) for eye health that may also help your brain health:

• **See an ophthalmologist regularly:** Correcting poor vision with eyeglasses or getting cataract surgery can help prevent diabetic eye disease through early detection and reduce the risk of cognitive impairment. A recent study concluded that one of the easiest ways to reduce the risk of dementia is by correcting poor vision.

• **Eat a healthy diet:** The American Academy of Ophthalmology (AAO) recommends regularly consuming green leafy vegetables, fish, and fruits to provide the nutrients that the eyes need, slow down the rate of cognitive decline, and reduce the risk for dementia.

• **Cardiovascular exercise:** Cardiovascular exercise can help manage chronic health conditions such as diabetes, which can damage the vessels in the retina, leading to visual impairment and, in some cases, even blindness and also increase the risk of dementia. Even in the absence of diabetes, studies have found that regular exercise can help maintain good cognitive function over time.

Sidebar 12.4 – Memory and mental health

Memories can be immensely powerful but, for people struggling with mental health conditions, that power can be a burden. Because memory has an important role in pathological thinking and behavior, however, what scientists and clinicians have learned about memory can also be key to helping people recover from mental illness.

Memory and common mental disorders

Widespread mental health conditions such as depression, substance use disorders, and anxiety disorders have complex causes that differ substantially. Yet it is clear that each is characterized, in some ways, by how memory works in the people who suffer from them.

Can stress impair memory?

Stressful situations can result in strong future memories about the experience. But, during a stressful event, remembering information can be more challenging than usual. Over time, chronic stress and elevated levels of stress hormones like cortisol may have a detrimental effect on the ability to remember. In addition, the experience of psychological stress is well established as a force affecting how we remember. Taking steps to reduce stress is one way people can seek to preserve memory ability.

Can depression make one forgetful?

Depression is associated with multiple kinds of cognitive impairment, including forgetfulness— though memory difficulties often resolve after a depressive episode is successfully treated. A depressed person may also show other memory differences, including relatively weak memory for positive events, stronger memory for negative ones, and relatively general (rather than specific) recollections about personal experiences. Depression has been linked with reduced volume in the hippocampus, a part of the brain that is important for memory.

13

Memory and the aging brain

Contents

13

Memory and the aging brain

It is important to understand that brains change over time, and it is helpful to be able to distinguish normal changes from those that require medical and psychological attention.

What brain changes are normal for older adults?

Although new neurons develop throughout our lives, our brains reach their maximum size during our early twenties and then begin very slowly to decline in volume. Blood flow to the brain also decreases over time. Fortunately, many studies have shown that **the brain remains capable of regrowth and of learning and retaining new facts and skills throughout life**, especially for people who get regular exercise and frequent intellectual stimulation. Although there are tremendous differences among individuals, some cognitive abilities continue to improve well into older age, some are constant, and some decline.

Is it typical to forget things as one ages?

Changes in the ability to remember are normal, even in the absence of dementia or other condition, and memory loss is a common concern among older adults. Declines in certain types of memory (such as **working memory** and **episodic memory**) mean that a person might occasionally forget the word they had intended to say or where they left a frequently used object. Other forms of memory, including **semantic memory** (knowledge about the world) and **procedural memory**, seem to be less affected by normal aging.

At what age does memory decline?

Memory ability, at least for some kinds of memory (such as **working memory**), can begin to gradually decline as early as age in the twenties or thirties, with downward trends extending into later life. Research indicates that **episodic memory** ability (memory for experiences) tends to decrease after age 60. For some individuals, memory is preserved to a greater extent and for longer.

Some types of memory improve or stay the same

It is well known that some forms of memory ability tend to become less sharp with age. Just like other parts of the body, the brain also changes with age, with accompanying differences in the ability to recall information. But not everyone experiences such declines to the same degree as they get older, and some forms of memory (such as the memory for familiar physical tasks) seem largely unhindered by age.

Semantic memory (the ability to recall concepts and general facts that are not related to specific experiences) continues to improve for many older adults (see Chapter 12). For example, understanding the concept that clocks are used to tell time is a simple example of semantic memory. This type of memory also includes vocabulary and knowledge of language. In addition, **procedural memory** (the memory of how to do things, such as how to tell time by reading the numbers on a clock) typically stays the same.

Other types of memory decline somewhat

Episodic memory is the memory which captures the "what," "where," and "when" of daily lives. Both episodic and **longer term memory** decline somewhat over time.

Other types of brain functions that decrease slightly or slow down include:

- Information processing and learning something new.
- Doing more than one task at a time and shifting focus between tasks.

Memory and aging

Age-related memory loss, sometimes described as "normal aging" is qualitatively different from memory loss associated with types of dementia such as Alzheimer's disease dementia (ADD), and has a different brain mechanism. It is believed to originate in the dentate gyrus, whereas AD is believed to originate in the entorhinal cortex.

Mild cognitive impairment

Mild cognitive impairment (MCI) is a condition in which people face memory problems more often than that of the average person their age. These symptoms, however, do not prevent them from carrying out normal activities and are not as severe as the symptoms for AD. Symptoms often include misplacing items, forgetting events or appointments, and having trouble finding words.

MCI is the transitional state between cognitive changes of normal aging and AD. Several studies have indicated that individuals with MCI are at an increased risk for developing AD, ranging from 1% to 25% per year. In one study, 24% of MCI patients progressed to AD in two years and 20% more over three years, whereas another study indicated that the progression of MCI subjects was 55% in four and a half years. Some patients with MCI, however, never progress to AD.

Studies have also indicated patterns that are found in both MCI and AD. Much like patients with AD, those with MCI have difficulty accurately defining words and using them appropriately in sentences when asked. While MCI patients had a lower performance in this task than the control group, AD patients performed worse overall. The abilities of MCI patients stood out, however, due to their ability to provide examples to make up for their difficulties. AD patients failed to use any compensatory strategies and therefore exhibited the difference in use of **episodic memory** and executive functioning.

Normal aging

Normal aging is associated with a decline in various memory abilities in many cognitive tasks; the phenomenon is known as 'age-related memory impairment' (ARMI) or 'age-associated memory impairment' (AAMI). The ability to encode new memories of events or facts and **working memory** show decline in both cross-sectional and longitudinal studies. Studies comparing the effects of aging on **episodic memory, semantic memory, short-term memory** and priming find that **episodic memory is especially impaired in normal aging** and **some types of short-term memory are also impaired**.The deficits may be related to impairments seen in the ability to refresh recently processed information. The chart of Figure 13.1 gives a detailed overview of the term "memory" as used in various branches of academia".

Figure 13.1 - Overview of the forms and functions of memory

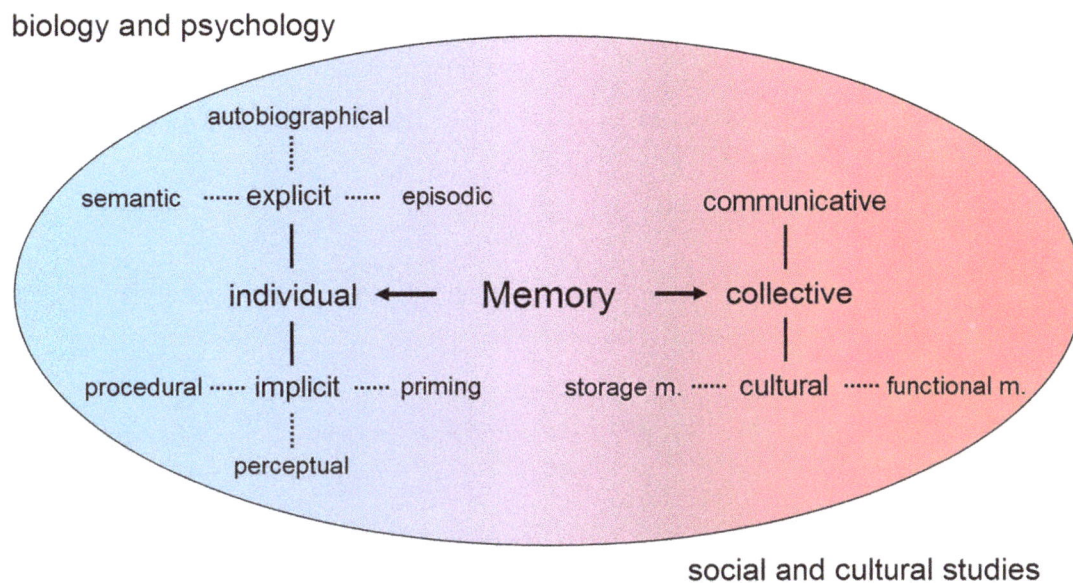

Source: Bernhard Wenzi

Some types of memory are further elaborated upon below as the brain ages.

Implicit or procedural memory

Typically, **implicit or procedural memory shows no decline with age**.

Episodic memory

Episodic memory is supported by networks spanning frontal, temporal, and parietal lobes. The interconnections in the lobes are presumed to enable distinct aspects of memory, whereas the effects of grey matter lesions have been extensively studied, less is known about the interconnecting fiber tracts. In aging, degradation of white matter structure has emerged as an important general factor, further focusing attention on the critical white matter connections.

Exercise affects many people young and old. For the elderly, especially those with AD or other diseases that affect the memory, when the brain is introduced to exercise, the hippocampus is likely to retain its size and improve its memory.

It is also possible that the years of education a person has had and the amount of attention they received as a child might be a variable closely related to the links of aging and memory.There is a positive correlation between early life education and memory gains in older age. This effect is especially significant in women.

In particular, **associative learning**, which is another type of **episodic memory**, is vulnerable to the effects of aging, as has been demonstrated across various study paradigms. This has been explained by the 'associative deficit hypothesis' (ADH), which states that aging is associated with a deficiency in creating and retrieving links between single units of information. This can include knowledge about context, events or items. The ability to bind pieces of information together with their episodic context in a coherent whole has been reduced in the elderly population. Furthermore, the older adults' performances in free recall involves temporal contiguity to a lesser extent than for younger people, indicating that associations regarding contiguity become weaker with age.

Three reasons have been speculated as to why older adults use less effective encoding and retrieval strategies as they age:

- **The "disuse" view:** It states that memory strategies are used less by older adults as they move further away from the educational system.
- **The "diminished attentional capacity" hypothesis:** It means that older people engage less in self-initiated encoding due to reduced attentional capacity.
- **The "memory self-efficacy" view:** It indicates that older people do not have confidence in

their own memory performances, leading to poor consequences. It is known that patients with AD and patients with semantic dementia both exhibit difficulty in tasks that involve picture naming and category fluency. This is tied to damage to their semantic network, which stores knowledge of meanings and understandings.

One phenomenon, known as "senior moments", is a memory deficit that appears to have a biological cause. When an older adult is interrupted while completing a task, it is likely that the original task at hand can be forgotten. Studies have shown that the brain of an older adult does not have the ability to re-engage after an interruption and continues to focus on the particular interruption unlike that of a younger brain. This **inability to multi-task is normal with aging** and is expected to become more apparent with the increase of older generations remaining in the work field.

For super-aged people, a biological explanation for memory deficits in aging includes a *post-mortem* examination of five brains of elderly people with better memory than average. It was found that these individuals had **fewer fiber-like tangles of tau protein** than in typical elderly brains. However, a **similar amount of amyloid plaque** was found.

More recent research has extended established findings of age-related decline in executive functioning, by examining related cognitive processes that underlie healthy older adults' 'sequential performance'. Sequential performance refers to the execution of a series of steps needed to complete a routine. An important part of healthy aging involves older adults' use of memory and inhibitory processes to carry out daily activities in a fixed order without forgetting the sequence of steps that were just completed while remembering the next step in the sequence. A 2009 study examined how young and older adults differ in the underlying representation of a sequence of tasks and their efficiency at retrieving the information needed to complete their routine. Findings from this study revealed that when older and young adults had to remember a sequence of eight animal images arranged in a fixed order, both age groups spontaneously used the organizational strategy of 'chunking' to facilitate retrieval of information. However, older adults were slower at accessing each chunk compared to younger adults, and were better able to benefit from the use of memory aids, such as verbal rehearsal to remember the order of the fixed sequence. Results from this study suggest that there are age differences in memory and inhibitory processes that affect people's sequence of actions and the use of memory aids could facilitate the retrieval of information in older age.

Working memory

Working memory involves the manipulation and use of information that is being obtained to complete a task. It **declines as the aging process progresses. W**orking memory plays a role in the comprehension and production of speech.

Table 13.1 summarizes some known facts about memory decline with normal aging:

Table 13.1 – Fate of various types of memory with normal aging

Memory type	Fate with normal aging	Brain region affected
Autobiographical	o Declines somewhat o Decreases after age 60	
Episodic	o Declines somewhat o Decreases after age 60; preserved to a greater extent and for longer for some individuals	o Supported by networks spanning frontal, temporal, and parietal lobes. o Degradation of white matter medial-temporal regions, which contain the hippocampi

Implicit	o No decline o Less affected than working and episodic memories	
Kinesthetic		
Long-term	o Declines somewhat	
Procedural	o No decline	
Prospective		
Semantic	o Continues to improve or stays the same for many adults o Less affected than working and episodic memories	
Sensory - Auditory (or echoic) - Haptic - Olfactory - Visual spatial (or iconic)		
Short-term - Active - Working	o Somewhat impaired o Little decline for other types of short-term memory o Semantic knowledge (e.g. vocabulary) improves with age o Enhancement seen in memory for emotional events maintained with age. o Declines. Primary reason for decline in a variety of cognitive tasks and in comprehension and production of speech	

Possible causes of memory issues with aging

The causes for memory issues and aging are still unclear, even after the many theories have been tested. It is still difficult to determine exactly how each aspect of aging affects the memory and aging process. However, it is known that the **brain shrinks with age** due to the expansion of ventricles, restricting the room in the head. Unfortunately, **a solid link between the shrinking brain and memory loss has not been established** due to not knowing exactly which area of the brain has shrunk and what the importance of that area truly is in the aging process. Attempting to recall information or a situation that has happened can be very difficult since **different pieces of information of an event are stored in different areas**. During recall of an event, the various pieces of information are pieced back together again and any missing information is unconsciously filled up by our brains, which can account for ourselves receiving and believing false information.

Memory lapses can be both aggravating and frustrating but they are due to the **overwhelming number of information that is being taken in by the brain**. Issues in memory can also be linked to several **common clinical, psychological, and physical causes** (listed below), some of which may be reversible (see also Chapter 6 for full details of diseases that may cause memory problems). For example, the following common conditions can lead to memory problems:

- **Clinical issues:**
  - Blood clots in the brain
  - Chronic conditions (heart disease, diabetes, etc.)
  - Dehydration
  - Infections
  - Medication side effects.
  - Thyroid imbalance
  - Vitamin B12 deficiency

- **Psychological issues:**
  - Anxiety
  - Depression
  - Psychological stress

- **Lifestyle issues:**
  - Changes due to traumatic events (accidents, head injuries, past abuse, loss of loved ones, etc.)
  - Chronic alcoholism
  - Insufficient water drinking
  - Poor nutrition
  - Substance abuse

It is important to discuss these and other possible causes of memory problems with a medical professional and to have a complete medical workup. Also, a psychologist may perform a complete neuropsychological evaluation to rule out anxiety, depression, or other psychological stresses and to test for cognitive changes. Taking care of body and mind with appropriate medication, doctoral check-ups, and daily mental and physical exercise can prevent some of these memory issues. There is a possibility that the damage to the brain makes it harder for a person to encode and process information that should be stored in long-term memory. There is support for environmental cues being helpful in recovery and retrieval of information.

Memory loss theories

Is it typical to forget things as one ages?

Changes in the ability to remember are normal, even in the absence of dementia or another condition, and memory loss is a common concern among older adults. Declines in certain types of memory (such as working memory and episodic memory) mean that a person might occasionally forget the word they had intended to say or where they left a frequently used object. Other forms of memory, including semantic memory (knowledge about the world) and procedural memory, seem to be less affected by normal aging.

At what age does memory decline?

Memory ability, at least for some kinds of memory (such as working memory), can begin to gradually decline as early as age twenties or thirties, with downward trends extending into later life. Research indicates that episodic memory ability (memory for experiences) tends to decrease after age 60. Yet these are averages; for some individuals, memory is preserved to a greater extent and for longer.

Six theories have been advanced in attempts to explain memory loss. A helpful mnemonic is **ACIAP**, **which encompasses several effects (A**tttention deficit; **C**ontiguity; **I**nhibitory control decline; **A**ttentional resources limitation; **P**rocessing).

1. Associative deficit effect

In the 'associative deficit theory of memory, access to the memory performance of an elder person is attributed to their difficulty in creating and retaining cohesive episodes.

2. Contiguity effect

Tests and data show that as people age, the contiguity effect (stimuli that occur close together in the associated time) starts to weaken. This is supported by the associative deficit theory of memory. The supporting research shows that greater age is associated with lower hit and greater false alarm rates, and also a more liberal bias response on recognition tests even after controlling for sex, education, and other health-related issues,

3. Inhibition and inhibitory control effect

Older people have a higher tendency to make outside intrusions during a memory test. This can be attributed to the inhibition effect that causes participants to take longer time in recalling or recognizing an item, and also subjects them to making more frequent errors. For instance, in a study using metaphors as the test subject, older participants rejected correct metaphors more often than literally false statements.

Inhibitory control may account for the decline seen in working memory that prevents the suppression of irrelevant information in working memory and, correspondingly, the limited capacity for relevant information. Less space for new stimuli may be attributed to the declines seen in individuals' working memory as they age.

As we age, deficits are seen in the ability to integrate, manipulate, and reorganize the contents of working memory in order to complete higher level cognitive tasks such as problem-solving, decision- making, goal-setting, and planning. More research must be completed in order to determine what the exact cause of these age-related deficits in working memory are. It is likely that many or all of the above theories (associated deficit, contiguity, inhibition, memory decline, attentional resources limitation, processing speed, and inhibitory control) may play a role in these age-related deficits. The brain regions that are active during working memory tasks are also being evaluated, and research has shown that different parts of the brain are activated during working memory in younger adults as compared to older adults.

4. Working memory decline effect

Working memory demonstrates great declines during the aging process and less capacity to hold information. There have been various theories offered to explain why these changes may occur, which include:

> Fewer attentional resources;
> Slower speed of processing;
> Less capacity to hold information;
> Lower degree of integration and manipulation of information because the products of earlier memory processing are forgotten before the subsequent products; and
> Lack of inhibitory control.

All of these theories offer strong arguments, and it is likely that the decline in working memory is due to the problems cited in all of these areas.

5. Attentional resources limitation effect

Another theory that is being examined to explain age-related declines in working memory is that there is a 'limit in attentional resources' seen with aging. Older individuals are less capable of dividing their attention between two tasks so that tasks with higher attentional demands are more difficult to complete due to a reduction in mental energy. Tasks that are simple and more automatic, however, see fewer declines with aging. Working memory tasks often involve divided attention, thus they are more likely to strain the limited resources of aging individuals.

6. Processing speed effect

Speed of processing information decreases significantly and is then responsible for the inability to use working memory efficiently as we age. As processing slows, cognitive tasks that rely on quick processing speed become more difficult.

Preserving memory ability

Can memory be protected as people grow older?

While a person may not be able to prevent decreases in memory ability entirely, experts have studied various steps one can take to increase one's odds of maintaining a sharp memory into older age. There are also techniques for working around common memory issues if they arise.

What are some strategies for preserving memory ability?

Adopting aspects of a generally health-promoting lifestyle—such as a healthy diet, routine physical activity, and plenty of sleep—may help maintain memory as one ages. So might playing cognitively challenging games, such as chess, cards, and crossword puzzles, or exercising one's mind in other ways.

How can one manage normal, age-related memory loss?

Reducing stress and getting enough sleep could be helpful. Other ways to compensate for forgetfulness include organizing objects (such as car keys) so that their locations are always the same, making an extra effort to concentrate when taking in information to be remembered, minimizing distractions, and using simple memory aids such as planners, calendars, written lists, and reminder notes. In some cases, it may be worth considering medications to enhance memory.

Mechanisms research

Age-related memory loss has been associated with several possible mechanisms (see Chapter 10 for a fuller discussion). For the purpose of this chapter, the following two mechanisms are emphasized.

Deficiency of the RbAp48 protein

In 2010, experiments that have tested for the significance of the under-performance of memory for an older adult group as compared to a young adult group, hypothesized that the associated memory deficit with age could be linked with a physical deficit. It can be explained by the inefficient processing in the **medial-temporal regions** – an important region for episodic memory containing the hippocampi, which are crucial in creating memory association between items. It is to be noted that age-related memory loss is believed to originate in the dentate gyrus, whereas AD is believed to originate in the entorhinal cortex.

Oxidative DNA damage

During normal aging, oxidative DNA damage in the brain accumulates in the promoters of genes involved in learning and memory, as well as in genes involved in neuronal survival. It includes DNA single-strand breaks (SSBs), which can give rise to DNA double-strand breaks (DSBs). DSBs accumulate in neurons and astrocytes of the hippocampus and frontal cortex at early stages and during the progression to AD, a process that could be an important driver of neurodegeneration and cognitive decline.

Is it typical to forget things as one ages?

Changes in the ability to remember are normal, even in the absence of dementia or another condition, and memory loss is a common concern among older adults. Declines in certain types of memory (such as working memory and episodic memory) mean that a person might occasionally forget the word they had intended to say or where they left a frequently used object.

Other forms of memory, including semantic memory (knowledge about the world) and procedural memory, seem to be less affected by normal aging.

At what age does memory decline?

Memory ability, at least for some kinds of memory (such as working memory), can begin to gradually decline as early as age twenties or thirties, with downward trends extending into later life. Research indicates that episodic memory ability (memory for experiences) tends to decrease after age 60. Yet these are averages; for some individuals, memory is preserved to a greater extent and for longer.

Take-aways

- ➢ Brains change over time, and it is helpful to be able to distinguish normal changes from those that require medical and psychological attention.
- ➢ Although new neurons develop throughout life, brains reach their maximum size during the early twenties and then begin very slowly to decline in volume. Blood flow to the brain also decreases over time.
- ➢ The brain remains capable of regrowth and of learning and retaining new facts and skills throughout life, especially for people who get regular exercise and frequent intellectual stimulation.
- ➢ Some types of memory improve or stay the same. Semantic memory (which also includes vocabulary and knowledge of language) continues to improve for many older adults. In addition, procedural memory typically stays the same.
- ➢ Other types of memory (episodic and longer term memory) decline somewhat over time.
- ➢ Other types of brain functions that decrease slightly or slow down include: Information processing and learning something new; doing more than one task at a time and shifting focus between tasks.
- ➢ Age-related memory loss, sometimes described as "normal aging" is qualitatively different from memory loss associated with types of dementia such as Alzheimer's disease, and has a different brain

mechanism. It is believed to originate in the dentate gyrus, whereas AD is believed to originate in the entorhinal cortex.

➤ Mild cognitive impairment is the transitional state between cognitive changes of normal aging and Alzheimer's disease.

➤ Normal aging is associated with a decline in various memory abilities in many cognitive tasks. Studies comparing the effects of aging on episodic memory, semantic memory, short-term memory and priming found that episodic memory is especially impaired in normal aging and some types of short-term memory are also impaired.

➤ One type of episodic memory (source information) declines with old age. This deficit may be related to declines in the ability to bind information together in memory during encoding and to retrieve those associations at a later time.

➤ Typically, implicit or procedural memory shows no decline with age. Episodic memory is supported by networks spanning frontal, temporal, and parietal lobes. In aging, degradation of white matter structure has emerged as an important general factor, further focusing attention on the critical white matter connections.

➤ For the elderly, especially those with Alzheimer's or other diseases that affect the memory, when the brain is introduced to exercise, the hippocampus is likely to retain its size and improve its memory.

➤ There is a positive correlation between early life education and memory gains in older age. This effect is especially significant in women.

➤ Associative learning, another type of episodic memory, is vulnerable to the effects of aging has been explained by the associative deficit hypothesis, which states that aging is associated with a deficiency in creating and retrieving links between single units of information. This can include knowledge about context, events or items.

➤ Three reasons have been speculated as to why older adults use less effective encoding and retrieval strategies as they age: The "disuse" view, the "diminished attentional capacity" hypothesis, and the "memory self-efficacy" view.

➤ One phenomenon, known as "senior moments", is a memory deficit that appears to have a biological cause. This inability to multi-task is normal with aging and is expected to become more apparent with the increase of older generations remaining in the work field.

- Superaged people have fewer fiber-like tangles of tau protein than in typical elderly brains but a similar amount of amyloid plaque.

- An important part of healthy aging involves older adults' use of memory and inhibitory processes to carry out daily activities in a fixed order without forgetting the sequence of steps that were just completed while remembering the next step in the sequence.

- Working memory involves the manipulation and use of information that is being obtained to complete a task. It declines as the aging process progresses and plays a role in the comprehension and production of speech.

- The causes for memory issues and aging are still unclear. It remains difficult to determine exactly how each aspect of aging affects the memory and aging process. However, it is known that the brain shrinks with age due to the expansion of ventricles, restricting the room in the head. Unfortunately, a solid link between the shrinking brain and memory loss has not been established.

- Memory lapses are due to the overwhelming number of information that is being taken in by the brain. Issues in memory can also be linked to several common clinical, psychological, and physical causes, some of which may be reversible.

- Six theories have so far been advanced in attempts to explain memory loss: Associative deficit effect; contiguity effect; inhibition and inhibitory control effect; working memory decline effect; attentional resources limitation effect; processing speed effect; and inhibitory control effect.

- Age-related memory loss has been associated with several possible mechanisms, including particularly deficiency of the RbAp48 protein and oxidative DNA damage, which includes DNA single-strand breaks that can give rise to DNA double-strand breaks. DSBs accumulate in neurons and astrocytes of the hippocampus and frontal cortex at early stages and during the progression to Alzheimer's disease, a process that could be an important driver of neurodegeneration and cognitive decline.

Sidebar 13.1 – What causes cognitive decline with age

The mental process of thinking, learning, remembering, being aware of surroundings, and using judgment changes as we age. As nerve cells and synapses in the brain alter over time, the ability to quickly process information and make decisions declines. For most people, the decline is gradual, starting at around the age of 50. However, this slight drop in processing speed and **working memory** is generally accompanied by improvements in cumulative knowledge well into old age.

The S-nitrosylation process

A new study, in mice, suggests that alterations in a brain protein may impair synaptic plasticity (the ability of nerve cells to modify the strength of their connections), leading to **memory** decline. Another mice study suggests that we can help delay age-related cognitive decline, how social interaction, cognitive training, and physical exercise activate an enzyme that improves the functioning of nerve cells and synapses, resulting in enhanced cognitive performance.

In two other studies, researchers investigated CaM kinase II (CaMKII), an enzyme that is involved in, among other processes, synaptic plasticity and the transmission of nerve impulses across synapses. By altering this brain protein, they mimicked the cognitive effects that occur during normal aging. They suggested that nitric oxide (NO) affects the action of CaMKII and that a process called S-nitrosylation, which relies on NO, modifies CaMKII. The reduced nitrosylation of CaMKII causes a reduction in synaptic localization of CaMKII, which happens during normal aging, **memory,** and learning abilities are impaired. Put simply, a reduction in NO slows down the movement of nerve impulses across the connections between nerve cells, which may cause cognitive decline.

Lifestyle and cognitive decline

Researchers have long known that a healthy lifestyle (positive experiences such as social interactions, physical exercise, intermittent fasting, cognitive training, and critical thinking) is essential for optimal brain health throughout life and is associated with a slower rate of **memory** decline in adults with normal cognition. What is not known is how exactly these lifestyle factors have their effect.

Memory and the diseased brain

Contents

14

Memory and the diseased brain

With increasing lifespan in the developed world, dementia has emerged as an increasing public health concern. It was uncommon in pre-industrial times and relatively rare before the 20th century. As more people are living longer, dementia is becoming more common in the population as a whole due to a decrease in risk factors. *Global Health Estimates 2016* lists Alzheimer's and other dementias as fifth among the top 10 global causes of mortality, costing annually $818 billion (excluding the majority of care that is provided by family carers).

The demented brain

Dementia is an umbrella term for several brain diseases that manifest themselves by a group of symptoms affecting **memory**, other cognitive abilities, and behavior (Figure 14.1).

Figure 14.1 – Dementia is an umbrella term for several different conditions

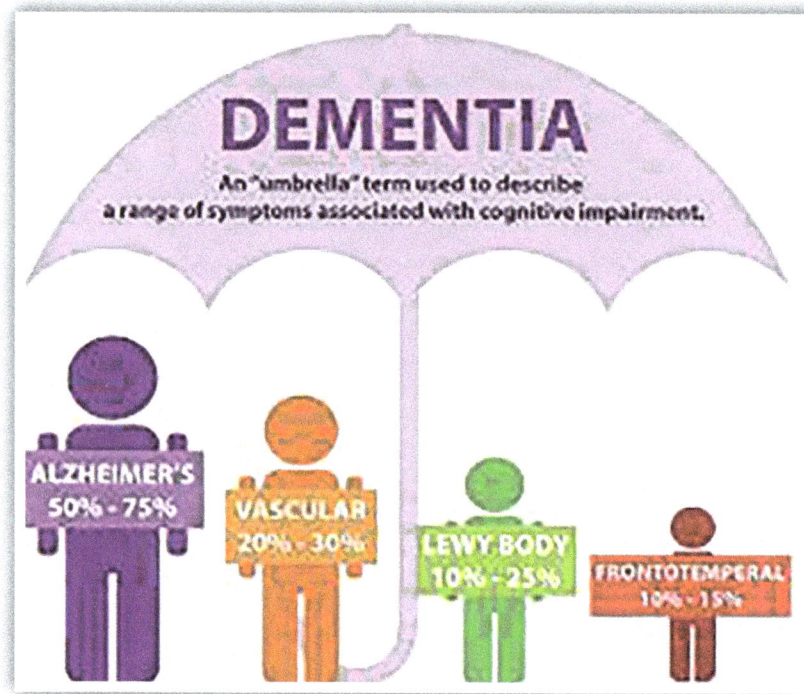

(Note: The umbrella shown is not wide enough as there are several other conditions that should also be included under it.)

But dementia is not an emerging disease! It has been referred to in medical texts since Antiquity (see the writings of Pythagoras, Solon, Plato, Cicero, Celsius, Galen, Bacon,...and others in Asia and China) although the disease was comparatively rare before the 20th century. Until the end of the 19th century, it was a much broader clinical concept that encompassed mental illness and any type of psychosocial incapacity. In the elderly, it was also believed to be the result of blockages of the major arteries supplying the brain or small strokes within the vessels of the cerebral cortex (two forms of cerebral atherosclerosis). It was only recently, on the basis of pathological examination of brain tissues, symptomatology, and different patterns of brain metabolic activity that a number of other types of dementia have been identified.

After all these past centuries, dementia remained (and continues to be) one of the most misunderstood diseases in medicine. It is only in the 1960s that the link between age-related cognitive decline and neurodegenerative diseases was established. Since then, the medical community maintained that Alzheimer's disease (AD) was the cause of the vast majority of mental impairments rather than vascular disease (VD), which is rarer than previously thought. It also thought that senility dementia (SD) could be linked to AD dementia, and that dementia is a mixture of both AD dementia and VD dementia. Since the beginning of the current century, a number of other types of dementia have been differentiated from these two.

Nonetheless, to this day, the causal etiology of many types of dementia, including AD, still remains unclear. While many theories (rather hypotheses) have been advanced, these are largely based on risk factors, associations or correlations, the cause of many types of dementia, including the most prevalent AD, remains unclear. But, risk factors, correlations, associations, and the like... are not causation! Likewise, risk management and symptomatic treatment... are not cure, only palliations! More recently (2017), I have posited that the *root cause* (not a risk factor) of Alzheimer's and other neurodegenerative diseases is but an autoimmune disease having gone rogue.

What is dementia?

Simply stated, dementia is really a general term for the process of decline in mental abilities. According to the definition provided by the World Health Organization (WHO, 2017), dementia is "...*an umbrella term for several diseases affecting* **memory**, *other cognitive abilities, and behavior that interfere significantly with a person's ability to maintain their activities of daily living. Although age is the strongest known risk factor for dementia, it is not a normal part of aging*". It is a broad category of brain diseases that cause a long-term and often gradual decrease in the ability to think and remember that is great enough to affect a person's daily functioning. Other common symptoms include emotional problems, language difficulties, and decreased motivation.

As pictured in part in Figure 14.1, many different diseases can cause dementia, including Alzheimer's disease (AD), vascular disease (VD), Lewy bodies (LB), frontotemporal disorders (FTD), syphilis, senility, and even stroke. Mixed dementia (MD) is the concurrence of two or more types of dementia. About

10% of individuals present with MD, usually the combination of AD and another type of dementia such as FTD or VD.

However, not being a specific disease, the above potential contributors do not reach to the primary cause of the disease. There lies our greatest shortcoming: Unable to pinpoint the root cause of the disease, we are powerless in curing it. Sure, drugs are available to treat some of the symptoms, but not the disease itself. They may improve symptoms or at best slow down the disease but there is no known cure for dementia. This is a sad observation on the state of the situation, which stems from our incomplete understanding of the deep biology of the contributing diseases and associated epigenetic/ecogenetic influences.

Risk factors and prevention

Although age is the strongest known risk factor for dementia, it is not an inevitable consequence of aging (see Table 14.1). Further, dementia does not exclusively affect older people – *young onset dementia* (YOD), defined as the onset of symptoms before the age of 65 years, accounts for up to 9% of cases. Some research has shown a relationship between the development of cognitive impairment and lifestyle-related risk factors that are shared with other noncommunicable diseases. These risk factors include physical inactivity, obesity, unhealthy diets, tobacco use, harmful use of alcohol, diabetes, and midlife hypertension. Additional potentially modifiable risk factors include depression, low educational attainment, social isolation, and cognitive inactivity.

Table 14.1 – Dementia variations with age of occurrence

Age	Contributor(s)	Treatment effects
< 40	o Rare without other neurological disease o Genetic disorders can cause true neurodegenerative dementia (NDD): - Alzheimer's disease dementia (ADD) - Spinocerebellar ataxia (SCA) type 17 dominant inheritance - X-linked adenoleukodystrophy (ADL) - Gaucher;s disease (GD) type 3 - Metachromatic leukodystrophy (MCLD) - Niemann-Pick disease (NPD) - Panthotenate kinase-associated neurodegeneration (PKAN) - Tay-Sachs disease (TSD) - Wilson's disease (WD)	o Treatment of underlying psychiatric illness, alcohol, drug abuse, or metabolic disturbance
< 65	o ADD is most frequent. Inherited forms account for higher proportion o Frontotemporal lobar degeneration (FTLD) o Huntington's disease (HD) accounts for the rest o Vascular disease dementia (VDD) in cases of repeated brain traumas o Chronic traumatic encephalopathy (CTE)	
> 65	o ADD o VDD o Dementia with Lewy bodies (DLB) occurring alongside either ADD or/and VDD o Hypothyroidism o Normal pressure hydrocephalus (NPH)	o Fully reversible with treatment o Treatment may prevent progression and improve other symptoms

Source: Fymat A. L., 2017 - 2019

Signs and symptoms

Most dementia types are slow and progressive. Symptoms vary across types and stages and also with the individual. A diagnosis requires a change from a person's usual mental functioning and a greater decline than one would expect due to aging. The signs and symptoms evolve in three consecutive phases (early, middle, and late phase) ending up in near total dependence and inactivity, serious **memory** disturbances, and more obvious physical signs and symptoms.

Behavioral and psychological symptoms of dementia occur almost always in all types of dementia and may manifest as agitation/aggression, anxiety, apathy, appetite changes, behavioral changes, delusions/hallucinations, depression, disinhibition, impulsivity, irritability, mood elations, motor abnormalities, psychosis, and sleep disturbances.

Each form of dementia has its own risk factors, but most forms have several risk factors in common. These are age (the biggest risk factor), family history, and other factors including lifestyle, high blood pressure, smoking, and diabetes. It is not known how treatment for these problems influences the risk of developing dementia. It seems as though people who remain physically active, socially connected, and mentally engaged are less likely to fall prey to dementia (or develop dementia later) than others.To compound things, more than one type of dementia may exist in the same person.

Dementias according to the affected brain areas

Figure 14.2 is a pictorial representation of the affected brain regions:

> - *Cortex:* Thought; perception and language; emotions and behavior. It devolves into three subcategories:
>   - *Cortical*: **Memory** (severe loss), language
>   - *Subcortical*: Ability to start activities, speed of thinking; and
>   - *Corticobasal degeneration. Hippocampus:* **Memory;**
> - *Midbrain* and *substantia nigra:* Movement;
> - *Brainstem:* **S**leep, alertness, and autonomic dysfunction;
> - *Hypothalamus:* Autonomic dysfunction; and

> **Olfactory cortex:** Smell.

Also affected are the:

> **Spinal cord** and **peripheral nervous system**: Autonomic dysfunction.

Let me briefly summarize these dementia types:

Cortical dementia

Cortical dementia (CD) occurs because of problems in the cerebral cortex, the outer layer of the brain. This type of dementia plays an important role in **memory** and *language*. People with cortical dementia usually have severe memory loss and cannot remember words or understand language.

Subcortical dementia

Subcortical dementia occurs because of problems in the part of the brain beneath the cortex. It affects the individual's *ability to start activities* and *speed of thinking.* Forgetfulness and language problems are typically not developed. Examples are Parkinson's disease dementia (PDD), Huntington's disease dementia (HDD), and HIV-associated dementia (HAD).

Corticobasal degeneration

Corticobasal dementia (CBD) is a rare form of dementia characterized by many different types of neurological problems that get progressively worse over time. The affected brain area is the posterior frontal lobe and parietal lobe, although many other brain parts can be affected.

It is a loss of nerve cells (atrophy) in the cerebral cortex and the basal ganglia areas of the brain. A corresponding illustrative brain is shown in Figure 14.2. It shares similar symptoms as Alzheimer's disease dementia (ADD) - **memory** loss, speech difficulty, and trouble swallowing.

Figure 14.2 – Brain areas affected by dementia

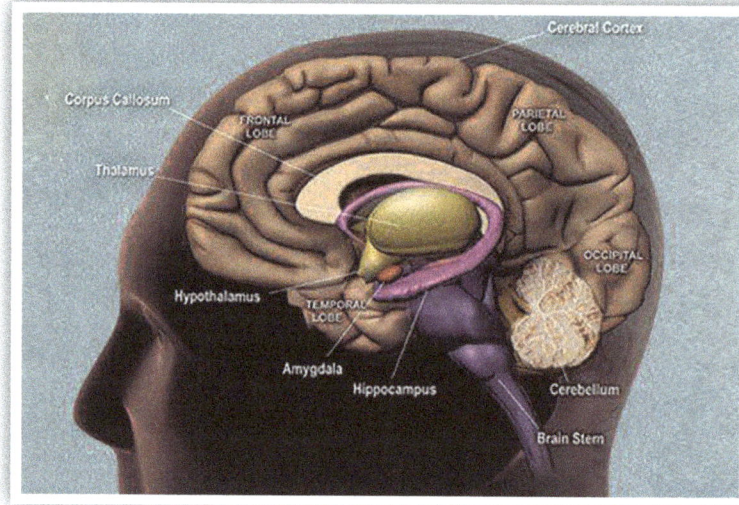

Table 14.2 is a categorization of the several dementia types, including their characteristics, symptoms, and disease examples.

Table 14.2 – Categorization of dementia types

Category	Characteristics	Symptoms	Disease examples
Affected brain area	Cortical (outer cortex)	o **Memory** o Thinking (thought, perception) o Language o Social behavior	o Alzheimer's disease dementia (ADD) o Creutzfeldt-Jacob disease dementia (CJD) o Dementia
	Subcortical (below the cortex)	o **Memory** (speed of thinking) o Emotions o Movement (ability to start activities)	o Parkinson's disease dementia (PDD) o Huntington's disease dementia (HDD) o HIV-associated dementia (HAD)
	Corticobasal	o Many types of neurological problems	o ADD o PDD o Parkinsonism o CJDD
	Hippocampus	o Memory	o ADD
	Midbrain and substantia nigra	o Movement	o PDD

	Brain stem	o Speed o Alertness o Autonomic dysfunction	o PDD
	Hypothalamus	o Autonomic dysfunction	o PDD
	Olfactory cortex	o Smell	o ADD
Progressive, irreversible	Becomes worse over time	o Interference with more and more cognitive abilities	o ADD o Lewy body dementias (LBD) o Vascular disease dementia (VDD) o Multi-infarct dementia (MID) o Frontotemporal disease dementia (FTDD) o Mixed dementia (MD)
Secondary to another disorder	Primary (does not result from any another disease)	o Dementia	o ADD
	o Secondary (peripheral to a pre-existing mental illness or condition, or injury) o The different symptoms depend on the seats of the lesions	o Brain infections o Multiple sclerosis (MS) o Some degree of paralysis, tremor, nystagmus, and speech disturbances. o Heterogeneous deterioration with nuchal dystonia and dementia	o Brain infections o Progressive supranuclear palsy (PSP) o Multiple sclerosis (MS)

Source: Fymat A. L., 2017 - 2019

As seen, Alzheimer's disease dementia occupies a special place as it originates in the cortex, is progressive and irreversible, and is a primary dementia. It also occurs in the corticobasal area, the hippocampus, and the olfactory cortex.

Creutzfeldt-Jakob disease dementia (CJDD) also takes place in the cortex and the corticobasal area whereas Parkinson's disease dementia (PDD) and features of parkinsonism (poor coordination, muscle rigidity, and shaking) occurs in the subcortical area, the corticobasal area, the midbrain and the substantia nigra, the brain stem and the hypothalamus.

Signs are difficulty using only one limb (named "alien limb") over which there seems to be no brain control, asymmetric symptoms including jerky movements of one or more limbs (myoclonus), strange repetitive movements (dystonia), speech difficulty (inability to move mouth muscles in a coordinated way), numbness and tingling of the limbs, and neglect of one side of the vision or senses. In neglect, a person ignores the opposite side of the body from the one that has the problem.

Patients with CBD deteriorate to the point where they can no longer care for themselves, and often die from secondary medical issues such as pneumonia or severe infection (sepsis).

Reversible and progressively irreversible dementias

Reversible dementias (RD)

There are four main causes of easily reversible dementia:

- ***Hypothyroidism;***
- ***Vitamin B12 deficiency;***
- ***Lyme disease (LD);*** *and*
- ***Neurosyphilis.***

All people with memory difficulty should be checked for hypothyroidism and B_{12} deficiency. For Lyme disease (LD) – see later in this Chapter - and neurosyphilis, testing should be done if there are risk factors for those diseases. Because risk factors are often difficult to determine, testing for LD and neurosyphilis, as well as other unmentioned factors, may be undertaken as a matter of course in cases where dementia is suspected.

Progressively irreversible dementias (PID)

Neurodegenerative disorders result in a progressive and irreversible loss of neurons and brain functioning. These PIDs become worse over time and patients eventually lose more of their abilities. Currently, there are no cures for these types of disorders. They include:

> *Alzheimer's disease dementia* (ADD);
> *Vascular disease dementia* (VDD) and *multi-infarct dementia* (MID) or contributions to cognitive impairment and dementia;
> *Lewy body dementias* (LBD) including Dementia with Lewy bodies (DLB); Frontotemporal disorders dementia (FTDD); and
> *Mixed dementia* (MD): A combination of two or more forms of dementia, at least one of which being ADD. In this context, "pure" dementia is ADD alone.

Dementia secondary to another disorder

This category includes both primary and secondary dementias.

Primary dementia (PD)

Primary dementia patients only show symptoms of dementia. ADD is a form of primary dementia, which accounts for 50%-75% of all dementia cases.

Reversible secondary dementia (RSD)

A secondary dementia is a form of dementia that develops as a peripheral condition to a pre-existing mental illness or condition. Brain infections, progressive supranuclear palsy (PSP), and multiple sclerosis (MS), whether disseminated, local or insular, are examples of such conditions. Unlike other types of dementias, many types of secondary dementias can be stopped or reversed,

Encephalopathy

Encephalopathy may develop relatively slowly and resemble dementia. Possible causes include:

- **Brain infection:** Viral encephalitis (VE); sub-acute sclerosing encephalitis (SASE); Whipple's disease (WD); or
- **Brain inflammation:** Limbic encephalitis (LE); Hashimoto's encephalopathy (HE); cerebral vasculitis (CV); tumors (lymphoma, glioma); drug toxicity (e.g., anticonvulsant drugs); metabolic causes (liver failure or kidney failure); and chronic subdural hematoma (CSH).

A preliminary look at the principal and common types of dementia

The principal types of dementia include ADD, VDD and MID; DLB; and frontotemporal dementias (FTDD) consisting of six variants.

For the principal types of dementia, I have charted in Table 14.3 their causes (or marks) and their symptoms:

Table 14.3 – The principal types of dementia

Types	Cause(s) or mark(s)	Symptoms
Alzheimer's disease dementia (ADD) (most common)	o Amyloid-beta plaques o Neurofibrillary-tau tangles o Loss of connections between neurons	o **Memory loss** o Severe **cognitive deficits**
Fronto-temporal disorders dementia (FTDD) (6 types)	o Progressive neuronal loss o Manifests in late adulthood (age 45-65 years) o Equally affecting men and women	o Changes in personal and social behavioral o Apathy o Blunting of emotions o Deficits in both expressive and receptive language) o **Memory problems** o Difficulty speaking

Lewy body dementia (LBD) including **dementia with Lewy bodies (DLB)** (much less common than ADD, comparable to VDD, but second to ADD in importance)	o Abnormal deposits of alpha-synuclein protein in the brain	o Impaired cognition o Delusions o Visual hallucinations o Sleep disorders, rapid eye movements (REM) o Behavioral disturbances
Mixed dementia (MD)	o Combination of 2 or more types of dementia, one of which is usually ADD	o Symptoms corresponding to those of the component dementias
Vascular disease dementia (VDD) (may overlap with ADD)	o Reduced blood flow to the brain	o Multiple small strokes

Source: Fymat A. L., Tellwell Talent Publishers 2017 - 2019

The main contributors to dementia are summarized in Table 14.4. Other minor contributors are also mentioned later in this section.

Table 14.4 – Contributors to dementia

Disease	Contribution	Characteristics & Symptoms
Alzheimer's disease dementia (ADD)	50% - 75%	CAUSES: o Runaway autoimmune disease (Fymat, 2017) SYMPTOMS: o Short-term **memory loss** o Repetitions o Getting lost o Difficulties keeping track of bills o Forgetting to take medications o Difficulties finding words o Trouble with visuo-spatial areas o Troubles with reasoning o Troubles with judgment o Troubles with insight SIGNS: o Death of nerve cells (neurons) in important parts of the brain o Hippocampus o Shrinkage of fronto-temporal parts

Vascular disease dementia (VDD)	20% - 30%	CAUSES: o Strokes o Blood vessels diseases o Hypertension o CVDs (particularly previous heart attacks, angina) o Diabetes SYMPTOMS: o Minor strokes SIGNS: o Lost or damaged ischemic brain areas
Dementia with Lewy bodies (DLB)	10% - 20%	CAUSES: o Abnormal protein structures within brain cells o Treatable with medication(s) SYMPTOMS: o PD (trembling, stiffness, slowness) o Visual hallucinations o Difficulties with visuo-spatial functions o Problems with attention, organization, executive functions o Parkinsonism (tremor, rigid muscles, stiffness, slowness, emotionless face, etc. SIGNS: o Vivid long-lasting hallucinations o "Act-out dreams" o Occipital hypoperfusion o Hypometabolism
Frontotemporal disorders dementia (FTDD)	10% - 15%	SYMPTOMS: o **Memory problems** (not a main feature) o Personality changes o Abnormal social behavior o Language difficulties SIGNS: o Nerve cell loss in frontal and temporal lobes (arise at earlier ages than AD) o Three types: Behavioral, temporal (or semantic), progressive non-fluent aphasia

Mixed dementia (MD)	10%	CAUSE: o More than one (often AD and vascular) SIGNS: o Over 80-years of age
Parkinson's disease dementia (PDD)	Unspecified	CAUSE: o During the corse of PD SYMPTOMS: o Very similar to PD
Progressive supranuclear palsy (PSP)	Unspecified	SYMPTOMS: o Eye movement problems o Movement problems: Balance problems, falling backwards, slow movements, rigid muscles o Behavioral problems: Irritability, apathy, social withdrawal, depression, progressive difficulty eating and swallowing, eventually talking o Misdiagnosed as PD SIGNS: o Atrophied mid-brain
Corticobasal degeneration (CBD)	Unspecified	SYMPTOMS: o Many different types of neurological problems, getting worse over time SIGNS: o Affected temporal lobes o Difficulty using only one limb ("alien" limb) o Numbness and tingling of limbs o Asymmetric symptoms (myoclonus or jerking movements of one pr more limbs) o Strange repetitive movements (dystonia) o Speech difficulties (inability to move mouth muscles in coordinated way) o Neglect one side of vision or senses
Creutzfeldt-Jakob disease (CJD)	Unspecified	CAUSE: o Prions SYMPTOMS: o Slow, at times rapid, progression

Encephalopathy	Unspecified	CAUSES: o Brain infection: Viral or sclerosing encephalitis and Whipple's disease (WD) o Brain inflammation: Limbic encephalitis (LE), Hashimoto's encephalitis (HE), cerebral vasculitis (CV) o Tumors: Lymphoma, glioma o Drug toxicity (anticonvulsants) o Metabolic causes: liver or kidney failure, chronic subdural hematoma (CSH)
Senility dementia (SeD)	Unspecified	
Normal pressure hydrocephalus (NPH)	Unspecified	
Syphilitic dementia (SyD)	Unspecified	
Immunologically-mediated dementia (IMD)	Unspecified	CAUSES: o Chronic inflammatory conditions (CID) o Behcet's disease (BD) o Multiple sclerosis (MS) o Sarcoidosis o Sjogren's syndrome (SJ) o Systemic lupus errhythematosus (SLE) o Celiac disease (CD) o Non-gluten celiac sensitivity SIGNS: o Can rapidly progress o Good response to early treatments (immunomodulators, steroids)

Inherited conditions	Unspecified	CAUSES: o Alexander's disease (AD) o Cerebrotendinous xanthomatosis (CX) o Dentatorubal pallidoluysian atrophy (DPA) o Epilepsy o Fatal familial insomnia (FFI) o Fragile X-associated tremor/ataxia syndrome (FXTAS) o Glutaric aciduria (GA) type 1 o Krabbe's disease (KD) o Maple syrup urine disease (MSUD) o Niemann-Pick disease (NPD) type C o Neuronal ceroid lupofuscinosis (NCL) o Neuroacanthocytosis o Organic acidemias o Pelizaeus-Merzbacher disease (PMD) o San Filippo's syndrome (SFS) type B o Spinocerebellar ataxia (SCA) type 2 o Urea cycle disorders
Other conditions including: o **Pugilistic dementia (PD)** o **Children's dementia (CD)**	Unspecified	CAUSES: o Cumulative damage in the brain (e.g., in chronic alcoholism, repeated head injuries, etc. o Dementia in children

Source: Fymat A. L., 2017 -2019

More details are provided in my books on these subjects (see Figures 7.1, 8.3, and Figures 14.12 through 14.18).

The Alzheimer-diseased brain

While we continue to unravel the complex brain changes involved in the onset and progression of AD, it seems likely that damage to the brain started a decade or more before **memory** and other cognitive problems appeared. During this preclinical stage of AD, people seem to be symptom-free but toxic changes are taking place in the brain. Abnormal deposits of proteins form amyloid plaques and fibrillary (tau) tangles throughout the brain and, once-healthy neurons stop functioning, they lose connections with other neurons and die.

Molecular and cellular changes in AD

Many molecular and cellular changes take place in the brain of a person with AD. These changes can be observed in brain tissue under the microscope after death. The damage initially appears to take place in the hippocampus, that part of the brain that is essential in forming memories. As more neurons die, additional parts of the brain are affected, and they begin to shrink.

By the final stages of AD, damage is widespread and brain tissue has shrunk significantly. Investigations are underway to determine which changes may cause AD and which may be a result of the disease.

Neuroradiological imaging

In Figure 14.3, I contrast a healthy brain (left side) with a severe Alzheimer-diseased one (right side). It is readily seen that the brain structure and convolutions are distorted with extreme shrinkage of the cerebral cortex and the hippocampus, and ventricles are severely enlarged. In fact, the extent of brain shrinkage may be used as a rough gauge for assessing the severity of the disease.

The brain ravages are further accentuated in Figure 14.4 where the shrinkage is highlighted (blue color) from preclinical AD to mild-to-moderate AD to severe AD. The anatomical pictures in Figures 14.3 and 14.4 can be better seen with different radiological imaging apparatuses. Such apparatuses include computerized tomography (CT) or computerized axial tomography (CAT); single photon emission computerized tomography (SPECT); magnetic resonance imaging (MRI) and its variants functional MRI (fMRI), magnetic resonance angiography (MRA) and magnetic resonance spectroscopy (sMRI); and positron emission tomography (PET). Each of these technologies yields different information and some may even be combined.

Figure 14.3 - Contrasting a healthy brain with a severe Alzheimer-diseased brain

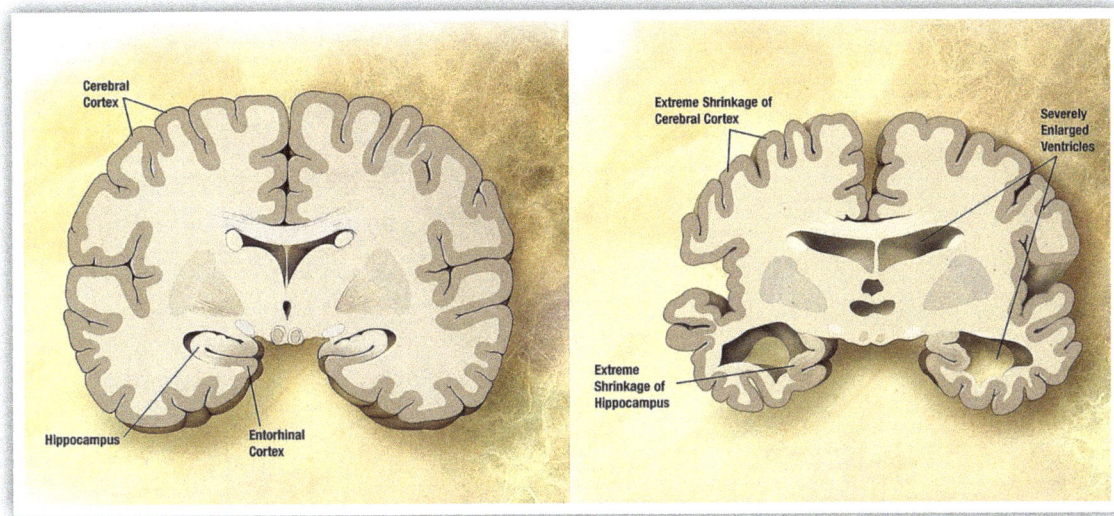

For example, MRI is a radiological imaging technique used to form pictures of the anatomy and the physiological processes of the body in both health and disease. The scanners employed to produce such images use strong magnetic fields, magnetic field gradients, and radio waves to generate the images.The technique does not involve X-rays or ionizing radiation, distinguishing it from CT or CAT.

PET is a nuclear medicine functional imaging technique that is used to observe metabolic processes in the brain (and more generally in the body) to aid in the diagnosis of disease. The system detects pairs of gamma-rays emitted indirectly by a positron -emitting radioligand, most commonly fluorine-18, which is introduced into the body on a biologically active molecule called a radioactive tracer. Metabolic trapping of the radioactive glucose molecule allows the PET scan to be utilized and different ligands may be used for different imaging purposes. Three-dimensional images of tracer concentration within the body region of interest are then constructed by computer analysis.

Figure 14.4 – Brain shrinkage from preclinical AD to mild-to-moderate AD to severe AD

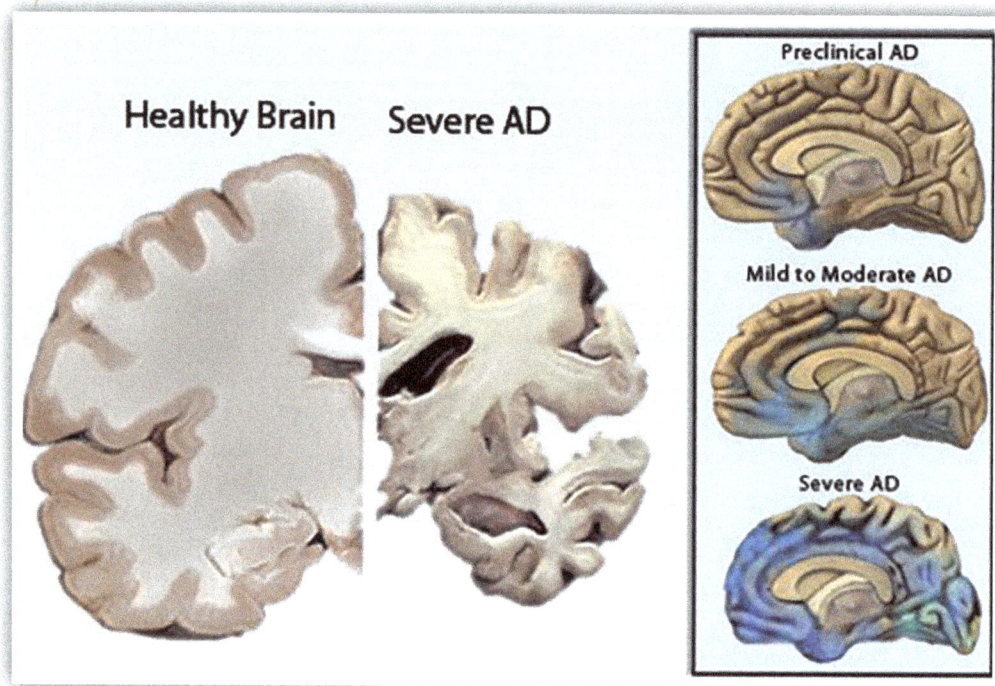

Figure 14.5 is an example of CT images showing cerebral atrophy with different grading systems (observe the decreased size of the gyri and the secondary increased size of the sulci).While the hazards of X-rays are nowadays generally well-controlled in most medical contexts, an MRI scan may still be seen as a better choice than a CT scan. It is widely used in hospitals and clinics for medical diagnosis, staging of disease, and follow-up without exposing the body to radiation. On the other hand, an MRI may yield different information compared with CT and there may be risks and discomforts associated with it. Further, compared with CT, MRI typically takes longer, is louder, and needs the subject to enter a narrow, confining tube. In addition, people with medical or/and dental implants or other non-removable metal inside their body may be unable to undergo an MRI examination safely.

Figure 14.5 – Head CT images of various grades of cerebral atrophy

(MTA=Medial temporal lobe atrophy; PA=Posterior atrophy; fGCA=Frontal cortical atrophy)

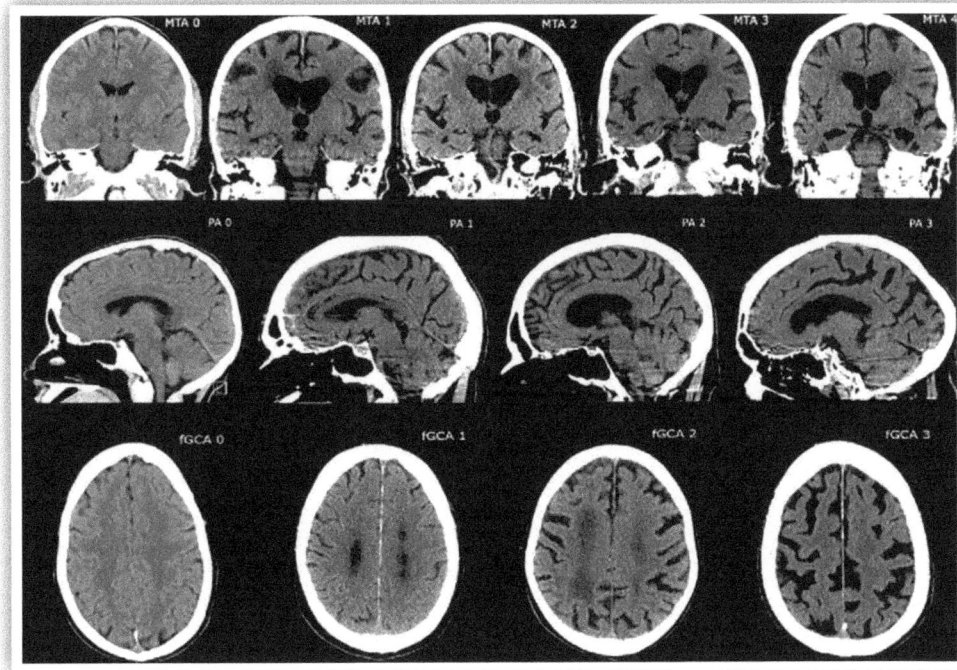

Considering the crucial importance of PET in the imaging of AD, I will provide several illustrations of it. Figure 14.6 is a sample PET brain image of a 56-year old patient (male). If the chosen biologically active tracer molecule is fludeoxyglucose, an analogue of glucose, the concentrations of tracer imaged will indicate tissue metabolic activity as they correspond to the regional glucose uptake. In the Figure, the red areas show more accumulated tracer substance whereas the blue areas are regions where low to no tracer have been accumulated. Use of this tracer to explore the possibility of cancer metastasis (i.e., spreading to other sites) is the most common type of PET scan in standard medical care (representing ~ 90% of current scans). The same tracer may also be used for PET investigation and diagnosis of types of dementia. Less often, other radioactive tracers, usually but not always labeled with fluorine-18, are used to image the tissue concentration of other types of molecules of interest.

Figure 14.7 illustrates AD effects in several brain areas (observe the several colored areas) and Figure 14.9 is the PET image of a diseased person's brain.

Figure 14.6 – A sample brain PET image

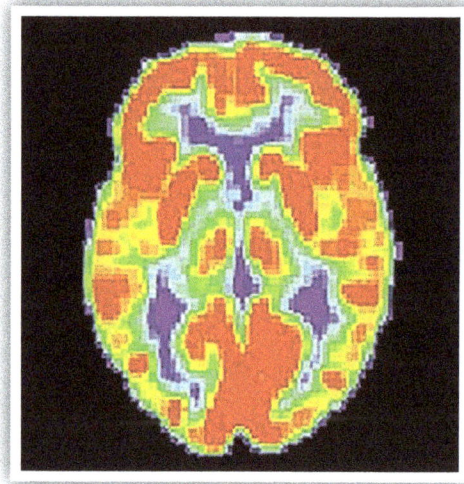

Figure 14.7 - PET images illustrating AD effects in several brain areas

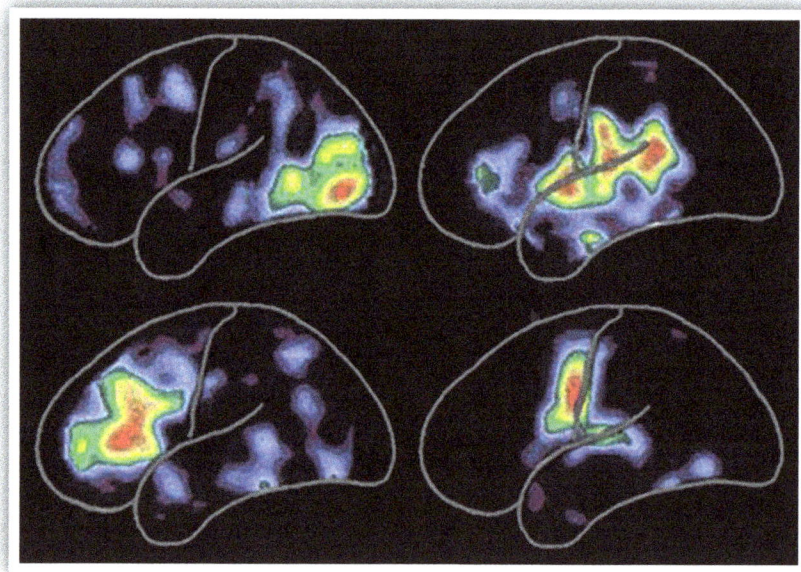

One of the disadvantages of PET scanners is their operating cost. SPECT, which is a similar imaging process to PET, also uses <u>radioligands</u> to detect molecules in the brain. I will not discuss or illustrate here SPECT or its use for imaging neurodegenerative diseases, including AD. Likewise, however useful they are, I will not consider fMRI, MRA and MRS that complement MRI and may respectively be employed to investigate brain physiology, blood circulation within the brain, and its metabolites. Figure 14.8 further contrasts a normal brain (left) to a brain with mild cognitive impairment (center) and an Alzheimer-diseased brain (right). Figure 14.9 further contrasts PET images of a normal brain (left) to a brain with mild cognitive impairment (center) and an Alzheimer-diseased brain (right)

Figure 14.8 – PET image of a diseased person's brain

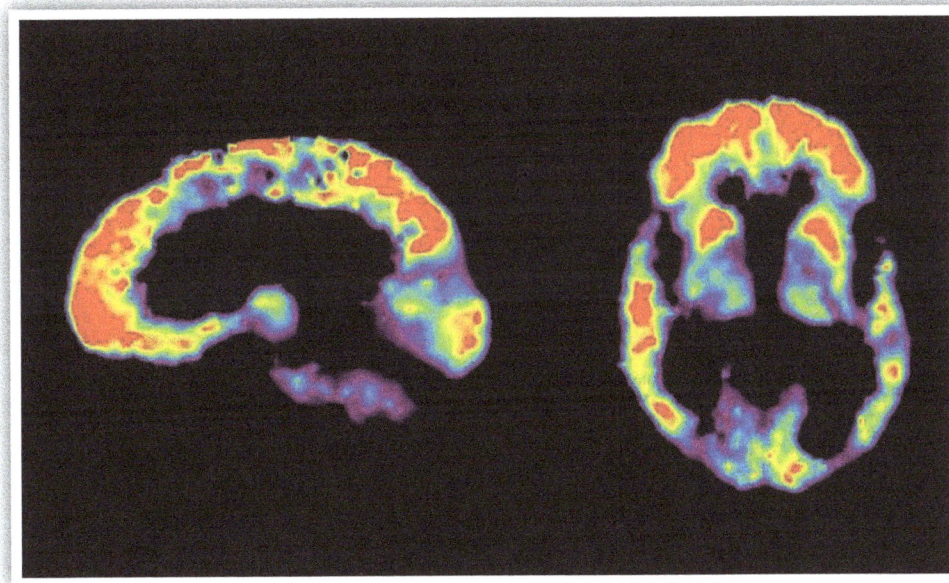

In this context, a few words of praise should be formulated regarding the United Kingdom Biobank. The biobank holds genetic, physical, and clinical data from a large cohort of individuals (by 2010, ~ 500,000 individuals age 40-69 at recruitment, and scheduled to increase to 5 million). Following this age group has enabled a focus on diseases of middle age and later including genetic influences on NDDs such as AD. In 2018, it reported a study of brain images of 10,000 individuals, which revealed genetic influences on brain structure and function, and showed correlations with neurodegenerative, psychiatric and personality traits. This trove of data is available free of charge to scientific researchers for the pursuit of a variety of research projects aimed at better understanding AD and other NDDs, and hopefully developing diagnostic and therapeutic procedures for such diseases. From such data, the cohort of axial brain MRI images of Figure 14.10 images was obtained.

At the Jülich Institute of Neurosciences and Biophysics in Germany, the world's largest and most powerful PET-MRI device began operation in April 2009. Presently, only the head and brain can be imaged at the high magnetic field strengths employed. For brain imaging, because of the absence of motions, registration of CT, MRI and PET scans may be accomplished without the need for an integrated PET-CT or PET-MRI scanner by using a device known as the N-localizer. Figure 14.11 shows fused PET/CT and PET/MRI technologies for brain imaging

Figure 14.9 - PET images contrasting a normal brain (left) to a brain with mild cognitive impairment (center) and an Alzheimer-diseased brain (right)

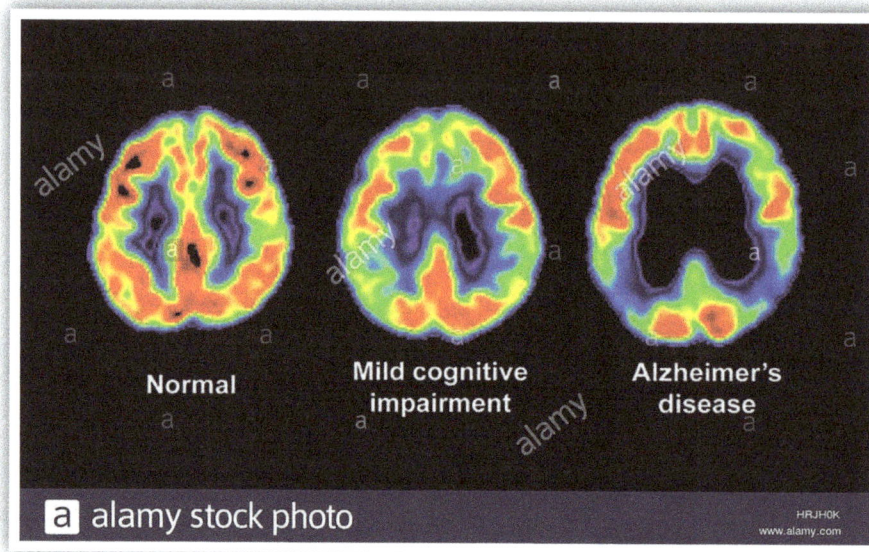

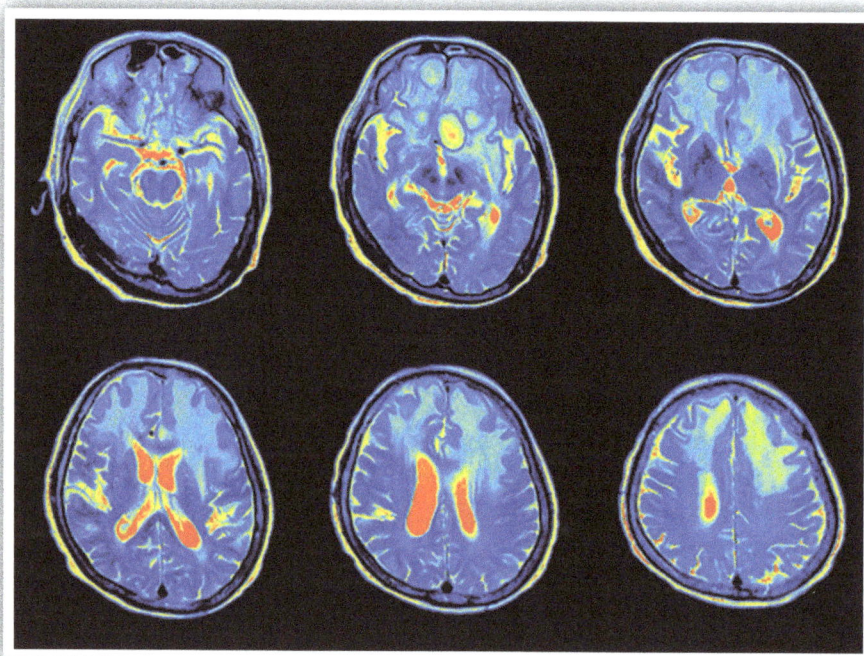

Figure 14.10 - A cohort of axial brain MRI images

Source: UK Biobank

With all these advanced technologies, whether singly or in combination, it is possible to accurately diagnose AD and monitor its ineluctable progression. When treatments and (hopefully) even a cure will be available, the same technologies will also enable us to follow their efficacy and personalize them to the patient

Figure 14.11 – Fused PET/CT and PET/ MRI technologies for brain imaging

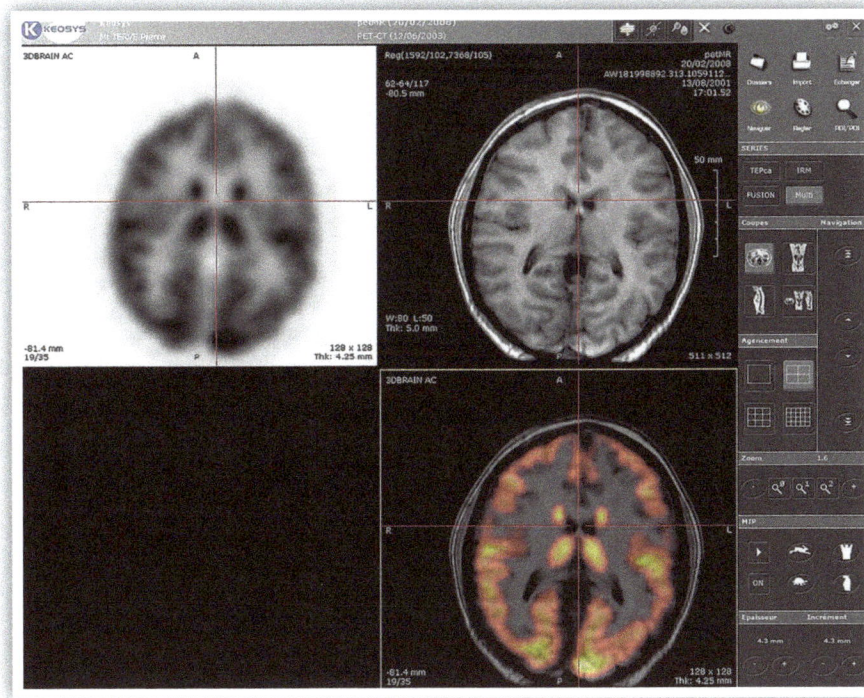

References are also made to my other books on Parkinson's disease (Figure 14.12), multiple sclerosis (Figure 14.13), multiple system atrophy (Figure 14.14), and epilepsy (Figure 14.15):

Figure 14.12 – Parkinson's disease: Elucidating the disease and what you can do about it

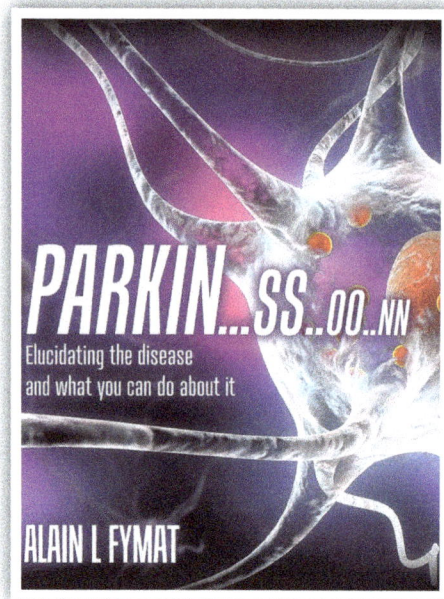

Source: Fymat A.L., Tellwell Talent Publishers, 2020

Figure 14.13 – Multiple sclerosis: The progressive demyelinating autoimmune disease

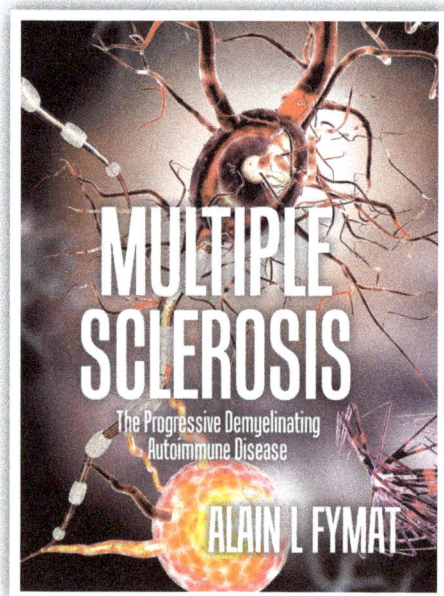

Source: Fymat A.L., Tellwell Talent Publishers, 2023

Figure 14.14 – Multiple system atrophy: The chronic, progressive, neurodegenerative, synucleopathic disease

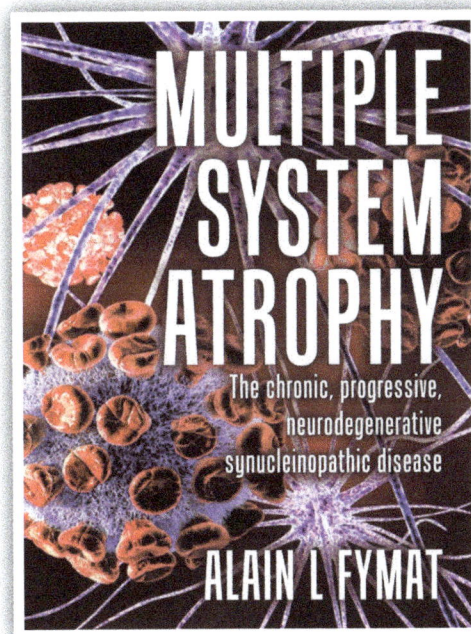

Source: Fymat A.L., Tellwell Talent Publishers, 2023

Figure 14.15 – Epilepsy: The electrical storm in the brain

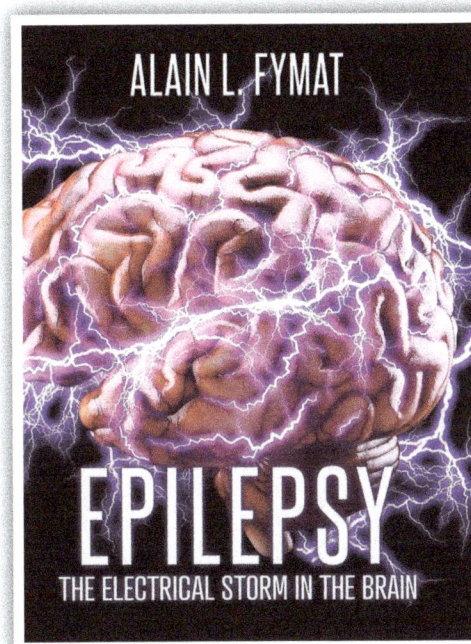

Source: Fymat A.L., Tellwell Talent Publishers, 2022

Component and related conditions

Symptoms are very similar in all types of dementia and, thus, cannot by themselves help in reaching the correct diagnosis of demential type(s). At present, the main contributors to dementia are Alzheimer's disease dementia (ADD; 50-75% of cases), vascular disease dementia (VDD; 25%), Lewy body dementias (LBD; 15%), others of unspecified contribution including Parkinson's disease dementia (PDD), frontotemporal disorders dementia (FTDD), and still others: mixed, senilitic, syphilitic, progressive supranuclear palsy (PSNP), corticobasal degeneration (CBD), encephalopathy, and Creutzfeldt-Jakob disease dementia (CJDD). (se Table 14.3.) Immunologically mediated, chronic inflammatory conditions include Behcet's disease (BD), multiple sclerosis (MS), sarcoidosis, Sjogren's syndrome (SS), systemic lupus errhythematosus (SLE), and celiac and non-celiac diseases. There are still many other medical and neurological conditions in which dementia only occurs late in the illness.

Inherited conditions include various pathologies:

> **Diseases:** Alexander's (AD), Krabbe's (KD), Niemann-Pick (NPD) type C, maple syrup urine (MSUD), and Pelizaeus-Merzbacher (PMD), epilepsy.
> **Syndromes:** Fragile X -associated tremor/ataxia, San Filippo's syndrome (SDS) type B.
> **Other disorders:** Cerebrotendinous xanthomatosis (CX), dentatorubal pallidoluysian atrophy DPA), fatal familial insomnia (FFI), glutaric aciduria (GA) type 1, neuronal ceroid lipofuscinosis (NCL), neuroacanthocytosis, organic acidemias, spinocerebellar ataxia (SCA) type 2, and urea cycle).

There are, nonetheless, some reversible conditions such as hypothyroidism, Vitamin B_{12} deficiency, Lyme disease, and neurosyphilis. Except for the treatable types of dementia listed above, and in the absence of a thorough understanding of the deep biology of this disease, there is currently no cure. Medical interventions remain heretofore palliative in nature with aim to alleviate pain and suffering.

The Lyme-diseased brain

What is Lyme disease (LD)?

Also known as Lyme *borreliosis*, LD is a tick-borne zoonotic disease that affects humans and animals. It is a bacterial, vector-borne infection due to *borrelia* (a helicoid spirochete) that is transmitted by bites from the *Ixodes* tick. *Borrelia* includes a dozen of species (36 as of the end of 2018, but others may still be discovered) that were named in their entirety after the French bacteriologist Amedee Borrel (1867-1936). Whereas *borrelia burgdorferi* is the best known of them for being primarily responsible for LD in the U.S., dozens of other *borrelias* had been identified in Europe and registered (under different names) since the beginning of the 20th century or long before the discovery of *borrelia burgdorferi* in the mid-1970s. The ticks are found in temperate forested regions of North America, Europe, and Asia, generally at elevations less than 1300 meters. (Figures 14.16 and 17.)

LD was identified in the U.S. in 1975 after a mysterious outbreak of what appeared to be juvenile rheumatoid arthritis (also called juvenile idiopathic arthritis) in children who lived in Lyme and Old Lyme, Connecticut. However, there is no relationship between juvenile rheumatoid arthritis and LD for which it was originally (mis)named. Until then, Rocky Mountain spotted fever had been the main concern.

Figure 14.16 – Pictorial illustrating the signs and symptoms of Lyme disease

LYME DISEASE

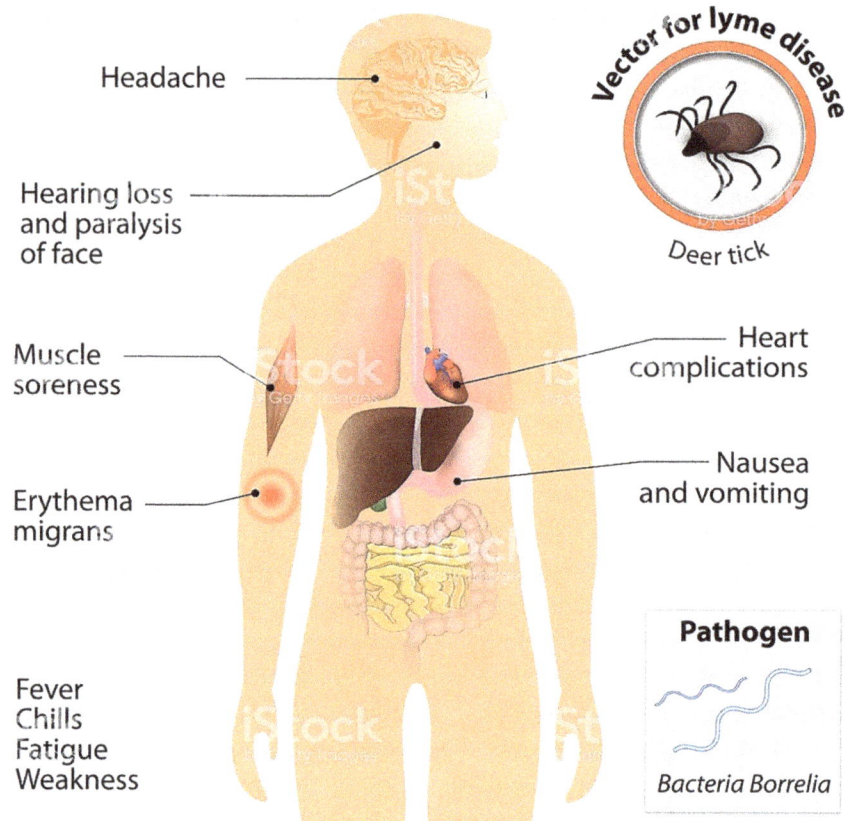

Headache

Hearing loss and paralysis of face

Muscle soreness

Erythema migrans

Fever
Chills
Fatigue
Weakness

Vector for lyme disease

Deer tick

Heart complications

Nausea and vomiting

Pathogen

Bacteria Borrelia

LD is a complex disease, which is often difficult to diagnose and treat effectively. Like other zoonoses, it is transmitted by a vector that picks up the pathogen during a blood meal from a vertebrate host. In the eastern and central U.S., the spirochete bacterium *borrelia burgdorferi* infects black-legged ticks, *Ixodes scapularis*, which feed on a wide variety of birds, lizards, and mammals including mice, deers, and humans. Since human risk is a function of the prevalence of infection among vectors, outbreak prevention depends in part on understanding what controls infection rates among the agents of transmission. Typical symptoms, which may appear in whole or in part, include fever, headache, fatigue, and a characteristic skin rash called *erythema migrans*. Symptoms may vary depending on the specific type of *borrelia.* In North America, the principal species is *borrelia burgdorferi sensu stricto*, which is particularly likely to also cause arthritis. In contrast, the European species *borrelia garinii* and *borrelia afzelii* are more often associated with **neurological** and chronic dermatologic manifestations, respectively. If left untreated, infection can spread to the joints, the heart, and the nervous system. Fortunately, most cases of Lyme disease can be treated successfully with a few weeks of antibiotics.

Figure 14.17 - *Borrelia* bacteria, the principal causative agents of Lyme disease

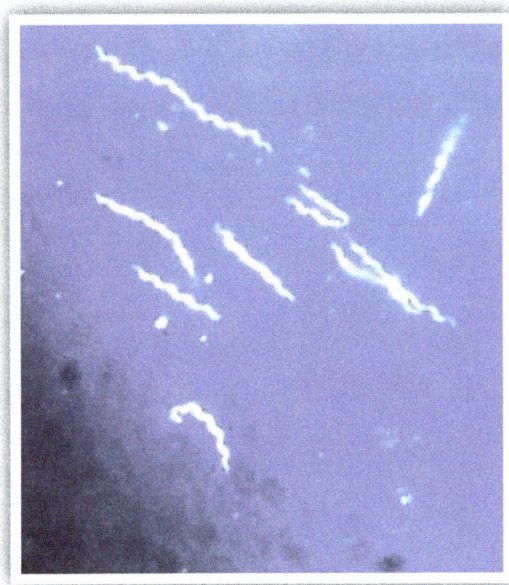

Source: Scott Bauer, U.S. Department of Agriculture, Agriculture Research Service

Of particular interest to us here are the neurological manifestations of Lyme and their effects on **memory.**

What is Lyme *neuroborrelliosis* (LNB)?

LNB is a disorder of the central nervous system (CNS). It is caused by a systemic infection of spirochetes of the genus *Borrelia.*It is often preceded by the typical symptoms of LD, which include the *erythema migrans* (EM) rash and flu-like symptoms such as fatigue, fever, headache, and muscle and joint pains. Its neurologic symptoms include meningo-radiculitis (more common in European patients), cranial nerve abnormalities, and **altered mental status**. **Sensory findings** may also be present. Rarely, a progressive form of encephalomyelitis may occur. In children, symptoms of *neuroborreliosis* include headache, sleep disturbance, and symptoms associated with increased intracranial pressure (such as papilledema) can occur. Less common childhood symptoms can include meningitis, myelitis ataxia, and chorea. Ocular LD has also been reported, as has *neuroborreliosis* affecting the spinal cord, but neither of these findings are common.

A number of diseases can produce symptoms similar to those of LNB, including: Alzheimer's disease (AD); acute disseminated encephalomyelitis (ADE); viral meningitis (VM); multiple sclerosis (MS); Bell's palsy (BP); and amyotrophic lateral sclerosis (ALS) (aka Lou Gehring disease).

Diagnosis is determined by clinical examination of visible symptoms. *Neuroborreliosis* can also be diagnosed serologically to confirm clinical examination via various assays (western blot, ELISA, and PCR).

What is brain fog and what can be done about it?

Brain fog is a lay term to describe fluctuating **mild memory loss** that is inappropriate for a person's age. It may include forgetfulness, spaciness, confusion, decreased ability to pay attention, inability to focus, and difficulty in processing information. This is more than the gradual cognitive decline taking place from early adulthood is a fact of life.

Brain fog can also occur in Sjögren's syndrome (SS). Recent scientific data show that longevity is associated with the successful management of chronic diseases, such as SS, not the absence of any disease! A major cause of cognitive dysfunction can be side effects of drugs and drug interactions, especially in patients over 65-70 years of age; but other factors that might be causing these symptoms should also be considered.

Managing one's lifestyle to optimize one's health and sense of well-being and developing a close working relationship with one's doctor(s) are recommended actions against brain fog. These include: Always reporting changes in **cognition/memory** and mood (depression, anxiety); training and boosting one's brain power. Considerably more details can be found in my book on this subject (Figure 14.18).

Trauma and memory

Memory extends the reach of traumatic experiences. Shocks they cause to the system such as acts of violence or abuse or a life-threatening accident allow them, in many cases, to continue to disrupt the lives of those who had them long after they occur. Post-traumatic stress disorder (PTSD) is marked, in part, by upsetting and uncontrolled memories, which trauma-focused therapies are used to help defuse.

How does trauma affect memory?

After someone suffers a traumatic experience, common reactions include mentally replaying the memory of the experience. Recurring, involuntary, and intrusive distressing memories are one symptom of PTSD. Sometimes, when the memory of a trauma is cued by an experience in the present, the individual may feel as though the traumatic experience is happening again—a reaction commonly called a 'flashback'.

Figure 14.18 – Lyme disease: The dreadful invader, evader, and imitator

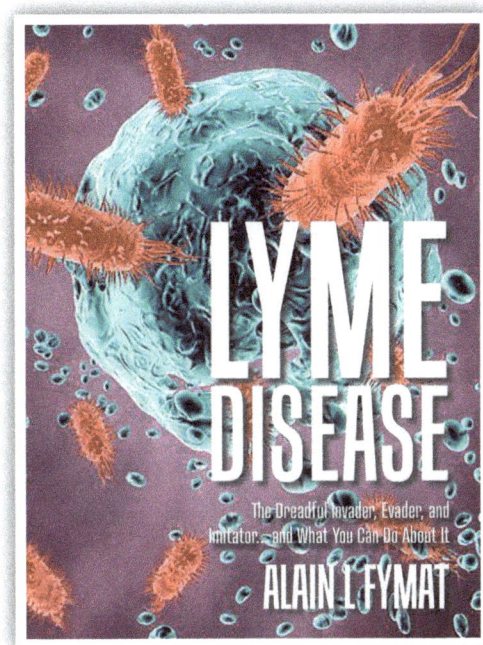

Reference: Fymat A. L., Tellwell Talent Publishers, 2020

Given that these forms of re-experiencing can be highly distressing, it is also common for someone who has lived through trauma to try to avoid thinking about the experience and to avoid cues that may trigger the memory of the experience.

What triggers traumatic memories?

A variety of things can remind someone of a traumatic experience and potentially cause distress or other forms of re-experiencing. These cues may include: Places, people, or other things related to the traumatic event(s) (such as a location close to where the event occurred, a person who looks like the one who caused the trauma, or a situation that resembles, in some way, that in which the traumatic experience occurred). They may also include internal physiological states associated with the experience.

Take-aways

> With increasing lifespan in the developed world, dementia has emerged as an increasing public health concern. But dementia is not an emerging disease! However, it is only in the 1960s that the link between age-related cognitive decline and neurodegenerative diseases was established.

> To this day, the causal etiology of many types of dementia, including Alzheimer's disease (AD), still remains unclear. While many theories (rather hypotheses) have been advanced, these are largely based on risk factors, associations or correlations. They are not the cause of many types of dementia, including the most prevalent AD, which remains remains unclear. In 2017, I had posited that the *root cause* (not a risk factor) of Alzheimer's and other neurodegenerative diseases is but an autoimmune disease having gone rogue, a theory that has garnered support among various research groups and has not been challenged so far.

> Dementia is a general term for the process of decline in mental abilities. It is a broad category of brain diseases that cause a long-term and often gradual decrease in the ability to think and remember that is great enough to affect a person's daily functioning. Other

common symptoms include emotional problems, language difficulties, and decreased motivation.

> Although age is the strongest known risk factor for dementia, dementia is not an inevitable consequence of aging. Further, dementia does not exclusively affect older people. Some research has shown a relationship between the development of **cognitive impairment** and lifestyle-related risk factors that are shared with other noncommunicable diseases. These risk factors include physical inactivity, obesity, unhealthy diets, tobacco use, harmful use of alcohol, diabetes, and midlife hypertension. Additional potentially modifiable risk factors include depression, low educational attainment, social isolation, and cognitive inactivity.

> Many different diseases can cause dementia, including AD, vascular disease (VD), Lewy bodies (LB), frontotemporal disorders (FTD), syphilis, senility, and even stroke. Mixed dementia (MD) is the concurrence of two or more types of dementia. However, not being a specific disease, the above potential contributors do not reach to the primary cause of the disease. There lies our greatest shortcoming:

> While we continue to unravel the complex brain changes involved in the onset and progression of AD, it seems likely that damage to the brain started a decade or more before **memory** and other cognitive problems appeared.

> Many molecular and cellular changes take place in the brain of a person with AD. They take place in the hippocampus. As more neurons die, additional parts of the brain are affected, and they begin to shrink. By the final stage of AD, damage is widespread and brain tissue has shrunk significantly.

> In AD, the brain structure and convolutions are distorted with extreme shrinkage of the cerebral cortex and the hippocampus, and ventricles are severely enlarged. In fact, the extent of brain shrinkage may be used as a rough gauge for assessing the severity of the disease.

> Anatomical pictures of the affected brain can be better seen with different neuroradiological imaging apparatuses.

> Also known as Lyme *borreliosis*, Lyme disease (LD) is a tick-borne zoonotic disease that affects humans and animals. It is a bacterial,

vector-borne infection due to *borrelia* (a helicoid spirochete) that is transmitted by bites from the *Ixodes* tick.

➤ LD is a complex disease, which is often difficult to diagnose and treat effectively. Like other zoonoses, it is transmitted by a vector that picks up the pathogen during a blood meal from a vertebrate host. Of particular interest here are its neurological manifestations and their effects on **memory.**

➤ Lyme neuroborreliosis (LNB) is a disorder of the central nervous system caused by a systemic infection of spirochetes of the genus *Borrelia.* Neurologic symptoms include meningo-radiculitis (more common in European patients), cranial nerve abnormalities, and **altered mental status**. **Sensory findings** may also be present. Rarely, a progressive form of encephalomyelitis may occur.

➤ A number of diseases can produce symptoms similar to those of LNB, including: AD, acute disseminated encephalomyelitis (ADE); viral meningitis (VM); multiple sclerosis (MS); Bell's palsy (BP); and amyotrophic lateral sclerosis (ALS) (aka Lou Gehring disease).

➤ Brain fog describes the fluctuating **mild memory loss** that is inappropriate for a person's age. It may include forgetfulness, spaciness, confusion, decreased ability to pay attention, inability to focus, and difficulty in processing information. This is more than the gradual cognitive decline taking place from early adulthood that is a fact of life.

➤ Managing one's lifestyle to optimize one's health and sense of well-being and developing a close working relationship with one's doctor(s) are recommended actions against brain fog. These include: Always reporting changes in **cognition/memory** and mood (depression, anxiety); training and boosting one's brain power.

➤ Memory extends the reach of traumatic experiences. Shocks they cause to the system may continue to disrupt the lives of those who had them long after they occur. Post-traumatic stress disorder (PTSD) is marked, in part, by upsetting and uncontrolled memories, which trauma-focused therapies are used to help defuse.

➤ After suffering a traumatic experience, common reactions include mentally replaying the **memory** of the experience. When the memory of a trauma is cued by an experience in the present, one may feel as though the traumatic experience is happening again (a 'flashback').

➤ A variety of things can remind someone of a traumatic experience and potentially cause distress or other forms of re-experiencing including internal physiological states associated with the experience.

➤ Also known as Lyme *borreliosis*, Lyme disease is a tick-borne zoonotic disease that affects humans and animals. It is a bacterial, vector-borne infection due to *borrelia* (a helicoid spirochete) that is transmitted by bites from the *Ixodes* tick.

➤ Lyme is a complex disease, which is often difficult to diagnose and treat effectively. Typical symptoms, which may appear in whole or in part, include fever, headache, fatigue, and a characteristic skin rash called erythema migrans. Symptoms may vary depending on the specific type of borrelia. The European species *borrelia garinii* and *borrelia afzelii* are more often associated with **neurological** and chronic dermatologic manifestations, respectively.

➤ The neurological manifestations of Lyme affect **memory.** Lyme neuroberriliosis is a disorder of the central nervous system caused by a systemic infection of spirochetes of the genus *Borrelia.* Neurologic symptoms include meningo-radiculitis, cranial nerve abnormalities, and altered mental status. Sensory findings may also be present.

➤ A number of diseases can produce symptoms similar to those of Lyme neuroberriliosis including: Alzheimer's disease; acute disseminated encephalomyelitis; viral meningitis; multiple sclerosis; Bell's palsy; and amyotrophic lateral sclerosis.

➤ Brain fog is a lay term to describe fluctuating **mild memory loss** that is inappropriate for a person's age. It may include forgetfulness, spaciness, confusion, decreased ability to pay attention, inability to focus, and difficulty in processing information. This is more than the gradual cognitive decline taking place from early adulthood is a fact of life. It an also occur in Sjögren's syndrome.

➤ Memory extends the reach of traumatic experiences. Post-traumatic stress disorder is marked, in part, by upsetting and uncontrolled memories, which trauma-focused therapies are used to help defuse.

➤ After someone suffers a traumatic experience, common reactions include mentally replaying the memory of the experience.

PART F
MEMORY TREATMENT
PORTFOLIO

15

Memory degradation: Prediction and prevention

Contents

15

Memory degradation – Prediction and prevention

"The best time to plant a tree was 20 years ago. The second best time is today"
(Chinese proverb)

Forgetfulness is common and happens to most people, including memory champions. Distraction, fatigue, depression, anxiety, absent-mindedness, and many other factors may contribute to it. Fortunately, most episodes of forgetfulness are simply temporary and not a harbinger of Alzheimer's disease (AD) or other memory disorder. Such episodes are frequently linked to situational factors and normal age-related changes. For most people, mental flexibility starts to become a bit less efficient with each passing decade from the late 20s onward, and memory starts to decline in the late 30s, so it is common to notice more memory problems with age.

Memory problems have reached historically high concerns

However, because memory impacts nearly every aspect of daily life, and because the rate of AD and other memory disorders also increases with age, it becomes important to distinguish between normal age-related memory changes and signs of a memory disorder. In the U.S. and other Western countries, this focus has surged in recent years as their population of older adults has reached historically high levels. Examples abound in the U.S.:

- **2011 survey by the Metropolitan Life Insurance:** It showed that America's 76 million baby boomers feared AD only second to cancer.
- **2015 U.S. Aging survey:** It found that 35% of people over age 60 (about 23 million people) were concerned about **memory loss.**
- **2017 West Health Institute survey:** It found that memory loss was the top concern of adults over age 60.
- The Alzheimer's Association (AA) refers to AD as "the defining disease of the baby boomers," and estimates that 10 million baby boomers will eventually have AD (representing a significant increase from the 5.4 million Americans who currently have the disease).

Prediction of memory degradation

How do we begin to tell apart the signs of normal versus abnormal memory changes when memory itself can be impacted by dozens of different variables? While numerous signs have been identified, the following may signal a potential memory problem:

- ➤ **Current memory is notably weaker than previous levels:** This is evidenced by increasing forgetfulness for well-known, frequently used information. Such forgetting goes well beyond related "brain blips".
- ➤ **Increasing forgetfulness for recent events:** For example, conversations, activities, and appointments.
  - ○ **New difficulty managing daily tasks due to memory problems:** For example, forgetting whether medications have been taken or having paid the bills.

The above is especially the case if it does not appear to be explained by a known medical, emotional, or situational issue. For example, some people experience temporary memory problems due to stress, lack of sleep, medication side effects, thyroid issues, or other medical problems, and memory bounces back after the underlying issue is corrected.

Note that forgetting childhood memories and other "remote" information from many years ago is not a common early sign of a memory problem (though it may occur in the later stages of a memory disorder), and waiting for this type of memory problem can result in a delay in seeking help.

- ○ **Others have noticed that memory is worsening:** It is not uncommon for someone with a memory problem to not be fully aware of it, because they may not remember their own forgetfulness. Often, those with whom we spend the most time are the first to notice a memory problem, and can comment on whether it has worsened over time.

Notice that the signs above have a few commonalities. Forgetfulness may be a potential problem if it:

- ➢ **Reflects a notable decline from previous levels.**
- ➢ **Does not improve when potential contributing factors are addressed** (and often worsens over time).
- ➢ **Involves forgetfulness for well-known information.**
- ➢ **Impairs performance of well-known tasks.**
- ➢ **Is noticeable to others.**

Some helpful steps to take

Because memory can be impacted by dozens of factors, the warning signs noted above do not definitely indicate a memory disorder is present, Rather, they suggest that helpful steps may be taken, such as:

- ➢ **Discussing memory concerns with a health-care provider:** This may lead to a "work-up" to investigate possible contributing factors, which may include:
  - ○ Laboratory tests to measure thyroid, vitamin, and other metabolic levels;
  - ○ Analysis of possible medication side effects;

- Brief memory screening (which provides a basic measure of thinking skills, though usually not enough detail to make a diagnosis or detect subtle memory problems);
- A neuropsychological evaluation which statistically analyzes memory, attention, visual functioning, reasoning, strategy formation, and other skills (i.e., the "software" of the brain) to determine if memory problems are present and how best to treat them; and
- Possible neuroimaging (e.g., head CT or brain MRI) to evaluate the "hardware" of the brain.

➤ **Cardiovascular exercising:** Multiple studies have shown that the most powerful treatment for mild memory problems is cardiovascular exercise, which can slow the rate of memory loss and even improve memory. Exercise also increases the density of brain tissue in the hippocampus (a core memory processing area) and the frontal lobes. Exercise can also slow the rate of memory loss for those who already have moderate AD.

Given that AD-related brain changes can start 10-30 years prior to diagnosis (in the *late-onset* variant, where symptoms begin after age 65), and given that there is no treatment to stop the progression of AD, it is most advantageous to exercise proactively. However, it is never too late to begin exercising.

➤ **Increasing neuronal density:** Increasing the number and density of neuronal pathways in the brain by building "cognitive reserve" has been shown to help the brain compensate for AD-related changes, and may even prohibit AD symptoms from being expressed!

Whether or not forgetfulness is a "brain blip" or a sign of a potential memory problem, it is never too late to start building better brain health.

Extraordinary memory abilities

The vast potential of the human brain becomes especially clear in the domain of memory. The most captivating instances of superior memory ability may be few and far between—e.g., the savant who memorizes a library's worth of books, the otherwise regular person who cannot help but remember what she did 10 years ago today, etc. But such cases show that, at its outer reaches, memory capacity can be far more immense than it is for most of us on even our most lucid day.

Hyperthymesia, savants, and photographic memory

> **Hyperthymesia:** A condition that leads people to be able to remember an abnormally large number of their life experiences in vivid detail. Some awe-inspiring individuals develop highly unusual abilities to remember particular kinds of information—personal experiences, historical facts, musical compositions, or others. These powers of memory can arise in the absence of extensive training, and the cause is often unclear. They can also appear in people who are otherwise intellectually ordinary or who show deficits in other areas of cognitive functioning.

> **Highly superior autobiographical memory (HSAM):** This is another name for hyperthymesia – the ability to remember far more about one's own life than is typical, including details of personal experiences and when they occurred. Someone with HSAM would likely be able to recount what h/she personally did, what the weather was like, or what the top news was on a randomly chosen date many years ago. H/she may also be able to recall the exact dates on which various events occurred. However, people with HSAM do not show such unusual memory for all kinds of information, their autobiographical memory is not perfect, and they may not stand out on other cognitive characteristics.

HSAM is thought to be very rare. As of the mid-2010s, according to an expert report, fewer than 100 people with HSAM ability had been found.

> **Memory champion:** Someone who can accomplish impressive feats of memory not because of a radical difference in cognitive functioning relative to other people, but through training and the use of techniques for enhancing memory. The examples of these memory champions suggest that even relatively ordinary minds can take memory to extraordinary levels. Some of the feats performed by memory

champions include memorizing long strings of digits, series of random words, sequences of cards in decks, and names and faces. Memory champions regularly set new world records: In 2019, for example, a contender memorized a sequence of 335 random words in 15 minutes. Another memorized 1,168 digits in the same amount of time.

➢ **Memory athlete:** Someone who participates in memory competitions, which can involve a variety of tests of memory ability. Competitors train their ability to recall information with the aid of mental techniques called mnemonics. Memory sport includes international competitions (the World Memory Championships launched in 1991) as well as national and lower-level contests.

Take-aways

➢ Forgetfulness is common and happens to most people, including memory champions. Distraction, fatigue, depression, anxiety, absent-mindedness, and many other factors may contribute to it.

➢ Most episodes of forgetfulness are simply temporary and not a harbinger of AD or other memory disorder. Such episodes are frequently linked to situational factors and normal age-related changes.

➢ Because memory impacts nearly every aspect of daily life, and because the rate of AD and other memory disorders also increases with age, it becomes important to distinguish between normal age-related memory changes and signs of a memory disorder. To do so, helpful steps may be taken, such as: Discussing memory concerns with a health-care provider; cardiovascular exercising: and increasing the number and density of neuronal pathways in the brain by building "cognitive reserve".

➢ The vast potential of the human brain becomes especially clear in the domain of memory. The most captivating instances of superior memory ability may be few and far between.

➢ Hyperthymesia is a condition that leads people to be able to remember an abnormally large number of their life experiences in vivid detail. These powers of memory can arise in the absence of extensive training, their cause is often unclear, and they can appear in people who are otherwise intellectually ordinary or who show deficits in other areas of cognitive functioning.

➢ Highly superior autobiographical memory is the ability to remember far more about one's own life than is typical, including details of personal experiences and when they occurred. A memory champion can accomplish impressive feats of memory not because of a radical difference in cognitive functioning relative to other people, but through training and the use of techniques for enhancing memory. A memory athlete is someone who participates in memory competitions, which can involve a variety of tests of memory ability.

➢ Whether or not forgetfulness is a "brain blip" or a sign of a potential memory problem, it is never too late to start building better brain health.

16

Treatment portfolio:
I. Nutrition and supplementation

16

Treatment portfolio: I. Nutrition and supplementation

Nutrition in general

The following properties and health benefits of various food types are standard in the dietary and nutrition literature (Table 1). More will be said in the following sections regarding nutrition for brain health:

Table 16.1 – General properties and health benefits of various food types

Food type	Examples	Properties	Health benefits
Avocados	Avocado	Antioxidants	o **Memory** improvement o Cholesterol lowering o Arthritis prevention o Skin protection

Blueberries	Blueberries	o **A**nthocyanins (**p**olyphenols) o Anti-inflammatory	o Brain protection o Inflammation reduction o Strengthens **short-term memory** o DNA damage lessening o Cell communication improvement <u>Dietary aim</u>: Fresh berries: Better
Cruciferous vegetables	o Broccoli o Brussel sprouts o Cauliflower	Sulforaphane	o Immune booster o Cancer risk lowering
Dairy products	o Cheese o Milk o Yogurt <u>Alternatives:</u> o Orange juice (fortified) o Rice o Soy drinks o Tofu	Calcium	o Bone health o Osteoporosis risk lowering o Cancer (colon) risk lowering o High-blood pressure lowering <u>Dietary aim</u>: 1,200[mg]/day
Dark leafy greens	o Collard greens o Kale o Spinach	Antioxidants	o Anti-cataract o Anti macular degeneration o **Memory** improvement o **Cognition** betterment <u>Dietary aim</u>: 1 serving/day
Fiber	o Fruits o Legumes o Nuts o Oatmeal o Veggies	High in fibers	o Blood sugar lowering o Cholesterol levels lowered o Constipation eased o Weight controlled <u>Dietary aims</u>: o Men (50+); 30[g]/day o Women: 21[g]/day

Fish	Fatty fish: o Herring o Salmon o Trout (farmed) o Tuna Alternatives: o Algae o Chia seeds o Flaxseed o Walnuts	o High in DHA (omega-3 fatty) acid o Low DHA linked to Alzheimer's disease	o Brain enhancement o **Memory** enhancement o Learning improvement Dietary aim: 2 x day
Lean protein	o Dairy products o Eggs o Meat (lean)	Rich protein	o Muscle lessening of natural loss Dietary aim: Avoid powdered protein
1. Red- and orange colored produce	o Bell peppers (red, orange) o Strawberries o Tomatoes o Watermelon	Lycopene	o Cancer risk lowered o Stroke risk lowered
Spices	o Cinnamon o Garlic o Turmeric	Antioxidants	o Cinnamon: Lowers cholesterol and triglycerides o Garlic: Keeps blood vessels open o Turmeric: Protects from depression and Alzheimer's disease; and against cancer Dietary aim: Fresh or dried
Sweet potato	Sweet potato	o Beta carotene	o Converts beta carotene into vitamin A o Protects eyesight o Protects skin o Keeps strong immune system o Slows down brain changes Dietary aim: o Use purple variety

Tree nuts	o Almonds
	o Cashews
	o Pecans
	o Pistachios
	o Walnuts
	o Other nuts
		Anti-aging powers	o Aging brain
			  protection
			Delay or/and prevent:
			o Age-related heart
			  disease
			o Cancer (some types)
			o Diabetes type 2
			o Nerve disease
			o Stroke

Water	Water	Food for health	o Cushions joints Helps control: o Body temperature o Mood Dietary aim: 8 glasses/day

Whole grains	o Quinoa
	o Wheat berries
	o Whole-wheat
	  bread
	o Whole-wheat
	  couscous
		o Fibers
		o Vitamins: B6,
		  folate
			o Brain health
			o Cancer risk lowered
			o Diabetes risk lowered
			o Heart disease
			  lowered risk

Mediterranean diet	o Green veggies
	  (specifically
	  spinach, Swiss
	  chard, and kale
	  rich in nitrates)
			o Helps dilate the
			  arteries
			o Optimal diet for
			  heart health
			o Improves blood flow
			o Improves vascular,
			  heart, and cognitive
			  function

In brief, as per the above Table, good foods for memory improvement include especially: avocados, blueberries, dark leafy greens (also for cognition betterment), and fish.

Nutrition for brain health

Blueberry consumption

In randomized, double-blind, placebo-**controlled trials, researchers found that a daily dose of blueberries ameliorates brain health in that**

it improves executive function, **strengthens** short-term memory, **and speeds up reaction times. However, they do not seem to ameliorate delayed recall.**

It appears that the blueberries' anthocyanins (the blue pigments) are responsible for improving cerebral (and vascular) blood flow - the likely mechanisms behind healthy cognitive function. Anthocyanins are polyphenols, a family of plant-based compounds that are increasingly associated with health benefits. There are about 8,000 different types of polyphenols (some also present in strawberries, raspberries, red grapes, and purple vegetables) provide health benefits.** They can also provide a brain boost, lower blood pressure, **and contribute to better cardiovascular health.** Some other types of foods that have beneficial polyphenols include green tea, broccoli, pears, and spices like turmeric and cinnamon.

Polyphenols mechanism

The mechanism behind the beneficial effects of polyphenols is not yet fully understood. **One theory is that their metabolites may "*act as signaling molecules, acting through several cell-signaling pathways, modulating nitric oxide bioavailability and different enzymes*".** **However, w**hile blueberries improve cerebral and vascular blood flow, they do not reduce arterial stiffness. It has been hypothesized that polyphenols may act via enhancing the abundance of butyrate-producing beneficial bacteria, and therefore the production of butyrate in the gut microbiota.

Other foods

According to the American Heart Association (AHA), a better cardiovascular and cognitive health is promoted by a diet rich in vegetables, fruits, whole grains, healthy proteins, minimally processed foods, and moderate oil and salt intake. A Mediterranean diet (green veggies, specifically spinach, Swiss chard, and kale rich in nitrates) can help dilate the arteries and may be the optimal diet for heart health. It helps to improve blood flow and improve vascular, heart, and cognitive function.

There are numerous other foods linked to cognitive health (Table 16.1) such as omega-3 fats (wild salmon and sardines), which are linked to better cognition because of their rich DHA content and potent anti-inflammatory properties. In addition, unsaturated fats may also help lower levels of beta-amyloid, a component in the development and progression of Alzheimer's disease (AD).

Supplementation for memory and mental health

Brain creatine

In a 1999 research paper, it was shown that *creatine (Cr) was also present in the human brain and that* oral Cr intake increased brain Cr levels, suggesting that at least some Cr passed through the blood-brain barrier (BBB). Like muscle, human brain function is highly energy intensive. Therefore, it made sense that the brain would also use Cr as a supplemental energy source. *In fact, research revealed that "creatine is so important to human brain function that the brain even synthesizes its own creatine".*

Cr is most commonly known as a sports supplement to enhance physical performance. It is a powdery non-steroidal supplement sold in most health food stores and used by bodybuilders or weightlifters to increase strength and muscle size. Although small amounts of Cr can be obtained directly from food (primarily fish and beef), muscles also readily absorb Cr from oral supplementation because muscles can use Cr to create adenosine triphosphate (ATP), the life-enabling energy source vital to cellular and muscular function. *Muscle cells containing more Cr can produce more energy for physical activities.* Thousands of studies support the safety and efficacy of Cr for muscle function. New research indicates that Cr is also important to brain function, affecting mood and cognition and early trials have suggested that Cr supplementation can improve stress resilience, depression, and brain functions such as **memory**.

Improvements to memory function and other brain conditions

Given that it is a bioactive substance in the brain, and proven it improves muscle function, does Cr also improve brain function? If so, which brain functions and which people are most likely to benefit? After more two decades of Cr research, it now appears that:

- Cr supplementation **moderately improves memory function in healthy adults**. On average, improvements are larger for older adults and smaller for younger adults.
- Cr supplementation may be **more beneficial for people experiencing acute/chronic stress or who consume smaller amounts of creatine through diet** (e.g., vegans and vegetarians).
- There are **higher depressive symptoms among people with lower Cr levels**.
- Because anxiety, PTSD, and depression symptoms are associated with metabolic dysfunction and impaired energy levels in the brain - all mechanisms improved by Cr - Cr supplementation can be beneficial. Further, initial human Cr interventional trials have reliably shown small to **moderate symptom improvements for individuals with these mental health conditions**.
- Animal studies and initial human trials likewise indicate **potential benefits of Cr supplementation in people with mild traumatic brain injury** (mTBI). Indeed, impaired metabolic function is a common side effect of TBI. This process could potentially be improved by higher Cr intake.
- However, at this point, **the optimal dosing schedule** (i.e., how much Cr? how often to take it? how long to take it?) **for brain benefits remains unclear.** Most brain Cr trials borrow from protocols established for studies testing Cr for physical performance, where consistent regimens of 5 grams of creatine/day are consumed or "pre-loading" regimens of 10-20 grams of Cr/day for 1-2 weeks followed by a 5-gram/day "maintenance" dose are used. But, these doses for physical performance may not necessarily be the appropriate ones for brain function and performance.

(Note: As with all health supplements, if considering creatine use, preference should be given to brands that submit to third-party testing to ensure product quality. There is also no scientific basis to use any form other than Cr monohydrate—the cheapest and most proven form of Cr.)

Vitamin B-12 deficiency

If memory loss is due to vitamin B-12 deficiency, taking the vitamin through diet or nutritional supplement can help correct the condition.

Sidebar 16.1 provides more details on Cr; sidebar 16.2 looks into the question as to whether tweaking memories can improve mental health; sidebar 16.3 is interested in the care for mental health; and sidebar 16.4 examines whether digital puzzle gaming improves memory.

Take-aways

- **A daily dose of blueberries ameliorates brain health, improving executive function, strengthening short-term memory, speeding up reaction times, but not ameliorating delayed recall.**
- **A better cardiovascular and cognitive health is promoted by the Mediterranean diet, which can help dilate the arteries, and improve blood flow and vascular, heart, and cognitive function.**
- **The mechanism behind the beneficial effects of polyphenols is not yet fully understood.**
- Creatine supplementation moderately improves memory function in healthy adults, may be more beneficial for people experiencing acute/ chronic stress or who consume smaller amounts of creatine through diet, ameliorate depressive symptoms, and moderately improve mental health conditions and mild traumatic brain injury.
- The optimal dosing schedule (i.e., how much creatine/how often to take/how long to take) of creatinine supplementation for brain benefits remains unclear.
- If memory loss is due to vitamin B-12 deficiency, taking the vitamin through diet or nutritional supplement can help correct the condition.

- Researchers are exploring ways to manipulate memories to discover novel methods to treat post-traumatic stress disorder (PTSD), depression, and Alzheimer's disease.
- Digital puzzle strategic gaming improves working memory more for older adults than for younger adults who play action games.
- For older people, puzzle games have the surprising ability to support mental capabilities to the extent that memory and concentration levels are the same as for 20 year-olds who had not played puzzle games.

Sidebar 16.1 – Creatine

A brief history

In 1832: Michel Eugène Chevreuil isolated and first identified creatine (Cr) from the basified water- extract of skeletal muscle.

In 1912: Otto Folin and Willey Glover Denis found evidence that ingesting Cr can dramatically boost the Cr content of the muscle.

In the 1920s: Consumption of large amounts of Cr did not result in its excretion, pointing to the ability of the body to store Cr which, in turn, suggested its use as a dietary supplement.

In 1927: Phosphocreatine (PCr, creatine phosphate) is discovered.

In 1928: Cr is shown to exist in equilibrium with creatinine.

In the late 1920s: After finding that the intramuscular stores of Cr can be increased by ingesting Cr in larger than normal amounts, and having discovered PCr, scientists determined that Cr, naturally formed in vertebrates, is a key player in the metabolism of skeletal muscle.

In the 1960s: Creatine kinase (CrK) is shown to phosphorylate ADP using PCr to generate ATP. It follows that ATP, not PCr is directly consumed in muscle contraction. CK uses Cr to "buffer" the ATP/ADP ratio.

Since the early twentieth century: Cr's influence on physical performance has been well documented.

In 1992: Following the 1992 Olympics in Barcelona, an August 7, 1992 article in The Times reported that Linford Christie, the gold medal winner at 100 meters, had used Cr before the Olympics. (Christie was found guilty of doping later in his career.) Further, an article in Bodybuilding Monthly named Sally Gunnell, the gold medalist in the 400-meter hurdles, as another Cr user. Still further, The Times also noted that 100-meter hurdler Colin Jackson began taking Cr before the Olympics.

In 1993: Cr supplements designed for strength enhancement became commercially available when a company called Experimental and Applied Sciences (EAS) introduced the compound to the sports nutrition market under the name *Phosphagen*. Research performed thereafter demonstrated that the consumption of high glycemic carbohydrates in conjunction with Cr increases Cr muscle stores.

Metabolic role

Cr is a naturally occurring non-protein compound and the primary constituent of PCr, which is used to regenerate ATP within the cell. 95% of the human body's total Cr and PCr stores are found in skeletal muscle, while the remainder is distributed in the blood, brain, testes, and other tissues.

Cr is not an essential nutrient. It is an amino acid derivative, naturally produced in the human body from the amino acids glycine and arginine and subsequently methylated. Cr itself can be phosphorylated and used as an energy buffer in skeletal muscles and the **brain**. A cyclic form of Cr, called creatinine, exists in equilibrium with its tautomer and with Cr.

Phosphocreatine systems

Cr is transported through the blood and taken up by tissues with high energy demands, such as the brain and skeletal muscle, through an active transport system. Cr has the ability to increase muscle stores of PCr, potentially increasing the muscle's ability to resynthesize ATP from ADP to meet increased energy demands. Cr supplementation appears to increase the number of myonuclei that satellite cells will 'donate' to damaged muscle fibers, which increases the potential for growth of those fibers.

Genetic deficiencies

Genetic deficiencies in the Cr biosynthetic pathway lead to **various severe neurological defects.** Clinically, there are three distinct disorders of Cr metabolism. Deficiencies in the two synthesis enzymes are inherited in an autosomal recessive manner. A third defect, Cr transporter defect, is caused by mutations in SLC6A8 and inherited in a X-linked manner. This condition is related to the transport of Cr into the brain.

(Note for vegetarians: Some studies suggest that total muscle Cr is significantly lower in vegetarians than non-vegetarians, probably due to an omnivorous diet being the primary source of Cr. Supplementation is needed to raise the concentration of Cr in the muscles of lacto-ovo vegetarians and vegans up to non-vegetarian levels as they have lower Cr concentrations in muscle and blood, but not brain.)

Pharmacokinetics

Most of the research to-date on Cr has predominantly focused on its pharmacological properties and not into its pharmacokinetics. Studies have not established pharmacokinetic parameters for clinical usage of Cr such as volume of distribution, clearance, bioavailability, mean residence time, absorption rate, and half life. A clear pharmacokinetic profile would need to be established prior to optimal clinical dosing.

Dosing

> **Loading phase:** Approximately 0.3 g/kg/day divided into 4 equally-spaced intervals has been suggested since Cr needs may vary based on body weight. Also, taking a lower dose of 3 grams a day for 28 days can increase total muscle Cr storage to the same amount as the rapid loading dose of 20 g/day for 6 days. However, a 28-day loading phase does not allow for ergogenic benefits of Cr supplementation to be realized until fully saturated muscle storage. Supplementing Cr with carbohydrates or carbohydrates and protein has been shown to augment Cr retention. Higher doses for longer periods of time are being studied to offset CR synthesis deficiencies and mitigating diseases.

> **Maintenance phase:** After the 5–7 day loading phase, muscle Cr stores are fully saturated and supplementation only needs to cover the amount of Cr broken down per day. This maintenance dose was originally reported to be around 2–3 g/day (or 0.03 g/kg/day), however,

some studies have suggested 3–5 g/day maintenance dose to maintain saturated muscle Cr.

Absorption

Endogenous serum or plasma Cr concentrations in healthy adults are normally in a range of 2–12 mg/L. A single 5 gram (5000 mg) oral dose in healthy adults results in a peak plasma Cr level of approximately 120 mg/L at 1–2 hours post-ingestion. Cr has a fairly short elimination half-life, averaging just less than 3 hours, so to maintain an elevated plasma level it would be necessary to take small oral doses every 3–6 hours throughout the day.

Clearance

It has been shown that once supplementation of Cr stops, muscle Cr stores return to baseline in 4–6 weeks.

Exercise and sport

Cr supplements are marketed in ethyl ester, gluconate, monohydrate, and nitrate forms. For sporting performance, they are considered safe for short-term use but there is a lack of safety data for long term use. Cr monohydrate might help with energy availability for high-intensity anaerobic exercise, but has no significant effect on aerobic endurance.

Research

Cognitive performance

Cr is reported to have a beneficial effect on brain function and cognitive processing, although the evidence is difficult to interpret systematically and the appropriate dosing is unknown. The greatest effect appears to be in individuals who are stressed (due, for instance, to sleep deprivation) or cognitive impairment.

A 2018 systematic review found that "*generally, there was evidence that short term memory and intelligence/reasoning may be improved by creatine administration*", whereas for other cognitive domains "the results were conflicting". Another 2023 review initially found evidence of improved memory function. However, it was later determined that faulty statistics led to the statistical significance and after fixing the "double counting", the effect was only significant in older adults.

Some mitochondrial diseases

Parkinson's disease (PD)

Cr's impact on mitochondrial function has led to research on its efficacy and safety for slowing PD. As of 2014, the evidence did not provide a reliable foundation for treatment decisions, due to risk of bias, small sample sizes, and the short duration of trials.

A National Institutes of Health (NIH) study suggests that caffeine interacts with Cr to increase the rate of progression of PD.

Huntington's disease (HD)

Several primary studies have been completed but no systematic review on HD has been completed yet.

Adverse effects of supplementation

Side effects include:

- Weight gain (within the first week of the supplement schedule), likely attributable to greater water retention due to the increased muscle Cr concentrations by means of osmosis.
- Potential muscle cramps / strains / pulls.
- Upset stomach.
- Diarrhea.
- Dizziness.

Sidebar 16.2 - Can tweaking memories improve mental health?

Can replacing bad memories with good ones or even erasing certain memories improve mental health? Researchers are exploring ways to manipulate memories to discover novel methods to treat post-traumatic stress disorder

(PTSD), depression, and Alzheimer's. National Geographic is actually conducting public events that feature thought-provoking presentations on this topic by today's leading explorers, scientists, photographers, and performing artists.

Sidebar 16.3 – Caring for mental health

Mental health includes emotional, psychological, and social well-being. It affects how we think, feel, act, make choices, and relate to others. Mental health is more than the absence of a mental illness—it is essential to overall health and quality of life. Self-care can play a role in maintaining mental health and help support treatment and recovery.

About self-care

Self-care means taking the time to do things that help live well and improve both physical health and mental health. Although it is not a cure for mental illnesses, understanding what causes or triggers mild symptoms and what coping techniques work can help manage mental health. When it comes to mental health, self-care can help manage stress, lower risk of illness, and increase energy. Even small acts of self-care in daily life can have a big impact such as:

- ➢ **Getting regular exercise.**
- ➢ **Eating healthy, regular meals, and staying hydrated.**
- ➢ **Making sleep a priority**.
- ➢ **Trying a relaxing activity (**wellness programs or apps, which may incorporate meditation, muscle relaxation, or breathing exercises).
- ➢ **Setting goals and priorities.**
- ➢ **Practicing gratitude.**
- ➢ **Focusing on positivity**.
- ➢ **Staying connected.**

Sidebar 16.4 - Can digital puzzle gaming improve memory?

Since aging has a negative impact on working memory, are certain types of games connected with improvements in memory among younger and older adults? Certain experiments showed that young adults who play strategy games show a greater working memory capacity compared to young adults who play action games. This may be surprising because other experiments showed that action games have been associated with superior performance in various measures of attention, perception, and executive function.

For older people, puzzle games have the surprising ability to support mental capabilities to the extent that memory and concentration levels are the same as for 20 year-olds who had not played puzzle games. Older adults who play digital puzzle games may have a higher working memory capacity than older adults who play either other game types or do not play games at all. In addition, older adults who play digital puzzle games can ignore distractions better than other older adults. It seems that the strategy elements of the games (planning, problem solving, etc.) stimulate better memory and attention in younger rather than older people.

17

Treatment portfolio: II. Pharmacotherapy

Contents

17

Treatment portfolio: II. Pharmacotherapy

It is typical for people to have mild memory lapses over time; these may be age-related and should not cause concern. However, people with memory loss experience greater than expected levels of forgetfulness, may have difficulty with both short- and long-term memory recall. When memory loss occurs more frequently and affects a person's daily activities, a doctor should be consulted to discuss symptoms and effects of memory loss. Without medication, symptoms of memory loss can become severe.

There are presently no disease-modifying medications for memory loss. Cholinesterase inhibitors and N-Methyl-D-aspartic Acid (NMDA) glutamate regulators can only stop memory loss symptoms for a short time. They can help manage a person's memory loss symptoms and modify the progression of their condition. However, they cannot stop or reverse that progression. Additional research can help scientists understand the effectiveness of amyloid clearing therapies and produce novel drug therapies. The treatment will depend on the cause of memory loss, but various drugs have been suggested in recent years. For the treatment of AD, five drugs are currently FDA-approved, all acting on the cholinergic system: Donepezil, Galantamine, Rivastigmine, Tacrine, and Leqembi (this last medication approved only in

July 2023). Although these medications are not a cure, AD symptoms may be reduced for up to eighteen months for mild or moderate dementia but do not forestall the ultimate decline to full AD.

This chapter outlines the various medications for memory loss, their indications, and potential side effects as well as their management.

Can medication help slow memory loss?

How memories are formed has been a puzzle that has perplexed researchers for over a century, and there are still many questions that remain about the biological mechanisms that underpin them. Perhaps because of this gap in understanding, there are no pharmacological interventions that can be taken to improve memory. No drug treatment can effectively cure memory loss. The National Institute on Aging (NIA) states that "*people should avoid any treatment that promises to restore brain function and improve memory*". It further notes that these medications are typically unsafe and can cause negative drug interactions with other medications. However, certain medications can help individuals ease the symptoms and manage the condition's progression. Health experts recommend that those with memory loss follow doctor-approved prescriptions only.

Types of medication for memory loss

Few medications are available to help manage memory loss. The severity of a person's memory loss and the underlying cause will indicate the most suitable drug therapy. Table 17.1 summarizes memory loss medications, including drug information and side effects. For most people with memory loss, a doctor will recommend one of the types of drugs therein listed.

Table 17.1 – Memory loss medications, including drug information and side effects

Generic/brand name	Drug type	Drug indication	Side effects
Donepezil/ Aricept	Cholinesterase inhibitor	o Alzheimer's disease dementia (ADD) ==>Can be prescribed off-label for: o Parkinson's disease dementia (PDD) o Lewy body dementia (LBD) o Vascular disease dementia (VDD) o Traumatic brain injury (TBI)	o Anorexia o Diarrhea o Edema o Fatigue o Hyper/hypotension o Insomnia o Muscle cramps o Nausea o Vomiting
Galantamine/ Razadyne	Cholinesterase inhibitor	o ADD	o Atrioventricular blockage o Gastrointestinal bleeding o Headache o Low appetite o Sinus bradychardia o Skin reactions o Slow heart rate o Stomach ulcer o Weight loss o Other common side effects
Rivastigmine/ Exelon	Cholinesterase inhibitor	o ADD o PDD	o General irritability o Increased risk of death from long-term use o Involuntary movements o Muscular contractions o Sleep disturbances o Tremors
Memantine/ Namenda	Glutamate regulator and NMDA receptor antagonist	o Moderate-to-severe memory loss due to AD	o Confusion o Constipation o Dizziness o Headache o High stomach acid level
Donepezil+Memantine/ Namzaric	Cholinesterase inhibitor + Glutamate regulator	Moderate-to-severe memory loss due to AD	o Anorexia o Breathing difficulty o Diarrhea o Seizure o Slow heartbeat o Urinary hesitancy

Aducanumab/ Aduhelm*	Monoclonal antibody ==> Biologic drug comprising living cells. It destroys plaques of toxic beta-amyloid protein	First-line treatment for early stage AD or ADD ==> May be prescribed for mild cognitive impairment (withdrawn from market)	o Delirium o Edema o Falls o Hypersensitivity o Immunogenicity
Lecanumab/ Leqembi	Monoclonal antibody	o Alzheimer's disease dementia (ADD)	

Source: Fymat A.L. (2019)

Key: AD: Alzheimer's disease; ADD: AD dementia; PD: Parkinson's disease; PDD: PD dementia; TBI: Traumatic brain injury; VDD: Vascular disease dementia;

(* Note: Some hail human monoclonal antibodies that clear beta-amyloid deposits from the brain as the first disease-modifying treatments for the condition. However, they are not without controversy such as the one concerning the FDA-approved Aducanumab despite a lack of evidence for its efficacy and concerns about adverse effects.)

- ➤ **Cholinesterase inhibitors:** These medications can manage various conditions affecting memory, including AD and PD. They work by blocking the enzyme cholinesterase from breaking down acetylcholine, which is a chemical messenger that plays a vital role in memory and learning. Increasing the levels of acetylcholine in the brain can help maintain memory and delay worsening symptoms. They are the first choice treatment for memory loss. The treating physician may also prescribe the single-dose drug combination (cholinesterase inhibitor + glutamate regulator) to treat moderate-to-severe memory loss.
- ➤ **Glutamate regulators:** Glutamate regulators control the amount of glutamate in the central nervous system to an optimal level. Glutamate is the most common neurotransmitter in the brain. It can excite nerve cells to their death through a process known as 'excitotoxicity'. Excitotoxic cell death can cause neurodegenerative conditions that affect memory. One example of a glutamate regulator is Memantine (Namenda), an NMDA receptor antagonist that stops calcium from invading the neurons and causing nerve injury. Due to their minimal side effects, glutamate regulators may be prescribed either alone or alongside a cholinesterase inhibitor.
- ➤ **Combined cholinesterase inhibitor and glutamate regulator drug:** Combining the two classes of drugs is more effective than using

only one medication. While it is superior to single drug therapy, it can complicate treatment plans for patients and their caregivers.

Currently, there are no specifically approved drugs for improving memory formation. While some prescription medications are used to improve memory in conditions like AD, they are not recommended for general memory enhancement in healthy adults.

Table 17.2 summarizes the psychopharnacotherapy for Alzheimer-type and other dementias:

Table 17.2 – Psychopharmacotherapy for Alzheimer-type and other dementias

Pathology	Drugs	Precautions	Side effects
Memory problems (Monitored over an 8-week course)	Provide no cure: o Cholinesterase inhibitors*: Donepezil (Aricept®), Rivastigmine (Exelon®), Galantamine (Razadyne®) o Glutamate regulators: - Memantine (Namenda®): o Used in combination with anti-cholinesterase - N-Methyl D-Aspartate (NMDA) receptor blockers o Folate or Vitamin B-12 o Statins o Blood pressure medications	o Symptoms may worsen if the treatment is stopped or after treatment o Periodic evaluation of the treatment is required o May cause increase in cardiovascular-related events	o Aggression o Diarrhea o Dizziness o Difficulty sleeping with very vivid dreams (when taken at bedtime) o Fainting spells in people with heart problem(s) o Gastro-intestinal upset o Hallucinations o Muscle cramping o Nausea o Slow heart rate o Vomiting o Weight loss o No benefit o No clear link with dementia o No improved outcomes
Behavioral symptoms	o Environment change, physical exercise, avoiding triggers that cause sadness, socializing with others, engaging in pleasant activities o Antipsychotics:		o Agitation o Anxiety o Irritability o Not usually recommended due to little benefits, side effects, increased risk of death

Depression	o Behavioral therapy and/or medications o Selective serotonin re-uptake inhibitors (SSRI): - Citalopram** (Celexa®) - Escitalopram (Lexapro®) - Fluoxetine (Prozac®) - Paroxetine (Paxil®) - Sertraline** (Zoloft®)		
Anxiety & Aggression	Medications		Can be caused by several factors: o Confusion o Depression o Disorientation o Frightening o Hallucinations o Medical conditions (such as difficulty urinating or severe constipation) o Misunderstanding o Paranoid delusions o Sleep: disorders, Reduced altered sleep/wake cycles o Other causes of physical pain or discomfort
Sleep problems	o Medications or/and behavior changes o Benzodiazepines (Diazepam) and non-benzodiazepine hypnotics To be avoided: o Melatonin, Ramelteon, Trazodone		o Increased cognitive impairment o Falls: Increased o Worsened confusion o Little evidence to improve sleep in dementia patients
Pain	Medications		o Ambulation decrease o Appetite impaired o Cognitive impairment exacerbated o Falls o Functional implications profound o Functional psychosocial implications o Mood depression o Quality of life implications o Sleep disturbances

| Eating difficulties | Assisted feeding, gastrostomy, feeding tube | | o Pressure ulcers worsening o Fluid overload
o Diarrhea
o Abdominal pain
o Complications local
o Aspiration risk |

Source: Fymat A.L. (2019)

Key: NMDA: N-Methyl D-Aspartate; SSRI: Selective serotonin re-uptake inhibitors

(**Notes:**

* Precautions: Donepezil should be used with caution in people with: (a) cardiac problems: heart disease, cardiac conduction disturbances, chronic obstructive pulmonary disease (COPD), severe cardiac arrhythmias; (b) asthma; (c) sick sinus syndrome (SSD); (d) peptic ulcer disease (PUD) or taking non-steroidal anti-inflammatory drugs (NSAID); and (e) in case of predisposition to seizures.

** Sertraline and Citalopram do not reduce symptoms of agitation compared to placebo and do not affect outcomes.)

Role of melatonin in memory formation

Melatonin is a hormone naturally produced by the pineal gland in the brain's center in response to darkness. It helps regulate the circadian clock and sleep. Synthetic forms can be taken as a supplement to help induce sleep. According to the National Center for Complementary and Integrative Health (NCCIH), the role of melatonin in helping treat the symptoms of jet lag and insomnia in humans is the focus of research.

Sleep having been linked to improved retention of memory for over a century, it is thought that the brain state during sleep is optimized for memory consolidation. However, the exact mechanisms underlying this link are unclear.

Mechanism linking melatonin and improved memory

To determine the mechanism underlying the link between melatonin and improved memory, and explore whether melatonin and its derivatives had any effects on memory, researchers conducted a series of experiments on male mice. The aim was to establish whether the activation of melatonin receptors, or phosphorylation of other proteins, is involved in memory formation. The experiment was designed to measure long-term memory by modulating the phosphorylation levels of memory-related proteins. (Phosphorylation is the addition of a chemical group to a protein, which affects its activity levels in biochemical reactions.) These proteins are involved in receptor binding-related memory formation pathways and pathways not associated with receptor binding.

Changes in medication management

Dementia is a life-limiting disease with an average survival time of less than 5 years from diagnosis. Co-morbidities and polypharmacy are common, though evidence is scarce for medication safety, tolerability, and efficacy. Compared to their peers (i.e., cognitively intact people of a comparable age), people with dementia have many co-morbidities, take a mean of five or more medications daily, and are more likely to use certain medication classes (antihypertensives, laxatives, diuretics, antidepressants, and antipsychotics). This medication use may reflect risk factors for dementia and common co-morbidities such as cardio- and reno-vascular disease.

Age-related pharmacokinetic changes occur in all older people, and an altered blood-brain barrier (BBB) permeability in people with dementia renders them more sensitive to neurological and cognitive effects of medications than their peers. These pharmacokinetic changes are additional to drug-disease interactions that occur in dementia. The safety profile and efficacy of many medications in people with dementia are undetermined due to their active exclusion from 85% of published clinical trials. Furthermore, the tendency for people with dementia to under-report disease-related symptoms means that it is likely they also under-report side-effects.

Research in people with dementia focuses on treatments that prevent or delay dementia onset and/or progression and manage dementia-specific neuropsychiatric or behavioral symptoms. Evidence for the efficacy of these medications is conflicting and the harms of some, such as antipsychotics and benzodiazepines, make them potentially inappropriate in this population.

Despite the frequency of co-morbidities and medication use among people with dementia, appropriate medication management in this life-limiting condition is infrequently studied and poorly understood. For example, studies of antihypertensives, hypoglycemics, statins, and anti-inflammatories mainly assess their ability to delay dementia onset. After dementia onset, medication appropriateness to manage co-morbidities is complicated by a relative absence of evidence.

Preventive treatments may require a treatment time to benefit that exceeds life expectancy, or may target treatment goals that are not relevant to the individual or their families. This is combined with a shifting focus on the priorities of healthcare in this patient cohort and the balance between the benefits and harms of medicines.

Medication management is subsequently complicated for people with dementia so that careful consideration should be given to initiation and continuation of all medications. Medication management decisions for people with dementia are often based on data collected in younger adults or peers, which may not be generalizable or relevant to this population. The existing explicit prescribing criteria developed for older people do not account for the additional complexities of dementia or its life-limiting nature. Specific guidance for people with dementia would assist clinicians with decision-making in this population.

For people living with dementia, medication management remains a complex task as it is unclear what constitutes optimal medication management in this population due to the shifting focus of health priorities and the balance between the benefits and harms of medications. A study was conducted by a large panel of mltidisciplinary experts in geriatric therapeutics (including pharmacists, doctors, nurse practitioners, a patient advocate, and a psychologist) to define the appropriate medication management of co-morbidities. It developed the Medications Appropriateness Tool for Co-Morbid Health – Dementia (MATCH-D), including criteria that can help identify ways in which a diagnosis of dementia changes medication management for other health conditions. More information on MATCH-D is provided in Sidebar 17.1. Sidebar 17.2 provides some information on the FDA accelerated drug approval process, specifically for the latest drug Leqembi.

Take-aways

> It is typical for people to have mild memory lapses over time; these may be age-related and should not cause concern. However, people with memory loss experience greater than expected levels of forgetfulness and may have difficulty with both short- and long-term memory recall. Without medication, symptoms of memory loss can become severe.

> Medications can help manage a person's memory loss symptoms and eventually modify the progression of their condition. However, they cannot stop or reverse the progression of the condition. For the treatment of Alzheimer's disease, five drugs are currently FDA-approved: Donepezil, Galantamine, Rivastigmine, Tacrine and, as of July 2023, Leqembi. Nonetheless, while helping ease symptoms and manage the condition's progression, medications are typically unsafe and can cause negative drug interactions with other medications.

> The severity of a person's memory loss and the underlying cause will indicate the most suitable drug therapy. The particulars of available memory loss medications, including drug information and side effects, have been provided. These include cholinesterase inhibitors, glutamate regulators, or their combination.

> The link between sleep and improved memory retention has still not been elucidated. It is thought that the brain state during sleep is optimized for memory consolidation. However, the exact mechanisms underlying this link are unclear.

> Melatonin and its derivatives may have effects on memory formation by modulating the phosphorylation levels of memory-related proteins, which are involved in receptor binding related to memory formation pathways and pathways not associated with receptor binding.

> Co-morbidities and polypharmacy in dementia are common, though evidence is scarce for medication safety, tolerability, and efficacy. People with dementia are likely to use daily five or more medications on the average (antihypertensives, laxatives, diuretics, antidepressants, and antipsychotics), reflecting risk factors for dementia and common co-morbidities such as cardio- and reno-vascular disease.

> Age-related pharmacokinetic and changes in additional drug-disease interactions occur in older people. Further, an altered blood-brain

barrier permeability in people with dementia renders them more sensitive to neurological and cognitive effects of medications.

➤ The safety profile and efficacy of many medications in people with dementia are undetermined due to their active exclusion from 85% of published clinical trials. Furthermore, the tendency for people with dementia to under-report disease-related symptoms means that it is likely they also under-report side-effects.

➤ Research in people with dementia focuses on treatments that prevent or delay dementia onset and/or progression and manage dementia-specific neuropsychiatric or behavioral symptoms. Evidence for the efficacy of these medications is conflicting.

➤ Despite the frequency of co-morbidities and medication use among people with dementia, appropriate medication management in this life-limiting condition is infrequently studied and poorly understood.

➤ Preventive treatments may require a treatment time to benefit that exceeds life expectancy, or may target treatment goals that are not relevant to the individual or their families.

➤ Medication management is complicated for people with dementia so that careful consideration should be given to initiation and continuation of all medications. Medication management decisions for people with dementia are often based on data collected in younger adults or peers, which may not be generalizable or relevant to this population.

➤ For people living with dementia, medication management is a complex task as it is unclear what constitutes optimal medication management for them due to the shifting focus of health priorities and the balance between the benefits and harms of medications.

➤ The Medications Appropriateness Tool for Co-Morbid Health – Dementia (MATCH-D) criteria can help identify ways that a diagnosis of dementia changes medication management for other health conditions.

Sidebar 17.1 - Medication appropriateness tool for co-morbid health conditions in dementia (MATCH-D)

The MATCH-D study aimed to elicit opinion and gain consensus on appropriate medication management of co-morbidities in people with dementia. The intended outcome was to create a consensus-based list of statements to define appropriate medication management of co-morbidities in people with dementia. For this purpose, it convened a large panel of multidisciplinary experts in geriatric therapeutics including pharmacists, doctors, nurse practitioners, a patient advocate, and a psychologist.

The participants generated a list of statements that provided guidance on appropriate treatment goals in people with dementia and important discussion points for patient-centered care. The statements gave specific consensus-based advice in the broad themes of preventive medication, symptoms management, prescribing to reduce the risk of future events, behavioral and psychological symptoms management, treatment goals, principles of medication use, medications to slow dementia progression, psychoactive and other medications, the experience of side-effects, and medication reviews in people living with dementia.

The MATCH-D study complements existing dementia guidelines by describing appropriate pharmacological management of co-morbidities as dementia progresses. One of its strong messages was the importance of a person-centered approach to pharmacological management. Such management needs to focus on treatment goals that are relevant to the individual and their families, as older adults vary in their preferences for treatment when they consider the potential risks and benefits of medication management. Regretfully, general prescribing criteria for older adults do not specifically consider the particularities of the progressive, life-limiting nature of dementia.

Sidebar 17.2 – On FDA's accelerated approval of Leqembi

The FDA, an agency within the U.S. Department of Health and Human Services (DHHS), *"protects the public health by assuring the safety, effectiveness, and security of human and veterinary drugs, vaccines and other biological products for human use, and medical devices. The agency also is responsible for the safety and security of... dietary supplements, ..."*

The accelerated approval program

The FDA instituted its Accelerated Approval Program *"to allow for earlier approval of drugs that treat serious conditions, and fill an unmet medical need based on a surrogate endpoint if a drug is shown to have an effect on a surrogate endpoint that is reasonably likely to predict a clinical benefit to patients"*. A surrogate endpoint is a marker (such as a laboratory measurement, radiographic image, physical sign or other measure) that is thought to predict clinical benefit but is **not** itself a measure of clinical benefit. The use of a surrogate endpoints can considerably shorten the time required prior to receiving FDA approval.

Drug companies are still required to conduct studies to confirm the anticipated clinical benefit. If the confirmatory trial shows that the drug actually provides a clinical benefit, then the FDA grants traditional approval for the drug. If the confirmatory trial does not show that the drug provides clinical benefit, FDA has regulatory procedures in place that could lead to removing the drug from the market.

The Agency's use of that shortcut approach has come under increasing scrutiny from government watchdogs and congressional investigators.

On Leqembi approval

On January 6, 2023, FDA approved the drug Leqembi via the Accelerated Approval pathway for the treatment of AD. The FDA granted this application *Fast Track, Priority Review, and Breakthrough Therapy designations* to (Japan) Eisai R&D Management Co., Ltd (Biogen is its U.S. partner).

Leqembi is the second of a new category of AD-approved medications that target the fundamental pathophysiology of the disease. **This treatment option is the latest therapy to (presumably)** ***"target and affect the underlying disease process of AD, instead of only treating the symptoms of the disease"***.

Researchers initially evaluated Leqembi's efficacy in a double-blind, placebo-controlled, parallel-group, dose-finding study of 856 patients with AD. Patients' selection criteria included: (1) Mild cognitive impairment (MCI) or mild dementia stage (MDS) of disease and the (2) confirmed presence of amyloid-beta pathology. Every two weeks, subjects received an approved dose of 10 mg/kg of Lecanemab. Compared to controls, subjects showed a *"statistically significant reduction in brain amyloid plaque* (a marker of AD) *from baseline to Week 79"*. The accelerated approval was based on the observed reduction of amyloid beta-plaque, which was quantified using positron emission tomography (PET) imaging. The results of a Phase-3 randomized, controlled clinical trial, a larger 1,800-patient study, is under review by the FDA to confirm the drug's benefit, paving the way for full approval later this year.

Of particular note: The prescribing information for Leqembi includes a warning for amyloid-related imaging abnormalities (ARIA), which are known to occur with antibodies of this class. Usually, the drug does not have symptoms but may present the following side effects: (1) Infusion-related reactions such as a temporary swelling in areas of the brain that usually resolves over time and may be accompanied by (2) small spots of bleeding in or on the surface of the brain, though some people may have symptoms such as (3) headache, confusion, dizziness, vision changes, nausea, and seizure. Another warning for Leqembi is for a risk of infusion-related reactions, with symptoms such as flu-like symptoms, nausea, vomiting, and changes in blood pressure. Serious and life-threatening events may rarely occur.

Criticisms of the approval

While the drug has not yet received regular approval, the following criticisms have already been levied:

On the drug itself

> ➤ The drug may only modestly slow the brain-robbing disease, *albeit* with potential safety risks that patients and their doctors will have to carefully weigh.
> ➤ The (apparent) delay in cognitive decline brought about by the drug likely amounts to just several months, but could (perhaps) still meaningfully improve people's lives.
> ➤ The drug is not a cure. It does not stop the disease from getting worse, but may measurably slow its progression.

- Scrutiny of the new drug, will likely mean most patients will not start receiving it for months, as insurers decide whether and how to cover it.
- The larger (1800 subjects) study tracked patients' results on an 18-point scale that measures **memory**, judgment, and other cognitive abilities. Doctors compile the rating from interviews with the patient and a close contact. After 18 months, patients receiving Leqembi declined more slowly — a difference of less than half a point on the scale — than patients who received a dummy infusion. The delay amounted to just over five months. There is little consensus on whether that difference translates into real benefits for patients, such as greater independence. For some neurology researchers, that is really quite a small effect and probably below the threshold of what would be called clinically significant. A meaningful improvement would require at least a difference of one full point on the 18-point scale.
- There are no safety or effectiveness data on initiating treatment at earlier or later stages of the disease than were studied.

On the drug's side effects and adverse events

- The medicine comes with downsides, including the need for twice-a-month infusions and possible side effects like brain swelling.
- About 13% of patients in the larger study had swelling of the brain and 17% had small brain bleeds, side effects seen with earlier amyloid-targeting medications. In most cases those problems did not cause other symptoms such as dizziness and vision problems. Also, several Leqembi users died while taking the drug, including two who were on blood-thinning medications. Although the manufacturer argued that these deaths cannot be attributed to the drug, the FDA label warns doctors to use caution if they prescribe Leqembi to patients on blood thinners.

On the approval process

- The drug has only been specifically approved for patients with Alzheimer's, mild cognitive impairment, or in mild dementia stage.

- The FDA approval came via its accelerated pathway, which allows drugs to launch based on early results before they are confirmed to benefit patients.
- On December 2022, a congressional report found that FDA's approval of a similar Alzheimer's drug called Aducanumab/Aduhelm (also from Eisai and Biogen) was "rife with irregularities", including a number of meetings with drug company staffers that went undocumented.
- Aduhelm/Aducanumab, the similar drug previously marketed but withdrawn by the same pharmaceutical company, was marred by controversy over its effectiveness. The FDA approved that drug in 2021 against the advice of the agency's own outside experts. Doctors hesitated to prescribe the drug and insurers restricted coverage. The FDA did not consult the same expert panel before approving Leqembi.

On cost and insurance reimbursement

- The drug will cost about US $26,500 for a typical year's worth of treatment. The company pegged its value at over US $37,000 per year but said it priced it lower to reduce costs for patients and insurers. An independent group that assesses drug value recently said the drug would have to be priced below US $20,600 to be cost-effective.
- Some neurology researchers seriously doubt whether the measurable benefit of the drug is worth the hefty price tag and the side effects patients may experience.
- Insurers are likely to only cover the drug for people like those in the company study — patients with mild symptoms and confirmation of amyloid buildup. That typically requires expensive brain scans. A separate type of scan will be needed to periodically monitor for brain swelling and bleeding.
- A key question in the drug's rollout will be the coverage decision by Medicare (the U.S. federal health plan that covers 60 million seniors and other Americans). The agency severely restricted coverage of Aduhelm/Aducanumab, essentially wiping out its U.S. market and prompting Biogen to abandon marketing plans for the drug. Regarding Leqembi, coverage is not expected until after the FDA confirms the drug's benefit, likely later this year.

Treatment portfolio: IV. Brain electromagnetic neurostimulation

Contents

18

Treatment portfolio: IV. Brain electromagnetic neurostimulation

In rare cases where patients may not improve using standard approaches, surgery can be an option. Surgeries include electroconvulsive therapy (ECT), transcranial electrotherapy stimulation (tETS), continuous theta burst stimulation (cTBS), repetitive transcranial magnetic stimulation (rTMS), vagus nerve stimulation (VNS), magnetic seizure therapy (MST), and deep brain stimulation (DBS). Brain stimulation is a means to potentially remediate symptoms in a range of neurological and psychiatric diseases, however, precise targeting of stimulation is necessary to ensure efficacy. In this chapter, I will discuss the principle and application of these several procedures, which still need to be further investigated and used only at centers with expertise in them.

Brief chronicle of the development and modeling of brain circuits

Understanding the brain circuitry underlying movement-related symptoms, particularly Parkinson's disease (PD) and other movement disorders, contributed significantly to the development of the above procedures. It can be traced back several decades:

In 1947: Development of the stereotactic frame apparatus to target specific brain areas based on the knowledge of brain anatomy and function known at the time and refinement through trial- and-error.

In the 1950s: Various movement disorders including PD, essential tremors (ET), and dystonia were treated surgically by inactivating or lesioning brain regions involved in motor control. Overall, surgical lesions improved motor symptoms for many patients, though sometimes at the expense of irreversible deficits in other functions.

In the 1960s: Several reports noted that high-frequency stimulation of target regions mimicked surgical lesions, while lower-frequency stimulation worsened motor symptoms.

In 1972: Russian neurophysiologist Natalia Bekhtereva suggested that brain stimulation might itself be used as a treatment for movement disorders instead of permanent lesions.

In the mid-1970s: Mahlon DeLong used electrical stimulation to meticulously characterize the functions of neurons in different brain areas as animals performed movements.

In the 1980s: Technological advances made chronic stimulation suitable for broad clinical application.

During the 1980s: French physician-scientist Alim Louis Benabid and others developed the deep brain stimulation (DBS) procedure, involving the surgical implantation of electrodes into parts of the brain.

In the mid-1980s: Investigators supported by the (U.S.) National Institute for Neurological Disorders & Stroke (NINDS) were among the first to use an implanted device for deep brain stimulation in the thalamus as a treatment for chronic pain.

In 2000: Deep brain stimulation is introduced as an alternative and promising treatment option for patients suffering from severe Tourette's syndrome (TS).

In 2001: The magnetic stimulation therapy procedure is introduced.

In 2008: The (U.S.) FDA clears the first repetitive transcranial magnetic stimulation (rTMS) device to treat several types of depression, including depression with comorbid anxiety and depression with suicidality.

In 2018: The FDA cleared rTMS for severe obsessive compulsive disorder and, more recently, a rapid- acting form of it for treatment-resistant depression.

In 2022: Deep brain stimulation received an FDA's Breakthrough Device Designation (BDD) to investigate its use for treatment-resistant depression.

With growing evidence for the safety of neurostimulation and results suggesting earlier intervention may be beneficial, researchers further examined its use for targeting different brain areas. Further innovations are emerging with advances in neuroscience and technology. For example, while traditional DBS delivers constant stimulation, newer adaptive devices can self-tune stimulation in response to certain features of a person's brain activity or behavior. One such closed-loop device had been approved for the treatment of medically-refractory epilepsy. Nonetheless, questions remain about exactly how some such procedures work, and new directions are likely to emerge through research on the mechanisms that underlie their benefits.

What are brain stimulation therapies?

Brain stimulation therapies (BSTs) treat serious mental illnesses and can play an important role in treating mental disorders. They are often used when a person with a serious mental illness is experiencing dangerous circumstances, such as not responding to the outside world or being at risk of self-harm. The therapies operate by activating or inhibiting the brain with electricity, which can be given directly through electrodes implanted in the brain or indirectly through electrodes placed on the scalp. The electricity can also be induced by applying magnetic fields to the head. Research is ongoing to determine the best use of these therapies and if they are effective treatments for other disorders and conditions. The FDA has authorized certain such therapies to treat specific mental disorders, including depression, bipolar disorder, and obsessive-compulsive disorder (OCD). Other newer therapies may still be considered experimental.

The authorized therapies covered in this Chapter are:

> Electroconvulsive therapy (ECT);
> Repetitive transcranial magnetic stimulation (rTMS); and
> Vagus nerve stimulation (VNS)

whereas the experimental therapies covered are:

> Magnetic seizure therapy (MST); and
> Deep brain stimulation (DBS).

Other brain stimulation therapies may also hold promise for treating mental disorders, including:

> Transcranial direct current stimulation (tDCS);
> Transcranial alternating current stimulation (tACS);
> Transcranial random noise stimulation (tRNS); and
> Transcranial ultrasound stimulation (tUSS).

(See the FDA website for the latest information, warnings, and guidance on brain stimulation devices and announcements about new ones.)

The FDA commonly gives two types of authorization to devices like BSTs:

> **Approved:** This means that the FDA has decided that the benefits of the device outweigh the known risks, as demonstrated by the results of clinical testing. Approval is usually required for devices that might have a significant risk of injury or illness, including devices implanted in the body.

> **Cleared:** It means that the device is substantially equivalent to a similar device that the FDA has already cleared or approved. Clearance is usually given to lower-risk devices used outside of the body.

How do brain stimulation therapies work?

In most cases, BSTs are used only after other treatments have been tried. Although less frequently used than medication or psychotherapy, BSTs hold promise for people with certain mental disorders who have not responded to other treatments. They should be prescribed and monitored by a health care provider with specific training and expertise together with a trained medical team. Most BSTs involve using anesthesia to sedate the patient and a muscle relaxant to prevent the patient from moving. If so, an anesthesiologist will monitor breathing, heart rate, and blood pressure throughout the procedure.

A BST treatment plan is based on a person's individual needs and medical situation, and usually also includes medication, psychotherapy, or both, which should usually be continued during and after therapy to maintain clinical improvement.

Electroconvulsive therapy

Electroconvulsive therapy (ECT) is a noninvasive procedure that treats serious mental disorders by using an electric current to induce seizure activity in the brain. It has the longest history of use for depression and is one of the most widely used BSTs. The procedure has been cleared to treat severe depressive episodes in people aged 13 years and older with depression or bipolar disorder and, in some cases, to treat schizophrenia, schizoaffective disorder, and mania. ECT is still considered the "gold standard" for treatment-resistant depression.

ECT is usually considered only if a person's illness has not improved after trying other treatments like medication or psychotherapy. To be eligible for ECT, a person must have severe, treatment-resistant depression or require a rapid response due to life-threatening circumstances, such as being unable to move or respond to the outside world (e.g., is catatonic), being suicidal, or being malnourished. ECT can be effective when medications have not worked, cannot be tolerated, or are undesirable due to physical illness, which is often the case in older adults. ECT also begins working more rapidly than antidepressant medications, usually taking effect within the first week of treatment.

How does ECT work?

A typical course of ECT is administered three times a week until a patient's symptoms improve (usually within 6–12 treatments). Frequently, a patient who undergoes ECT also takes an antidepressant or mood-stabilizing medication. Before a doctor performs ECT, the patient is sedated with a short-acting general anesthetic and given an intravenous muscle relaxant to prevent movement. During the procedure:

> Electrodes are placed at precise locations on the patient's head.
> An electric current is sent through the electrodes into the brain, causing seizure activity that lasts under a minute. Anesthesia ensures that the patient does not experience pain or feel the electrical pulses. Often, a blood pressure cuff is used on an arm or leg to block the muscle relaxant and allow movement of that limb to confirm that the seizure activity is adequate.
> The patient awakens 5–10 minutes after the procedure ends, feeling groggy at first as the anesthesia wears off, but after about an hour, be usually alert and able to resume normal activities.

Modern ECT devices can deliver electrical signals using brief or ultra-brief pulses. These short pulses are as effective as the traditional form of ECT but are given at a lower dose, helping further reduce cognitive side effects.

Although ECT is effective in treating depressive episodes, follow-up treatment—either antidepressant medication or 'maintenance ECT' —is usually required to sustain clinical improvement and reduce the chances that symptoms return. Maintenance ECT varies depending on the patient's needs and may range from one session per week to one session every few months.

ECT side effects

The most common side effects associated with ECT include:

> ➤ Aches (head, muscles).
> ➤ Disorientation or confusion.
> ➤ **Memory loss.**
> ➤ Upset stomach.

Some patients may experience memory loss, especially of memories around the time of treatment. The memory problems are more severe, but usually improve over the days and weeks following the end of a treatment course. Also, memory problems are more common with the traditional form of ECT, known as 'bilateral ECT', in which electrodes are placed on both sides of the head. In comparison, 'unilateral ECT' involves placing an electrode on only one side of the head, typically the right side, because it is opposite the brain's learning and memory areas, with another electrode placed on top of the head.

Repetitive transcranial magnetic stimulation

Repetitive transcranial magnetic stimulation (rTMS) is a noninvasive therapy that uses a magnet to deliver repeated low-intensity pulses to stimulate the brain. The magnetic field it creates is about the same strength (1 Tesla) as an MRI scan.

rTMS uses

The FDA cleared the first rTMS device in 2008 to treat several types of depression, including depression with comorbid anxiety and depression with suicidality in people who did not respond to at least one antidepressant medication in the current depressive episode. Although ECT is still considered the "gold standard" for treatment-resistant depression, strong clinical evidence supports the effectiveness of rTMS in reducing depressive symptoms. rTMS is now used to treat moderate-to-severe depression in cases where medications have proven ineffective or intolerable. In 2018, the FDA also cleared rTMS for severe obsessive compulsive disorder (OCD) and, more recently, a rapid-acting form of rTMS for treatment-resistant depression. Accelerated protocols that act more quickly than standard rTMS show similar effectiveness while shortening treatment length. Thus, patients benefit from receiving an entire course of treatment in much less time and getting relief from their symptoms more rapidly. Newer rTMS forms involving magnetic pulses with other parameters are also under investigation to treat depression, OCD, and other mental disorders.

How does rTMS work?

Rather than electric currents, rTMS uses low-intensity magnetic pulses to stimulate the brain. Unlike ECT, in which stimulation is generalized, in rTMS, magnetic stimulation is targeted to a specific brain site. Also, in contrast to ECT, the procedure does not require anesthesia and can be performed in a clinical or office setting. A typical rTMS session lasts 30–60 minutes. A typical course of rTMS treatment consists of daily sessions 5 days per week for 4–6 weeks. Accelerated rTMS protocols work much faster (within seconds to minutes). In this case, multiple sessions are delivered on a single day, with short breaks in between.

During the procedure:

> An electromagnetic coil is held against the head near an area of the brain thought to be involved in mood regulation, cognitive control, or both. These brain areas include the left prefrontal cortex (for depression) and the dorsomedial prefrontal cortex or anterior cingulate cortex (for OCD). In deep TMS, two coils may be used to deliver more stimulation to the region and target larger structures deep in the brain.
> Short electromagnetic pulses are repeatedly administered through the coil or coils. The patient usually feels a slight knocking or tapping on the head as the pulses are administered.
> The magnetic pulses pass easily through the skull and cause small electric currents that stimulate nerve cells in the targeted brain region.

There is not consensus on the best way to position the coil on the head or deliver the electromagnetic pulses. It has also yet to be determined if rTMS works best when delivered as a single treatment or when combined with medication, psychotherapy, or both. Research is underway to establish the safest and most effective uses of rTMS, the optimal brain sites to target, and the best follow-up approach to sustain clinical improvement.

rTMS side effects

Despite being considered a safe technique, rTMS carries the risk of inducing seizures among other milder adverse events, and thus, its safety should be continuously assessed. Several research groups conducted studies of the safety and tolerability of rTMS in patients. They estimated the risk of seizures and other adverse events during or shortly after rTMS application. They concluded that the atypical seizure happened during high-frequency rTMS with maximum stimulator output for speech arrest, clinically arising from the region of stimulation. Further, the risk of seizure induction in patients undergoing rTMS is small whereas the risk of other adverse events is similar to that of rTMS applied to other conditions and to healthy subjects. Nonetheless, these results should be interpreted with caution. The similarity between the safety profiles of rTMS supports further investigation of rTMS as a therapy. Overall, rTMS is safe and well tolerated by patients. Its side effects include:

> Discomfort at the site on the head where the magnet is placed.
> Contraction or tingling of scalp, jaw, or face muscles during the procedure.
> Mild headaches or brief lightheadedness.
> Dizziness.

Using magnetic pulses and targeting a specific brain site results in a milder stimulation than in ECT, avoiding most seizure activity. Although it is possible for the procedure to cause seizures, the risk is rare. Most side effects appear to be mild and short-term when expert guidelines are followed. Long-term side effects have not been determined, and more research is needed to establish the long-term safety of rTMS.

Vagus nerve stimulation

Vagus nerve stimulation (VNS) is a surgical procedure that involves a device implanted under the skin. The device sends electrical pulses through the left vagus nerve that runs from the brainstem through the neck and down the side of the chest and abdomen. The nerve carries messages from the brain to the body's major organs, including the heart, lungs, intestines, and between areas of the brain that control mood, sleep, and other functions. More recently, this therapy has been simplified by the introduction of noninvasive VNS (known as transcutaneous VNS [tVNS]), which uses a portable device to send electrical stimulation through the skin to activate the vagus nerve. Although tVNS is still experimental, the approach may offer advantages over surgical VNS, such as greater accessibility and affordability, while avoiding surgical complications.

VNS to improve behavioral control

Non invasive electrical stimulation of the vagus nerve via tVNS has been studied for its effects on cognitive functions, and inhibitory control in patients. Taking into account the role that gamma-aminobutyric acid (GABA) plays in inhibitory control, the alteration of GABA neurotransmission and the possibility to increase its release with tVNS may improve behavioral control in movement disorders.

VNS other uses

VNS was initially developed as a treatment for epilepsy. Research using brain scans showed that the procedure also affected areas of the brain involved in mood regulation, with favorable effects on depression symptoms. In 2005, the FDA approved surgical VNS for depression when the following conditions are met:

- ➤ The patient is 18 years of age and older.
- ➤ The depression has lasted for 2 or more years.
- ➤ The depression is severe or recurrent.
- ➤ The depression has not eased after trying at least four other treatments.

However, despite FDA approval for depression, VNS is not intended as a first-line treatment and remains infrequently used. The results of studies examining its effectiveness for depression have been mixed. Whereas a review of clinical trials of VNS for treatment-resistant depression found a sustained reduction in depression symptoms and enhanced quality of life, other studies did not report meaningful improvements. A portable VNS device has been cleared by the FDA to treat post-traumatic stress disorder (PTSD) under a 'Breakthrough Device Designation (BDD)", given to medical devices with preliminary evidence of clinical effectiveness compared to other available treatments. Research is ongoing to test the efficacy and safety of tVNS for depression, PTSD, and other mental disorders.

How does VNS work?

VNS is traditionally a surgical procedure:

> A device about the size of a stopwatch called a pulse generator is implanted in the upper left side of the chest while the patient is under anesthesia.
> Connected to the pulse generator is an electrical lead wire, which is then connected from the generator to the left vagus nerve.
> Typically, 30-second electrical pulses are sent every five minutes from the generator to the vagus nerve. The duration and frequency of the pulses may vary depending on how the generator is programmed.
> The vagus nerve, in turn, delivers those electrical signals to the brain.

The pulse generator, which operates continuously, is powered by a battery that lasts around 10 years, after which it must be replaced. Patients usually do not feel pain or discomfort as the device operates. It may be several months before a patient notices any benefits, and not all patients respond to VNS. Some patients have no improvement in symptoms, and some may even get worse.

The device can be temporarily deactivated by placing a magnet over the chest where the generator is implanted. A patient may want to deactivate the device if side effects become intolerable or before engaging in strenuous activity or exercise because it can interfere with breathing. The device reactivates when the magnet is removed.

Noninvasive forms of VNS consist of a device worn around the neck or ears or a handheld device. There are many questions about the most effective stimulation sites, parameters, and protocols for tVNS, and research is ongoing to determine the optimal conditions to achieve the greatest clinical benefits.

VNS side effects

VNS is not without risk. There may be complications, such as infection or pain from the implant surgery, or the device may come loose, move around, or malfunction, all of which can require additional surgery to correct. Other potential side effects include:

- ➢ Discomfort or tingling in the area where the device is implanted.
- ➢ Voice changes or hoarseness.
- ➢ Cough or sore throat.
- ➢ Neck pain or headaches.
- ➢ Breathing problems, especially during exercise.
- ➢ Difficulty swallowing.
- ➢ Nausea or vomiting.

If cleared by the FDA, tVNS devices may help overcome some of these surgical issues. Nonetheless, mild side effects of tVNS have been reported, including:

- ➢ Tingling, pain, or itchiness around the stimulation site.
- ➢ Nausea or vomiting.
- ➢ Dizziness.

The long-term side effects of all forms of VNS are unknown.

Other brain stimulation therapies are actively being explored for specific mental disorders. The following therapies are still considered experimental and have not yet been authorized by the FDA to treat mental disorders.

Magnetic seizure therapy

Magnetic seizure therapy (MST) is a noninvasive procedure that uses high-powered magnetic stimulation to induce seizures. The seizures are targeted to a specific site in the brain. In the U.S., MST is available only as part of a clinical trial or research study.

How does MST work?

MST combines aspects of both ECT and rTMS. Like rTMS, MST uses magnetic pulses to stimulate a specific brain site. The pulses are given at a higher intensity and frequency than in rTMS to induce a seizure. Like in ECT, the patient is anesthetized and given a muscle relaxant to prevent movement during the procedure. The goal is to retain the effectiveness of ECT while reducing the risk of cognitive side effects.

During the procedure:

> ➢ An electromagnetic coil is held against the head, typically targeting the brain's prefrontal area.
> ➢ Rapidly alternating strong magnetic pulses pass through the coil into the brain to induce a seizure. Anesthesia is used to ensure that the patient does not experience pain or feel the electrical pulses.
> ➢ The magnetic dosage is individualized for each patient by finding the patient-specific seizure threshold.

There is not agreement on MST's optimal dosing, coil size, and stimulation site, and researchers are actively conducting studies to determine those specifications.

MST uses

Introduced in 2001, MST is currently in the early stages of investigation and clinical use for treating mental disorders. A review of randomized clinical trials (RCT) examining MST for treatment-resistant depression showed promising results. However, more confirmatory evidence is needed to draw conclusions about MST's effectiveness in treating depression and other mental disorders.

MST side effects

Like ECT, MST carries the risk of side effects caused by anesthesia and the induction of a seizure. These side effects can include the following:

- ➢ Headaches or scalp pain.
- ➢ Dizziness.
- ➢ Nausea or vomiting
- ➢ Muscle aches or fatigue.

A systematic review and meta-analysis found that MST produced **fewer memory problems** and other cognitive side effects and caused less confusion and shorter seizures compared to ECT.

Deep brain stimulation

At present time, deep brain stimulation (DBS) is still in its infancy. Due to differing legal jurisdictions and treatment facilities in different countries, guidelines issued by regulatory or/and other organizations and professional societies should be understood as recommendations of experts to be used in treatment- resistant, and severely affected patients. Further, it is highly recommended to perform DBS in the context of controlled trials (see Chapter 19).

DBS therapy is a surgical procedure that aims to improve **memory** that could not be accomplished with medication, and where surgery to treat the cause is not possible. It has become a valid option for individuals with severe symptoms that do not respond to conventional therapy and management, although it is an experimental treatment. It uses electricity to directly stimulate sites in the brain and can be used to treat severe OCD or depression in patients who have not responded to other treatments. It is available for other mental disorders only as part of a clinical trial.. Selecting candidates who may benefit from DBS is challenging, and the appropriate lower age range for surgery is unclear. It is potentially useful in less than 3% of individuals. The ideal brain location to target has not yet been identified.

How does DBS work?

DBS works by sending electrical pulses to specific brain areas. It requires surgery to implant electrodes in the brain. The specific brain area depends on the disorder being treated. For depression, the brain area was initially the subgenual anterior cingulate cortex, which can be overactive in depression and other mood disorders, and now includes several brain areas. For OCD, the brain area is usually the ventral capsule/ventral striatum or the bed nucleus of the stria terminalis.

Prior to the procedure, scans of the brain are taken using MRI as a guide to determine where to place the electrodes during surgery. Once a patient is ready for surgery:

> The head is numbed with a local anesthetic so the patient does not feel pain.
> The surgeon drills one or two small holes into the patient's head; threads a thin insulated wire, usually a pair of wires, through the hole(s) and into the brain; and places electrodes into a specific brain area (Figures 18.1-3).
> The patient is awake while the electrodes are implanted to provide feedback on their placement but does not feel pain because the head is numbed and the brain itself does not register pain.
> After the electrodes are implanted, the patient is put under general anesthesia.
> The electrodes are attached to wires that run inside the body from the head, through the neck and shoulder, and down to the chest where a small battery-operated generator (about the size of a pacemaker) is implanted. The pulse generator is placed under the skin in the upper chest. Whereas early DBS models used two pulse generators, one wired to each of the two implanted electrodes, most newer models use a single pulse generator to stimulate both electrodes.
> From the pulse generator, electrical pulses are delivered through the wires to the electrodes in the brain. Stimulation is applied continuously, and its frequency and level are customized to each patient. Although it is unclear exactly how DBS works to reduce symptoms, researchers

believe that the pulses help "reset" the malfunctioning area of the brain so that it works normally again.

After the procedure, the patient may be given a device-based tool (like a hand-held controller or smart phone app) to help them monitor and manage their symptoms at home or provide feedback to their clinical care team.

Once the system is in place, and after a period of post-surgery healing, the device is programmed and tuned to sets of parameters that work best for each person over several visits with a neurologist. The therapy works by delivering electrical pulses from the implantable pulse generator (IPG) along the extension wire and the lead, and into the brain. These pulses change the brain's electrical activity pattern at the target site to reduce motor symptoms.

The DBS system

The DBS system consists of three components: the lead, the extension, and the IPG. The "lead" (also called an electrode)—a thin, insulated wire—is inserted through a small opening in the skull and implanted into the brain (Figures 18.1-3). The tip of the electrode is positioned within the specific brain area depending on the disorder. The "extension" is an insulated wire that is passed under the skin of the head, neck, and shoulder, connecting the lead to the IPG. The IPG is a surgically-implanted, battery-operated medical device (the "battery pack") that is similar to a heart pacemaker and has the approximate size of a stop-watch. It delivers electrical stimulation to specific areas in the brain, blocking the abnormal nerve signals that cause symptoms. The IPG is usually implanted under the skin near the collarbone; in some cases, it may be implanted lower in the chest or under the skin over the abdomen.

Figure 18.1 – Pictorial showing an inserted deep brain stimulation electrode

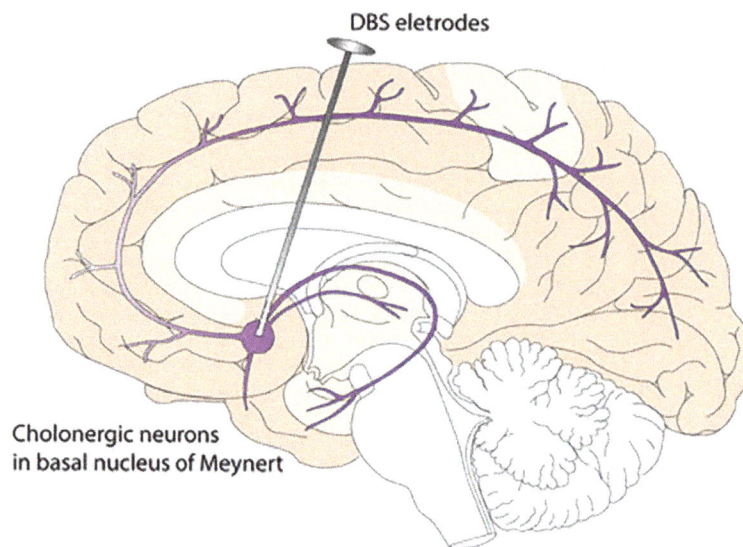

DBS eletrodes

Cholonergic neurons
in basal nucleus of Meynert

Treatment rationale

Patients with severe memory loss and resistant to medical and other therapy may benefit from the application of DBS. An important challenge and limitation in evaluating the evidence related to this procedure is that, even in expert DBS centers, extremely few if any operations per year are performed. Furthermore, there is limited information from randomized clinical trials for analysis and interpretation (see Sidebar 18.1).

Figure 18.2 - Placement of an electrode into the brain
(The head is stabilized in a frame for stereotactic surgery)

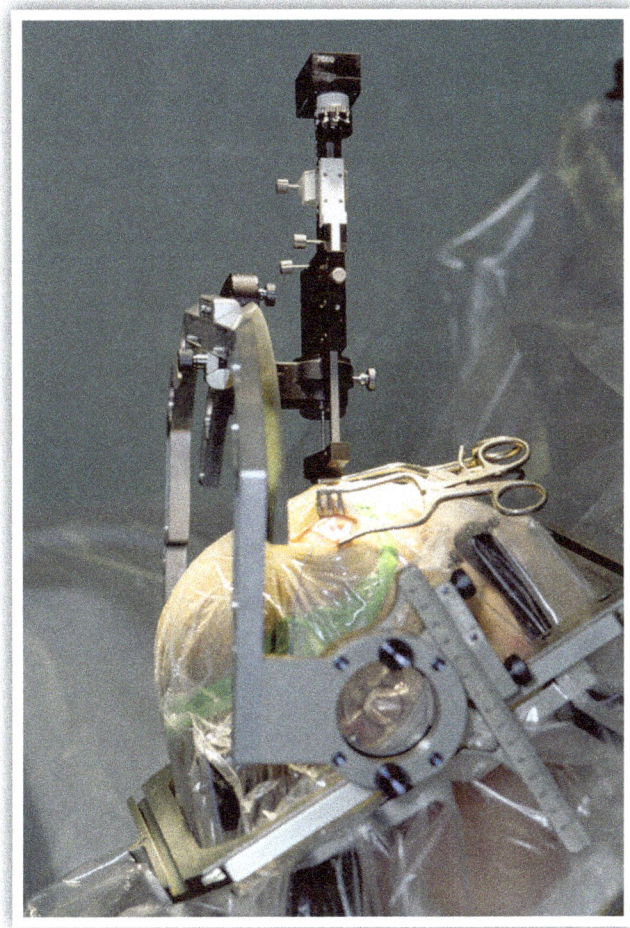

DBS uses

- DBS was first developed to treat movement disorders, including tremor and Parkinson's disease (PD).
- The FDA has since cleared DBS for severe OCD under a 'Humanitarian Device Exemption (HDE)',
- which is a provision for rare diseases or conditions experienced by relatively few patients among whom
- it has been difficult to gather evidence to demonstrate effectiveness. However, there is still much to be

- learned about optimizing DBS treatment. Similarly, in 2022, DBS received an FDA's Breakthrough
- Device Designation (BDD) to investigate its use for treatment-resistant depression.

Figure 18.3 - DBS-probes are shown in an X-ray of the skull

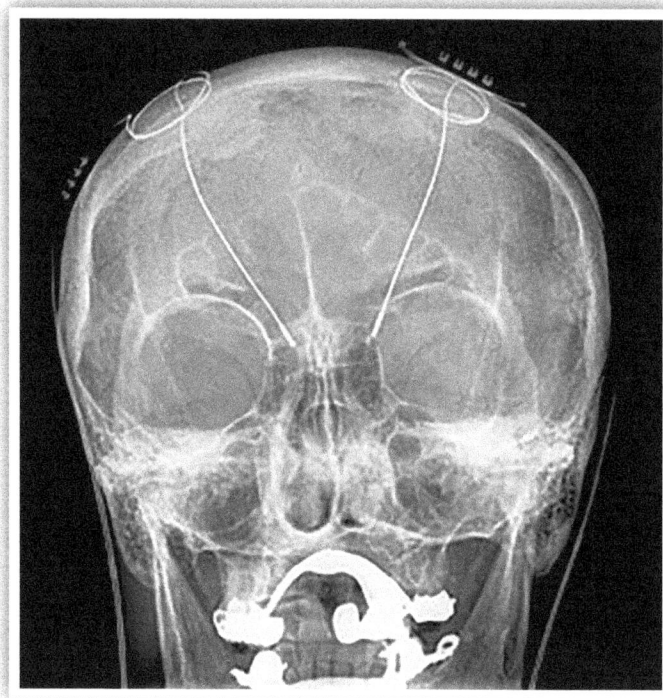

(Bright white areas around the maxilla and the mandibles represent metal dentures that are unrelated to the DBS device)

Although a systematic review found that DBS improves OCD symptoms, other review articles have called for more confirmatory evidence before drawing conclusions about its effectiveness. A systematic review and meta-analysis showed favorable effects of DBS in treating depression symptoms. Nonetheless, it remains an experimental treatment for depression until more data from high-quality studies are available.

DBS side effects

DBS carries risks associated with any brain surgery. For example, the procedure may lead to:

- ➢ Bleeding in the brain or stroke.
- ➢ Device-related discomfort, pain, or infection around the incision.
- ➢ Infection near the incision site.
- ➢ Headaches.
- ➢ Disorientation or confusion.
- ➢ **Cognitive impairment.**
- ➢ Lightheadedness, dizziness, nausea, or vomiting.
- ➢ Trouble sleeping, agitation, or restlessness.

Because the procedure is still being studied, other side effects not yet identified are possible. Long-term benefits and side effects are unknown.

Figure 18.4 - *Active DBS contact lesions in the bilateral atlas space* (*3D superior view*)

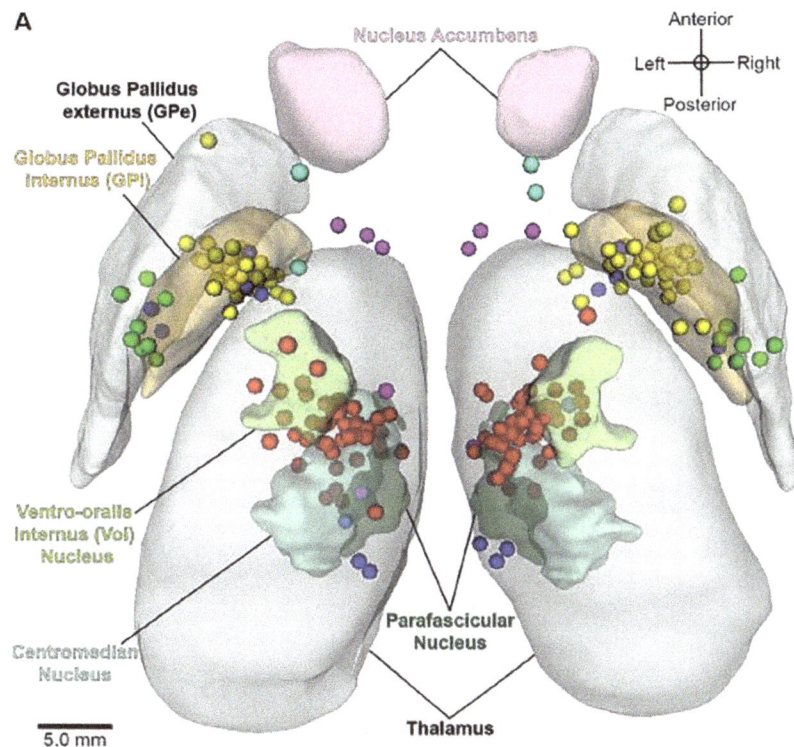

Source: Unknown

Surgery candidates and patients' selection

Surgery candidates should have the appropriate DSM-5 diagnosis with severe impairment despite exhaustive medical and other treatment trials. DBS should be offered to patients only by experienced DBS centers after evaluation by a multi-disciplinary team. Rigorous pre-operative and post-operative outcome measures and associated co-morbidities should be used. A local ethics committee (LEC) or institutional review board (IRB) should be consulted. While successes and failures have been reported for multiple brain targets, the optimal surgical approach remains unknown. Though still evolving, DBS is a promising approach for a subset of medication-refractory and severely-affected patients. Sidebar 18.1 retraces the surgical evaluation phases.

Appropriate patient selection is one of the most important predictors of success of DBS treatment, making multi-disciplinary evaluation essential. Because of the complexity of the patient population, centers performing DBS have been encouraged to screen candidates pre-operatively and to follow them post-operatively. There has been concern about high risk of suicide and other negative psychiatric sequelae in patients not screened and monitored for depression, anxiety, and bipolar tendencies.

Treatment recommendations

Treatment recommendations have been made by certain professional societies. For example, the Movement Disorders Society (MDS) recommends that best practices be followed, including: Confirmation of diagnosis; use of multidisciplinary screening; preoperative and postoperative visits for tuning the stimulation parameters and recording stimulation effects; and stabilization of psychiatric co-morbidities inclusive of active suicidality. In 2019, the American Academy of Neurology (AAN) had also issued its own recommendations.

In 2011, 63 patients have received DBS in 19 centers worldwide. As reported in the literature, 59 had a beneficial outcome following DBS with moderate-to-marked movement disorder improvement. However, randomized controlled studies including a larger number of patients are still lacking. Although persistent serious adverse effects (AEs) have hardly been reported, surgery-related (e.g., bleeding, infection) as well as stimulation-related AEs (e.g., sedation, anxiety, altered mood, changes in sexual function) may occur. Only two studies on just a few patients fulfill some of the evidence-based criteria. DBS for movement disorders such as, for example, Tourette's syndrome (TS) is therefore still highly experimental.

Stimulated brain regions

Different key structures and different brain targets have been defined for DBS:

> **Thalamus:** Centromedian-parafascicular complex region and subthalamic nucleus.
> **Globus pallidus:** Internus (ventral and dorsal), externus, and anteromedial (which is probably more likely than sham stimulation to reduce tic severity.
> **Nucleus accumbens:** Ventral capsular.
> **Basal ganglia.**
> **Vagus nerve.**

Figure 18.4 shows the *active DBS contact lesions in the bilateral atlas space (3D superior view). The circles represent an active DBS contact colored by its intended structural DBS target region. The active contacts are usually all found to be located relatively near the intended target nuclei.*

Treatment complications

Complications of treatment, including infection and removal of hardware, appear more common with DBS than with other neurologic conditions.

Benefits and risks of DBS

DBS is a surgical procedure that involves minimal permanent surgical changes to the brain and is minimally invasive. There is a low chance the placement of the stimulator may cause bleeding or infection in the brain. Nonetheless, it carries some associated risk. Complications may include bleeding and swelling of brain tissue, headaches, seizures, and temporary pain following the surgery. Such complications may result from mechanical stress from the device but are generally reversible. Also, the hardware may erode or break down with use, requiring surgery to replace parts of the device. If the DBS causes unwanted side effects or newer, more promising treatments develop in the future, the IPG can be removed and the DBS procedure halted. Also, stimulation from the IPG is easily adjustable—without further surgery—if the person's condition changes. Data on harms related to the use of DBS can be found in the complete and unabridged practice guideline.

The largest available randomized trials of DBS have revealed benefits on motor and phonic tics for the ventral globus pallidus internus and the centromedian thalamic region target (refer to Figure 18.4). However, these studies have raised methodological concerns that need to be addressed in future trials. Such concerns include intracerebral hemorrhage (a probability of 0.5%–2.0%), infection (1%–3%), as well as DBS-specific issues such as lead migration and fracture (1%–3%) and device malfunction (1%–3%). There is little information on the effects of DBS on psychiatric co-morbidities.

Prognosis following the procedure

DBS changes the brain firing pattern but does not slow the progression of the neurodegeneration. Despite small patient numbers, the procedure remains a valid option for medically intractable patients. Different brain targets result in comparable improvement rates, indicating a modulation of a common network. Future studies might focus on a better characterization of the clinical effects of distinct regions, rather than searching for a unique target.

International DBS Registry

An international DBS Registry has been developed to collect data on DBS outcomes in patients in various centers. The Registry also collects information about response to non-standardized selection criteria, various brain targets, differences in hardware, and variability in the programming parameters used.

Transcranial electrotherapy stimulation

Recent imaging data suggest that a disruption in the pattern of functional connectivity in cortico-basal ganglia networks could reflect a defect in brain maturation. However, it is difficult to capture on-line the cortical changes associated with tic generation using imaging techniques due to moving artifacts. The aims of the various TES studies relate to median nerve stimulation (MNS), continuous theta burst stimulation (cTBS), brain stimulation, and vagus nerve stimulation (VNS).

Brain stimulation may help with symptoms such as **memory**, concentration problems, movement symptoms, and mood in patients with a movement disorder who have mild-to-moderate problems with these mental abilities. The procedure does not involve any surgery or hair removal but places a small amount of electrode gel on the head to hold two electrodes while a small electrical current is generated. While occasionally leading to mild side-effects (e.g. headache, nausea, fatigue, exacerbation of scalp skin conditions), there are no known harmful long term effects. The positive benefits of brain stimulation can include **improving brain functioning with memory problems**. It is also possible that mood symptoms (e.g. depressive thoughts) could improve.

As a non-invasive therapy, cranial electrotherapy stimulation (CES) may be applied in various areas with few side effects.

Continuous theta burst stimulation

Continuous theta burst stimulation (cTBS) is relatively safe and effective, and its efficacy in psychiatric diseases has been gradually recognized. However, the results of current researches in the case of tic disorder treatment are varied and the evaluation method is relatively simple. cTBS under functional MRI-guided stimulation is employed in patients with tics to explore individualized cTBS treatment parameters, including stimulation frequency, intensity, type, time, and stimulation target. Based on DBS studies that reported that the medial globus pallidus internum (GPi) showed an obvious curative effect, a deep brain area can be modulated indirectly by a superficial target via functional connectivity. Therefore, cTBS stimulates the superficial target in the supplementary motor area (SMA) and the lateral motor area (LMA). Combined with clinical symptoms and neuroimaging, the therapeutic effect of cTBS may provide a new therapeutic method and a better therapeutic effect for the disease.

Other types of brain stimulation therapy

Other types of brain stimulation therapy are in development. Most are used in combination with other therapies or treatments to optimize clinical outcomes. One emerging therapy that shows promise for treating mental disorders is trigeminal nerve stimulation (TNS), which was FDA-approved to treat attention-deficit/hyperactivity disorder (ADHD) in children, but it has not yet been approved to treat other conditions or for adults.

The Neuromodulation and Neurostimulation Program and the Multimodal Neurotherapeutics Program at NIMH support researchers as they develop new therapies and refine existing therapies to treat mental disorders and conditions.

Table 18.1 is a summary of the several brain stimulation therapies including their therapeutic indication, the brain region(s) they stimulate, and their side effects.

Table 18.1 – The various brain stimulation therapies and their particulars

Brain stimulation therapy	Therapeutic indication	Brain region(s) stimulated	Benefits & Side effects
Generally Activating/inhibiting brain with electrical/ magnetic fields	o Serious mental illnesses o Authorized: Depression, bipolar disorder, and OCD		
Electroconvulsive therapy (ECT)* - Unilateral - Bilateral	o Bipolar disorder o Depression ("gold standard") o Rapid response due to life-threatening circumstances *In some cases:* o Mania o Schizophrenia o Schizoaffective disorder	Precise location(s) on patient's head	o Can be effective when medications have not worked, cannot be tolerated, or are undesirable Side effects: o Aches (head, muscles) - Confusion o Disorientation o **Memory loss** o Stomach upset

Transcranial electrotherapy stimulation (tETS)*	o **Memory** o Concentration problems o Movement symptoms o Mood symptoms (depressive thoughts)	Corticobasal ganglia networks	o Improvements in brain functioning with **memory problems** o Improvements in mood symptoms (e.g. depressive thoughts) Side effects: o Fatigue o Headache o Nausea o Scalp or/and skin conditions exacerbation o No known harmful long-term effects
Repetitive transcranial magnetic stimulation (rTMS)*	o Depression, including with comorbid anxiety and with suicidality ("gold standard") o Severe obsessive compulsive disorder o Other mental disorders	o Head near area of the brain involved in mood regulation, cognitive control, or both - Dorsomedial prefrontal cortex or anterior cingulate cortex (for OCD) - Left prefrontal cortex (for depression) o No consensus on the best approach	Side effects: o Contraction or tingling of scalp, jaw, or face muscles o Discomfort o Dizziness. o Mild headaches or brief lightheadedness o Risk of inducing seizures
Vagus nerve stimulation (VNS)*	o Behavioral control in movement disorders o Cognitive functions o Depression (not a first-line treatment) o Epilepsy o Inhibitory control o Mood regulation	o Electrical pulses through left vagus nerve from brainstem through neck, side of chest, and abdomen - Invasive (subcutaneous) - Non-invasive (transcutaneous)	Side effects: o Breathing problems o Cough or sore throat o Difficulty swallowing o Discomfort or tingling o Dizziness o Infection o Nausea or vomiting o Neck pain or headaches o Tingling, pain, or itchiness around the stimulation site o Voice changes or hoarseness Long-term side effects of all forms not known

Magnetic seizure therapy (MST)** (In U.S. only in clinical trials and research)	o Mental disorders o Treatment-resistant depression More confirmatory evidence needed	Specific brain site to induce seizure	o Less confusion o **Fewer memory problems** o Fewer other cognitive side effects o Shorter seizures compared to ECT. Side effects: o Dizziness o Headaches or scalp pain o Muscle aches or fatigue o Nausea or vomiting No agreement on optimal dosing, coil size, or stimulation site
Deep brain stimulation (DBS)** (Experimental)	o Depression in patients not responding to other treatments o Movement disorders (tremor, Parkinson's disease) o Severe **memory loss**, resistant to medical and other therapy o Severe OCD (need confirmatory evidence)	o Basal ganglia o Globus pallidus: Internus (ventral and dorsal), externus, and anteromedial o Nucleus accumbens: Ventral capsular o Thalamus: Centromedian-parafascicular complex region and subthalamic nucleus o Vagus nerve. Direct stimulation of specific brain areas o For depression: Subgenual anterior cingulate cortex o For OCD: Ventral capsule/ventral striatum or bed nucleus of stria terminalis	o Improves **memory** o Improves other mental disorders (only as part of a clinical trial) o Long-term benefits unknown Side effects: o Bleeding in brain or stroke o **Cognitive impairment** o Device-related discomfort, pain, or infection around incision o Disorientation or confusion o Headaches o Infection near incision site o Lightheadedness, dizziness, nausea, or vomiting. o Trouble sleeping, agitation, or restlessness. o Other side effects not yet identified o Long-term side effects not known
Transcranial alternating current stimulation (tACS)***			
Transcranial direct current stimulation (tDCS)***			
Transcranial random noise stimulation (tRNS)***			

Transcranial ultrasound stimulation (tUSS)***			

Key: *=Authorized; **=Experimental; ***=Other promising therapies

Take-aways

➢ Surgery can be an optional treatment in those rare cases of severely disabled patients who do not improve using standard approaches. It includes electroconvulsive therapy, transcranial electrotherapy stimulation, continuous theta burst stimulation, repetitive transcranial magnetic stimulation, vagus nerve stimulation, magnetic seizure therapy, and deep brain stimulation.

➢ Brain stimulation therapies treat serious mental illnesses and can play an important role in treating mental disorders. They operate by activating or inhibiting the brain with electricity. The FDA has authorized certain such therapies to treat specific mental disorders, including depression, bipolar disorder, and obsessive-compulsive disorder. Other newer therapies may still be considered experimental.

➢ The authorized therapies include: Electroconvulsive therapy, repetitive transcranial magnetic stimulation, and vagus nerve stimulation whereas the experimental therapies include: magnetic seizure therapy and deep brain stimulation. Other brain stimulation therapies may also hold promise for treating mental disorders, including: Transcranial direct current stimulation, transcranial alternating current stimulation, transcranial random noise stimulation, and transcranial ultrasound stimulation. Surgical procedures need to be further investigated and used only at expert centers.

➢ In most cases, brain stimulation therapies are used only after other treatments have been tried. Although less frequently used than medication or psychotherapy, they hold promise for people with certain mental disorders who have not responded to other treatments. The treatment plan is based on a person's individual needs and medical situation, and usually also includes medication, psychotherapy, or both.

➢ Electroconvulsive therapy is a noninvasive procedure that treats serious mental disorders by using an electric current to induce seizure activity in the brain. It treats severe depressive episodes in people aged 13 years and older with depression or bipolar disorder and, in some cases, to treat schizophrenia, schizoaffective disorder, and mania. It is still considered the "gold standard" for treatment-resistant depression.

➤ Continuous theta burst stimulation is relatively safe and effective in psychiatric diseases. Combined with clinical symptoms and neuroimaging, it may provide a new therapeutic method and a better therapeutic effect.

➤ Repetitive transcranial magnetic stimulation delivers repeated low-intensity pulses to stimulate the brain. It is used to treat moderate-to-severe depression in cases where medications have proven ineffective or intolerable. More recently, a rapid-acting form of it or treatment-resistant depression acts more quickly than the standard form and shows similar effectiveness while shortening treatment length. Despite being considered a safe technique, it carries the risk of inducing seizures among other milder adverse events, and thus, its safety should be continuously assessed.

➤ Vagus nerve stimulation, including its noninvasive transcutaneous form is still experimental but may offer advantages over surgery.

➤ Magnetic seizure therapy is a noninvasive procedure that uses high-powered magnetic stimulation to induce seizures targeted to a specific site in the brain. In the U.S., it is available only as part of a clinical trial or research study. It produces fewer memory problems and other cognitive side effects and caused less confusion and shorter seizures compared to electroconvulsive therapy.

➤ Deep brain stimulation therapy is a surgical treatment that has become a valid option for individuals with severe symptoms that do not respond to conventional therapy and management, although it is an experimental treatment. It delivers electrical stimulation to specific areas in the brain that control movement, blocking the abnormal nerve signals that cause symptoms.

➤ Deep brain stimulation therapy should be offered to patients only by experienced centers after evaluation by a multi-disciplinary team. The optimal surgical approach remains unknown. Though still evolving, it is a promising approach for a subset of medication-refractory and severely-affected patients.

- Appropriate patient selection is one of the most important predictors of success of deep brain stimulation treatment, making multi-disciplinary evaluation essential. There is no consensus on the optimal brain target. There is little information on the effects on psychiatric co-morbidities.
- An international deep brain stimulation Registry has been developed to collect data on DBS outcomes in implanted patients in various centers.
- Brain stimulation may help with symptoms such as **memory**, concentration problems, movement symptoms, and mood in patients with a movement disorder who have mild-to-moderate problems with these mental abilities.
- Of the well-known therapies, it would appear from Table 18.1 that convulsive therapy, transcranial electrotherapy stimulation, magnetic seizure therapy, and deep brain stimulation could be of use in the treatment of memory problems.

Sidebar 18.1 – Surgical evaluation phases

Pre-surgical non-invasive evaluation – Phase I

Pre-surgical evaluation consists of a one- or two-phase process to determine if surgery is the best option and can improve **memory** with minimal risk. Phase I involves all non-invasive (non-surgical) tests whereas Phase II involves invasive tests (requiring surgery) that are used in selecting patients.

Phase I evaluation is designed to find the area of the brain that is likely to be generating the memory disorder (the focus), to determine if that area can be safely treated, and to predict what kind of outcome might be expected.

There are generally six tests involved in Phase I, but not every patient requires every test available in this evaluation. For the selection of the necessary and appropriate tests, patients are evaluated by neurologists who determine such tests on an individualized basis. The tests provide separate independent information that can be correlated in order to zero-in on the location of origin of the memory disorder. These tests comprise:

Inpatient video-EEG monitoring

The aim of this test is to identify the likely location in the brain where memory disorders originate. As its name implies, inpatient video-EEG monitoring is a recording with simultaneous video and EEG. It is the most important pre-surgical test and is generally conducted in an inpatient setting in a specialized monitoring unit. It is performed with electrodes attached to the scalp (noninvasive monitoring). All the data are analyzed by a trained neurologist to evidence the likely location where the memory disorders might originate within the brain.

Magnetic resonance imaging (MRI)

The aim of this test is to detect abnormalities in the brain. The test may detect an abnormality that could be the cause of the memory disorders. With more powerful MRI machines and use of special protocols and software, subtle brain abnormalities are increasingly being identified.

Positron emission tomography (PET)

The aim of this test is to localize brain regions with decreased brain function. PET scans record the metabolic activity of the brain to determine if the brain is functioning normally. In patients with memory disorders, decreased brain function is seen in the region where they originate. On the other hand, the scan may show abnormalities even if the brain MRI is normal. PET scans are usually done in the outpatient setting.

Single-photon emission computed tomography (SPECT)

The aim of this test is to identify brain regions with increased blood flow. Single photon emission computed tomography (SPECT) scans can identify the brain regions where blood flow increases and thus indicate where the memory disorders might have begun. SPECT scans are performed when the patient is admitted to the hospital for video-EEG monitoring.

Neuropsychological evaluation and functional MRI

The aim of this combination test is to predict cognitive deficits after surgery. Neuropsychological evaluation and functional MRI (fMRI) are used to assess cognitive functions, especially language and **memory** function prior to surgery to determine which side of the brain is dominant for language and if there is decreased memory function. This allows prediction of cognitive deficits after surgery. Functional MRI measures blood flow changes in areas of the brain during the performance of specific cognitive tasks.

Intracarotid amobarbital/methohexital (Wada test)

The aim of this test is to predict language and **memory** function post surgery. Performed in selected cases, the test involves the injection of a medication such as sodium *Amobarbital* or *Methohexital* into one carotid artery at a time. The medication causes temporary (1-5 minutes) paralysis of one half of the brain allowing independent testing of language and memory function in the other half. This test is also used to predict post-operative deficits in language and memory function.

If all tests performed point to the same region of the brain, the patient is likely to be a good surgical candidate.

Based on the results of the Phase I evaluation, patients may be deemed good or poor surgical candidates. In some cases, despite all prior tests, surgical treatment may not be advisable so that more testing would be needed (called Phase II evaluation).

Presurgical invasive evaluation - Phase II

Phase II evaluation involves video-EEG monitoring with electrodes that are placed inside the skull (invasive monitoring). As there is more risk from invasive monitoring, the decision about the necessity for a Phase II evaluation is usually made by the neurological team as a whole and discussed in detail with the patient.

There are six surgical implantation options, each involving the implantation of electrodes either on the surface of the brain, or within the brain. The benefit of these electrodes is that they are closer to the area producing the **memory disorders** than those placed simply on the scalp. After surgical placement of electrodes, neurologists perform video-EEG monitoring in a similar fashion to the phase I monitoring.

The electrode types and implantation arrays differ and may include:

- **Subdural electrodes:** A subdural electrode grid is a thin sheet of material with multiple small (a couple of millimeters in size) recording electrodes implanted within it. The electrodes are placed directly on the surface of the brain. They have the advantage of recording the EEG without the interference of skin, fat tissue, muscle, and bone that may limit scalp EEG. Shapes and sizes of these sheets are chosen to best conform to the surface of the brain and the area of interest.

- **Depth electrodes:** These are small wires surrounded by electrodes, which are implanted within the brain itself through small skin pokes. The electrodes are able to record brain activity along the entire length of the implanted wire. They have the advantage of recording activity from structures deeper in the brain. They can be implanted.

- **Electrodes combination:** In a number of instances, it may be beneficial to implant a combination of subdural and depth electrodes.

Stereoelectroencephalography

Increasingly common, invasive monitoring may be done using stereoelectroencephalography (sEEG). Here, multiple depth electrodes are implanted in a specific pattern individualized to the patient. The three-dimensional space which is covered by the depth electrodes is designed to encompass the seizure focus.

Functional mapping

This is usually performed in patients with implanted subdural electrodes. Brief electrical stimulation is provided through each electrode separately to determine the normal function of the part of the brain underneath that electrode. It is a painless procedure. The purpose is to map out critically important areas of the brain such as those necessary for motor, sensory, and language functions. This allows tailoring of surgical resections to minimize the risk of major neurological deficits after surgery.

19

Treatment portfolio:
V. Participation in clinical trials

Contents

19

Treatment portfolio: IV. Participation in clinical trials

On clinical trials and research studies

Clinical trials (CTs) are prospective biomedical or biobehavioral research studies on human participants designed to answer specific questions about biomedical or biobehavioral interventions, including new treatments (such as novel vaccines, drugs, dietary choices, dietary supplements, and medical devices) and known interventions that warrant further study and comparison. They generate data on dosage, safety, and efficacy and look at new ways to prevent, detect, or treat diseases. Treatments might be new drugs or new combinations of drugs, new surgical procedures or devices, or new ways to use existing treatments. They can also look at other aspects of care such as improving the quality of life for people with chronic illnesses. Their overriding goal is to determine if a new test or treatment works and is safe.

People with memory problems may be able to take part in clinical trials. Healthy people with no memory problems and no family history of such conditions may also be able to participate. Joining a clinical trial or other research study is also a way to help fight such issues. To find out more about clinical trials:

- Check out www.ClinicalTrials.gov.
- See "NIH Clinical Research Trials and You" at www.nih.gov/health/clinicaltrials. This is a resource for people who want to learn more about clinical trials. (For answers to common questions about taking part in a clinical trial, refer to Chapter 22 of this book.)
- Visit the **Alzheimer's and related Dementias Education and Referral (ADEAR) Center** website at www.alzheimers.gov.
- Call the Alzheimer's and related Dementias Education and Referral (ADEAR) Center.
  Tel: 800-438-4380.

Sidebar 19.1 provides the main particulars of clinical trials. The following sections will briefly set forth the particulars and aims of 100 such trials on memory, which have been extracted from the 1908 clinical trials indicated on clinicaltrials.gov website as of the date of this writing (25 September 2023), Irrespective of its status, any trial having submitted results could be of interest to memory patients, their families, and carers if appropriate for the patient's medical condition.

Questions usually asked by potential memory participants

Can a memory patient participate in a clinical trial?

Yes, and it is encouraged for those eligible participants. The best way to find out about trials and to express interest in participating in one of them is to be referred by one's own neurologist or physician. That healthcare professional will be able to identify possible suitable trials for the existing medical condition, make a referral, and facilitate the enrollment process, as appropriate.

Is the list of clinical trials available?

It can be found on line: www.clinicaltrials.gov. This site lists all registered trials across the world and their status: New [N], Recruiting [R], Not Yet Recruiting

[NYR], Not Recruiting [NR]; Enrolling By Invitation [EBI]; Completed [C], Suspended [S], Terminated]T], Unknown [U], or Withdrawn [W].

Does it cost anything to participate in a clinical trial?

Participation is usually free.

Currently recruiting clinical trials

The number of clinical trials that are currently recruiting may vary depending on the particular date at which the website clinicaltrials.gov is searched.

Trials on memory functions and physiological processes

[C] Influence of Salbutamol on Emotional and Cognitive Functions in Healthy Subjects (Salmon-Basel) (ID NCT01957293) - Last update posted: 2014-12-16
Sponsor. University of Basel, Switzerland
Aim: To investigate the effect of beta-2 adrenergic stimulant salbutamol on **emotional and cognitive functions** in healthy humans.

[C] Influence of Cincalcet on Cognitive Functions in Healthy Human Subjects
(ID NCT01599962) - Last update posted: 2012-10-03
Sponsor: University of Basel, Switzerland
Aim: To investigate the effects of the calcimimetic agent Cincalcet on **cognitive functions** in healthy humans.

[NYR] Influence of Luteolin for Two Weeks on Memory in Healthy Subjects (LuMus2-2023)
ID NCT06047899 - Last update posted: 2023-09-21
Sponsor University of Basel, Switzerland
Aim: To learn if the dietary supplement Luteolin has a positive influence on memory functions in healthy people.

[T] Influence of Luteolin on Memory in Healthy Subjects (LuMus-Basel 20)

ID NCT04468854 - Last update posted: 2020-07-13

Sponsor University of Basel, Switzerland

Aim: To study the **physiological processes** (forgetting and **memory functions**, attention, **working memory**) in participants after multiple administration of the dietary supplement Luteolin.

[R] Communication Memory of Cancer Diagnosis Within the Pediatric Triangle

ID NCT04392908 - Last update posted: 2022-08-25

Sponsor Meyer Children's Hospital IRCCS, Florence, Italy

Aim: To investigate **memory functions** related to a cancer communication diagnosis in pediatric oncology.

[C] Brain-Derived Neurotrophic Factor (BDNF) Levels After Bacopa

ID NCT03974399 - Last update posted: 2021-03-02

Sponsor: Roskamp Institute Inc., Sarasota, Florida, USA

Aim: To investigate if level changes in BDNF (a well-known neurotrophic factor important for learning, **memory**, and synaptogenesis) in people after starting Bacopa enhances **cognition** and improves **mood.**

[C] Resveratrol for Improved Performance in the Elderly (RIPE)

ID NCT01126229 - Last update posted: 2013-12-11

Sponsor: University of Florida, USA

Aim: To determine whether a dietary ingredient Resveratrol supplementation is safe in the longer term and effective on age-related health conditions.and improves **memory** and physical performance in older adults.

[NR] Screening for Memory Studies

ClinicalTrials.gov ID NCT01123018 - Last update posted: 2022-04-27

Sponsor: VA Palo Alto Health Care System, Palo Alto, California, USA

Aim: To advertize, recruit, and do a preliminary screen for various clinical trials. Anonymous information collected will be entered in a database available to researchers connected with the Stanford/VA

Aging Clinical Research Center, located at VA Palo Alto Health Care System, Palo Alto Division.

[U] Functional Magnetic Resonance Imaging Study of Jaw-tapping Movement on Memory Function

ID NCT01873664 - Last update posted: 2013-06-10

Sponsor: Kyunghee University Medical Center, Gangdong, Republic of South Korea

Aim: To examine the possibility of using jaw-tapping training as a self-exercise for **developing memory** and preventing dementia in elderly subjects with memory disturbances using functional magnetic resonance imaging (fMRI).

[U] Multi-domain Versus Uni-Domain Training on Executive Control and Memory Functions of Older Adults (VIBAL)

ID NCT03823183 - Last update posted: 2019-02-01

Sponsor: Universidad Nacional de Educación a Distancia, Madrid, Spain

Aim: To examine the differential impact of multi-domain cognitive (video game training) and physical training (body-attack; a mix of dance, aerobic, strength, and muscular resistance) versus cognitive training and physical training separately on executive control and **memory functions** of healthy older adults in comparison with an active control group.

Trials on memory processes

[R] Decoding and Selective Modulation of Human Memory During Awake/Sleep Cycles

ID NCT05452122 - Last update posted: 2022-08-16

Sponsor: University of California, Los Angeles, USA

Aim: To elucidate **memory processes** and consolidation during sleep by leveraging the unique capability of direct recordings from the human brain at multiple levels of resolution-single neurons, localized neuronal assemblies, intracranial local field potentials during rich behavioral tasks with real-life narratives and extracting neural features that relate to different aspects of episodic experience. Further, to probe causal mechanisms of consolidation by application of auditory and electrical stimulations during sleep and its effect on modulating memory processes.

[U] Human Single Neuron Recordings in Epilepsy Patients
ID NCT04290416 - Last update posted: 2020-02-28

Sponsor: University of Birmingham, United Kingdom

Aim: To uncover the neural mechanisms underlying **memory formation and retrieval** using single neuron recordings in pre-surgical epilepsy patients and to improve diagnostic tools to identify epileptogenic tissue.

Trials on memory lapse / consolidation / reactivation

Memory consolidation is the transformation of recent experiences into stable, long-term memories.

[R] Toward a Real-time Access to Sleepers' Mental Content
ID NCT05452733 - Last update posted: 2023-05-08

Sponsor: Assistance Publique - Hôpitaux de Paris, Service des Pathologies du Sommeil, Hopital Pitie La Salpetriere, Paris, France

Aim: To provide real-time measures of the cognitive processes occurring within sleep using auditory stimulation in people with unique sleep peculiarities: sleepwalkers whose overt behaviors may enable to objectively visualize ongoing cognitive processes during non-REM (NREM) sleep.

[T] Autonomic Mechanisms of Sleep-dependent Memory Consolidation
(Terminated due to COVID-19)

ID NCT04021797 - Last Update Posted 2021-05-2

Sponsor: Langley Porter Psychiatric Institute, University of California, San Francisco, USA

Aim: To identify the impact vagal activity during sleep for memory formation and to examine the autonomic nervous system during sleep as a critical, causal pathway linking sleep to memory processing.

[NR] Mindful Attention to Variability in Everyday Memory
ID NCT03949868 - Last update posted: 2021-10-26

Sponsor: Harvard University, Massachusetts, USA

Aim: To investigate the 'attention to variability paradigm' through memory performance fluctuations throughout the day to provide **memory efficacy beliefs** and **memory performance** on a telephone task.

[C] Dietary Flavanols and Dentate Gyrus Function

ID NCT02312310 - Last update posted: 2020-06-11

Sponsor: New York State Psychiatric Institute, New York, USA

Aim: To assess the effect of differing amounts of a cocoa-derived dietary flavanol (epicatechin) on dentate gyrus function and corresponding **cognitive function.**

[R] The Impact of Reactivation During Sleep on the Consolidation of Abstract Information in Humans

ID NCT05746299 - Last update posted: 2023-04-14

Sponsor: University of Pennsylvania, Philadelpia, Pennsylvania, USA

Aim: To implement a "structure transfer" extension of a paradigm in which carefully designed graph structures govern the pattern of feature co-occurrences within individual categories in order to determine whether learning one structured category facilitates learning of a second identically structured category defined by a new set of features. Further, to provide evidence that structure representations are abstract to some degree.

[C] Neurophysiological Effects of Whole Coffee Cherry Extract in Older Adults

ID NCT03812744 - Last update posted: 2019-01-23

Sponsor:Auburn University, USA

Aim: To characterize the changes in the brain and body associated with whole coffee cherry extract, a source of naturally occurring nutrients.

[C] Effects Of Detrol LA On Memory And Cognition In Elderly Population

ID NCT00411437 - Last update posted: 2021-01-27

Sponsor: Pfizer's Upjohn/Mylan/Viatris Inc., tucson, Arizona, USA

Aim: To show that Tolterodine extended release has no effect on **memory** and other **cognitive abilities** in an elderly population.

[C] The Evaluation of the Efficacy and Safety of Donepezil Hydrochloride in Subjects With Mild Cognitive Impairment (MCI)

ID NCT00293176 - Last update posted: 2011-04-01

Sponsor: Eisai Inc.

Aim: To investigate the efficacy and safety of Donepezil in individuals with mild cognitive impairment on measures of **cognition**, global function and behavior.

[C] A Pilot Study to Assess the Amnesic Properties of Dexmedetomidine in Pediatric Patients

ID NCT02354378 - Last update posted: 2019-02-28

Sponsor: Boston Children's Hospital, Boston, Massachusetts, USA

Aim: To determine the effects of Dexmedetomidine on **memory and recall** of children who are receiving the standard Dexmedetomidine sedation administered for magnetic resonance imaging (MRI) studies.

Trials on memory delays, deficits, impairments, and disorders

[U] Attention and Memory Disorders Related to Acute Morphine (MEMOMORPH)

ID NCT03507985 - Last update posted: 2018-07-11

Sponsor: University Hospital, Toulouse, France

Aim: To determine if there are attention disorders related to acute morphine use in single-traumatized patients and whether there are immediate memory problems associated with acute morphine withdrawal in single-traumatized patients.

[C] Mechanisms of Insulin Facilitation of Memory

ID NCT01145482 - Last update posted: 2014-11-02

Sponsor University of Texas, Austin, USA

Aim: To test the hypothesis that Insulin-mediated facilitation of memory in Alzheimer's disease (AD) is achieved through enhanced glutamatergic neurotransmission due to improvements in cerebral glucose metabolism.

[C] Vilazodone for Corticosteroid-Induced Memory Impairment

ID NCT01828515 - Last update posted: 2019-04-11

Sponsor: University of Texas Southwestern Medical Center, Fort Worth, Dallas, Texas, USA

Aim: To examine whether Vilazodone attenuates the **memory and mood** effects of corticosteroids on the human hippocampus in 24 healthy controls.

[C] The Efficacy of Phosphatidylserine-Omega3 in Elderly Subjects With Memory Impairment

ID NCT00736034 - Last update posted: 2010-03-30

Sponsor: Enzymotec

Co-sponsor: Tel Aviv University Sourasky Medical Center, Israel

Aim: To assess the ability of Phosphatidylserine-Omega3 to improve cognitive performance in elderly subjects with **memory impairment**.

[C] The Effect of tES on a Cognitive Training

ID NCT03475446 - Last update posted: 2020-01-18

Sponsor: University of Bern, Switzerland

Aim: To investigate the effect of a transcranial electrical stimulation (tES) on a cognitive training in healthy elderly and **memory impaired** participants.

[R] Optimization of MRI Sequences Used in the Study of Neurodegenerative Diseases

ID NCT05929144 - Last update posted: 2023-07-03

Sponsor: University Hospital, Caen, France

Aim: To test the different MRI sequences obtained with 1 and 3 Tesla magnetic fields in order to optimize them with a view to integrating them in future studies of neurodegenerative diseases.

[U] Study of the Brain Stimulation Effect on Memory Impairment in Alzheimer Disease

ID NCT00947934 - Last update posted: 2011-12-08

Sponsor: Centre Hospitalier Universitaire de Nice, Nice, France

Aim: To assess the feasibility and safety of deep brain stimulation (DBS) of the fornix in the hypothalamus in Alzheimer's diseases (AD) patients with **mild cognitive and memory impairment**, and to evaluate the efficacy of DBS to slow down or stabilize this decline.

[T] Donepezil Memory Preservation Post ECT
(Terminated because of lack of subjects' recruitment.)
ID NCT02331771 - Last update posted: 2018-07-06
Sponsor: Porter Adventist Hospital, Denver, Colorado
Aim: To evaluate the use of Donepezil compared to placebo to reduce the risk of **memory impairment** after electroconvulsive therapy (ECT).

[C] Neuropsychological Rehabilitation of Spontaneous Confabulation: a Replica Study
ID NCT03183453 - Last update posted: 2018-05-29
Sponsor: San Rafael University Hospital, Granada, Spain
Aim: To replicate a treatment for confabulators with a larger sample of subjects.

[C] Hypnotic Medications and Memory: Effect of Drug Exposure During the Night
ID NCT01159652 - Last update posted: 2014-08-26
Sponsor: St. Luke's Hospital, Chesterfield, Missouri, USA
Aim: To determine the effect of two hypnotic medications (Zolpidem extended release and Zaleplon) on memory. It is expected that a hypnotic with shorter drug duration will allow greater **memory consolidation** than a hypnotic with longer drug duration.

[R] Predictive Factors of Autonomy Loss in Real-life Cohort
ID NCT03894254 - Last update posted: 2022-05-02
Sponsor: Hospices Civils de Lyon. Lyon, France
Aim: To study the predictive factors associated with change in functional autonomy level in Alzheimer's disease or related disorders (ADRD) patients and develop a regional database.

[R] Predictive Factors and Autonomy Level Change
ID NCT02302482 - Last update posted: 2021-06-28

Sponsor: Hospices Civils de Lyon, France

Aim: To develop a database for the predictive factors associated with change in functional autonomy level in Alzheimer's disease or related disorders (ADRD) patients and develop a regional database.

[C] Anti-Inflammatory Treatment for Age-Associated Memory Impairment: A Double-Blind Placebo-Controlled Trial
ID NCT00009230 - Last update posted: 2020-03-02
Sponsor: University of California, Los Angeles, USA

Aim: To study whether anti-inflammatory drugs, such as Celecoxib, may delay age-related mental decline and whether people with age-associated **memory impairment** who take Celecoxib show less evidence of mental decline than those receiving placebo.

[W] Comparison of the Panax Ginseng + Associations to Ginkgo Biloba in the Treatment of Cognitive Function Disorders (canceled by sponsor decision)
ID NCT01637168 - Last update posted: 2021-02-24
Sponsor: EMS, Sao Paulo, Brazil

Aim: Comparison of the Panax Ginseng + Associations to Ginkgo Biloba in the treatment of cognitive function disorders.

[R] Neural Correlates of Real World Spatial Navigation in Humans
ID NCT04874220 - Last Update Posted 2023-05-10
Sponsor: University of California, Los Angeles, USA

Aim: To understand the neural mechanisms that support real world spatial navigation in humans using deep brain recordings and stimulation during virtual reality, augmented reality, and real world memory tasks.

[U] Cerebrovascular and Cognitive Improvement by Resveratrol (resVida) and Fruitflow-II
ID NCT01766180 - Last update posted: 2015-04-21
Sponsor: Neurology Institute for Brain Health and Fitness, Baltimore, Maryland, USA

Aim: To determine whether Fruitflow-II, Resveratrol (resVida), alone or in combination, are effective in the treatment of memory problems in adult patients with **memory impairment.**

[C] AIT-082 Phase 1B Study

ID NCT00000180 - Last update posted: 2009-12-11

Sponsor: (U.S.) National Institute on Aging (NIA)

Aim: To study whether AIT-082 may delay age-related **mental decline**. (AIT-082 is a novel small molecule that crosses the blood-brain barrier (BBB) to enhance nerve function by increasing levels of neurotrophic growth factors and encouraging nerve sprouting in the brain.)

[C] Efficacy and Safety of Piracetam Taken for 12 Months in Subjects Suffering From Mild Cognitive Impairment (MCI)

ID NCT00567060 - Last update posted: 2013-12-16

Sponsor: UCB Pharma

Aim: To explore the relative potential and efficacy of Piracetam 9600 and 4800 mg daily.

[C] Age-related Longitudinal Changes in Aviator Performance

ID NCT01364753 - Last update posted: 2016-12-06

Sponsor: Stanford University, Stanford, California, USA

Aim: To evaluate whether there are significant age-related changes in flight simulator performance near age 60, and to assess whether there is an alternative model that can explain longitudinal flight simulator performance on the basis of measures of **cognitive function and expertise**.

[C] The Effects of Minocycline in Humans

ID NCT02193269 - Last update posted: 2019-09-19

Sponsor: Yale University, New Haven, Connecticut, USA

Aim: To determine the effects of Minocycline (a Tetracycline derivative antibiotic that also inhibits microglia activation and the release of pro-inflammatory cytokines, chemokines, and nitric oxide production) on **cognitive performance** and measures of mood in abstinent cocaine users.

Trials on memory and mental health

[C] Memory and Mental Health in Aging
ID NCT00043589 - Last update posted: 2013-12-05
Sponsor: Stanford University, Palo Alto, California, USA
Aim: To evaluate the effectiveness of Donepezil (Aricept®) and cognitive training in improving **memory performance** in elderly adults.

[C] Memory and Mental Health in Aging
ID NCT02988908 - Last update posted: 2017-02-10
Sponsor: Stanford University, USA
Aim: To evaluate the short-term and longer-term efficacy and effectiveness of a pharmacologic augmentation strategy (with Donepezil) for a nonpharmacologic treatment to improve **memory performance** in nondemented older adults.

[C] Reversing Corticosteroid Induced Memory Impairment
ID NCT01142310 - Last update posted: 2018-08-27
Sponsor: University of Texas Southwestern Medical Center, Dallas Fort Worth, Texas, USA
Aim: To explore the effects of corticosteroid therapy (Lamotrigine: a glutamate release inhibitor; Prednisone) on the human hippocampus following open-label, placebo-controlled, pilot data suggesting that Lamotrigine significantly improves **declarative memory** (a measure of hippocampal performance).

Trials on various types of memory

Autobiographical

[C] Autobiographical Memory
ID NCT04584138 - Last update posted: 2023-03-23
Sponsor: Nantes University Hospital, Nantes, France
Aim: To assess eye movement during **autobiographical retrieval** (i.e., retrieval of personal memories) in patients with Alzheimer's Disease.

Declarative

[T] The Effect of Feeding Infant Formula With Enriched Protein Fractions in the US (terminated due to lack of enrollment)
ID NCT02433600 - Last update posted: 2016-03-16
Sponsor: Mead Johnson Nutrition
Aim: To measure **declarative or stored memory** and behavior between infants who consume one of two infant formulas through approximately one year of age.

Emotional

[C] Losartan and Emotional Memory
ID NCT03763409 - Last update posted: 2018-12-06
Sponsor: University of Oxford, United Kingdom
Aim: To explore the effects of single-dose Losartan (50mg) versus identical placebo capsule on **emotional memory** and learning in healthy volunteers.

[C] Understanding Reactions to Emotional Material in the Media During COVID-19 - Study 2
ID NCT05063825 - Last update posted: 2021-12-23
Sponsor: Uppsala University, Sweden
Aim: To adapt a protocol usually run in the laboratory in the Psychology Department for healthy participants (including the trauma film paradigm and a simple cognitive task intervention) to remote (online) delivery because of restrictions to running in-person laboratory experiments during the COVID-19 pandemic.

Episodic

[C] Effect of Affective Content on Drug Induced Amnesia of Episodic Memory
ID NCT00142493 - Last update posted: 2015-12-24
Sponsor: Memorial Sloan Kettering Cancer Center, New York, NY, USA
Aim: To understand how some of the drugs commonly used in anesthesia (Propofol, Thiopental, Midazolam, and Dexmedetomidine, all of which

may have slightly differing effects) impair **episodic memory** and whether the emotion associated with a memory influences how well these drugs are able to block memory. Further, to understand how memory works, how these drugs affect memory, and possibly why some people don't have their memory blocked as easily as others.

[NYR] Episodic Memory Integration and Interference
ID NCT05974371 - Last update posted: 2023-08-03
Sponsor Boston College, Chestnut Hill, Massachusetts, USA
Aim: To assess how **emotional memories** integrate and interfere with one another over time.

[R] Influence of Temporo-occipital Transcranial Magnetic Brain Stimulation on Aversive Episodic Memory Performance (SAME)
ClinicalTrials.gov ID NCT05847933
Sponsor University of Basel, Basel, Switzerland
Aim: To examine the effect of repeated transcranial magnetic brain stimulation (rTMS) on the formation of **memories with negative valence** and develop a protocol to reduce memory performance for adverse events.

[C] Better Memory With Literacy Acquisition Later in Life
ID NCT04473235 - Last update posted: 2023-01-13
Sponsor: University of California, San Francisco, USA
Aim: To discover whether acquiring basic-literacy in adulthood can improve **episodic memory** and brain structural and functional connectivity.

[R] In-depth Investigation of Brain Network Interactions (BNI)
ID NCT04748146 - Last update posted: 2023-04-04
Sponsor:Northwestern University, Illinois, USA
Aim: To use recent advances in functional magnetic resonance imaging to delineate distributed brain networks within individuals, and use these network maps to guide selection of intracranial electrodes for stimulation during an **episodic memory** task.

[C] The Influence of Collective Schemas on Individual Memory
ID NCT02542800 - Last update posted:2017-12-27

Sponsor: Institut National de la Santé et de la Recherche Médicale, Caen, France

Aim: To ascertain the influence of collective schema on the neural substrates of individual memories using MRI brain imaging methods of subjects performing an encoding followed by **episodic memory**.

[N] Basic Experimental Study of Hippocampal Memory Functions

ID NCT05945628 - Last update posted: 2023-07-14

Sponsor: University of Chicago, IL, USA

Aim: To test the role of the human hippocampus (in individuals with epilepsy undergoing neurosurgical procedures as part of clinical care) in providing on-line representation of **episodic** content and providing the top-down signals to brain networks for visuo-spatial attention and visual processing needed to drive visual sampling for the formation of coherent episodic memories.

Intrusive

Intrusive memories are sensory memories of a traumatic event(s) that spring to mind involuntarily, and can evoke strong emotions and disrupt functioning in daily life. They are their debilitating core features and are triggered by certain clinical symptoms (PTSD, anxiety, depression, and insomnia). Little is known about the neurobiological formation of intrusions. Exposure therapy is amongst the most successful treatment of PTSD that is recommended by most of the current national and international guidelines. Research has indicated that a brief cognitive intervention can prevent the development of intrusive memories as well as reduce the number of intrusive memories of long-standing trauma.

[C] Behavioral Modulation of Intrusive Memories

ID NCT03227081 - Last update posted: 2022-03-10

Sponsor Charite University, Berlin, Germany

Aim: To examine whether sleep affects the development of **intrusive memories**.

[R] The Effect of Dronabinol on the Acquisition and Consolidation of Trauma-Associated Memories

ID NCT04871269 - Last update posted: 2023-04-04

Sponsor: Charite University, Berlin, Germany

Aim: To investigate the impact of an activation of the cannabinoid system with an exogenous cannabinoid Dronabinol (delta-9-tetrahydrocannabinol) on the formation of **intrusive memories** after analog trauma.

[C] Sleep's Influence on the Treatment of Intrusive Emotional

ID NCT05678361 - Last update posted: 2023-01-10

Sponsor University of Zurich, Switzerland

Aim: To test whether sleep as adjunct to written exposure sessions, a type of exposure- based treatment for PTSD's **intrusive memories**, may boost the effectiveness of the therapy.

[C] The Effect of Oxytocin on the Consolidation of Trauma-Associated Memories

ID NCT03875391 - Last update posted: 2023-04-04

Sponsor:Charite University, Berlin, Germany

Aim: To examine whether Oxytocin and certain polygenic risk scores affect the development of **intrusive memories**, a cardinal symptom of PTSD.

[C] Influence of the Noradrenergic System on the Formation of Intrusive Memories

ID NCT02541071 - Last update posted: 2015-09-04

Sponsor: Charite University, Berlin, Germany

Aim: To determine whether the activity of the noradrenergic system during an intrusion-inducing stressor influences subsequent **intrusive memories**.

[C] Cortisol and the Formation of Intrusive Memories

ID NCT02552654 - Last update posted: 2016-10-03

Sponsor:Charite University, Berlin, Germany

Aim: To determine whether Cortisol levels during an intrusion-inducing stressor influence subsequent **intrusive memories**.

[C] The Effect of Oxytocin on the Acquisition and Consolidation of Trauma-Associated Memories

ID NCT03031405 - Last update posted: 2018-08-21

Sponsor: Charite University, Berlin, Germany

Aim: To examine whether oxytocin and oxytocin receptor gene polymorphism affect the development of **intrusive memories**, a cardinal symptom of PTSD.

[C] Lóa Project: An Exploratory Pilot Randomized Controlled Trial of a Remotely-delivered Brief Cognitive Intervention to Reduce Intrusive Memories of Trauma for Women in Iceland

ID NCT05089058 - Last update posted 2022-11-17

Sponsor: University of Iceland

Aim: To compare remote delivery of the intervention (i.e. brief, digitally delivered imagery-competing task intervention) to an attention-placebo control condition (i.e., brief, digitally delivered relaxation exercise task). To explore whether (relative to the control condition) the intervention: (i) reduces the number of **intrusive memories** and (ii) improves other symptoms and functioning.

[NYR] The Lóa Study: A Brief Digital Intervention for Women With Intrusive Memories in the SAGA Cohort

ID NCT05849337 - Last update posted: 2023-09-15

Sponsor: University of Iceland

Aim: To investigate if access to a cognitive task - either a brief self-guided imagery-competing task or a brief self-guided psychoeducation and sign-posting task - versus treatment as usual, can reduce the number of **intrusive memories.**

[C] A Brief GAmeplay Intervention for NHS ICU Staff Affected by COVID-19 Trauma (GAINS Study) (GAINS)

ID NCT04992390 - Last update posted: 2023-09-08

Sponsor: P1vital Products Limited, Wallingford, Oxfordshire, United Kingdom

Aim: To optimize a brief digital intervention to help reduce the number of **intrusive memories** experienced by ICU staff and to explore if it can improve work functioning and well-being.

[R] A Brief Cognitive Task Intervention for NHS Staff Affected by COVID-19 Trauma (GAINS-2 Study) (GAINS-2)

ID NCT05616676 - Last update posted: 2023-04-28

Sponsor: P1vital Products Limited, Wallingford, Oxfordshire, United Kingdom

Aim: To test the effect of a digital imagery-competing task, a digital music-listening task, and treatment as usual for National Health Service (NHS) staff with **intrusive memories** of work-related traumatic events from the COVID-19 pandemic.

[R] Tackling Intrusive Traumatic Memories After Childbirth (ASTRAL)

ID NCT05381155 - Last update posted: 2023-05-12

Sponsor: Centre Hospitalier Universitaire Vaudois, Geneva, Switzerland

Aim: To investigate the efficacy of a single-session behavioral intervention composed of a brief evocation of the childbirth memory followed by a visuospatial task (the computer game "Tetris"), on childbirth-related **intrusive traumatic memories** (CB-ITM) and other childbirth-related post-traumatic stress disorder (CB-PTSD) symptoms.

[C] Tackling Intrusive Traumatic Memories After a Difficult Birth

ID NCT04286724 - Last update posted: 2021-06-22

Sponsor: Centre Hospitalier Universitaire Vaudois, Canton de Vaud, Lausanne, Switzerland

Aim: To investigate the effects of a brief behavioral procedure including a computerized visuospatial task (the computer game "Tetris") preceded by a reactivation of the traumatic memory of childbirth, on birth-related **intrusive traumatic memories** and other postpartum post-traumatic stress symptoms.

Motor

Motor skills require motor memories without which behavior is only reflexes and stereotypes. The way in which these memories form in the human brain constitute a major challenge for neuroscience research. Evidence suggests that any new motor skill is acquired in the cerebellum and then persists in the cortex. This vision seems however caricature as the formation of motor memories probably requires complex remodeling of cortico-cerebellar networks.

[U] Acquisition and Retention of Motor Memories in Adults and Typically Developing Children (MOTORMEMO)

ID NCT04598945 - Last update posted: 2020-11-17

Sponsor: University Hospital, Grenoble, France

Aim: To better understand the complex remodeling of cortico-cerebellar networks (cerebellar weakening and strengthening cortical) as a substrate for the formation of **motor memories**.

[C] Enhancing Motor Task Training by Action Observation Watching Others Perform the Task

ID NCT00393432 - Last update posted: 2017-07-02

Sponsor: (U.S.) National Institute of Neurological Disorders and Stroke (NINDS),Bethesda, Maryland

Aim: To determine how the brain learns a new **motor task** when the subject practices the task and watches others perform it (action observation) at the same time.

Prospective

[C] Prospective Memory in Parkinson's Disease

ID NCT00913640 - Last update posted: 2022-05-06

Sponsor: Washington University School of Medicine, Saint Louis, Missouri, USA

Aim: To test whether **prospective memory** is impaired in individuals with Parkinson's Disease (PD) compared to controls using reliable and validated experimental measures and to assess the impact of PD medication on prospective memory performance in PD to better estimate prospective memory function in PD patients' everyday (chronically treated) life.

Spatial

[NYR] Sevoflurane General Anesthetic and Spatial Memory in Humans

ID NCT05991817 - Last update posted: 2023-08-15

Sponsor: University of Chile, Santiago, Chile

Aim: To learn about the effect of general anesthetic on **spatial memory** in adults who will undergo an elective surgery, whether it transiently impairs spatial memory in humans, and induces an increase in inflammatory cytokines.

Subjective

[C] Efficacy of Cognitive Training in Subjective Memory Impairment
ID NCT02555774 - Last update posted: 2018-08-07
Sponsor: Asan Medical Center, Republic of Korea
Aim: To evaluate the efficacy of cognitive training in subjects with **subjective memory impairment**.

[C] Memory and Exercise Training Study in Older Adults With Subjective Memory Complaints
ID NCT02433691 - Last update posted: 2018-05-02
Sponsor: University of California, Los Angeles, USA
Aim: To contribute to combat age-related losses in cognitive function through preventive lifestyle strategies such as simultaneous exercise and memory training programs in non-demented volunteers with **subjective memory** complaints.Further, to assess the cognitive impact of 4-week memory training programs done twice weekly and to measure potential metabolic (e.g., glucose, lipid panel) and molecular (serum BDNF) mediators of observed cognitive changes.

[NYR] Investigation of Alzheimer's Predictors in Subjective Memory Complainers - Extension Study (INSIGHT-2)
ID NCT05806697 - Last update posted:2023-04-10
Sponsor: Institut National de la Santé et de la Recherche Médicale, Hopital Pitié Salpetriere, Paris, France
Aim: To follow subjects who previously participated in the INSIGHT study and who agree on an extension of their follow-up in the INSIGHT-2 research for additional 5-6 years. Further, to describe the natural history of preclinical Alzheimer's disease (AD).

Verbal and visual

[C] 26 Weeks' Dietary Supplementation With DHA- and EPA-enriched Oils on Memory Consolidation in Healthy Adults
ID NCT03592251 - Last update posted: 2019-01-24
Sponsor: Northumbria University, Newcastle Upon Tyne, United Kingdom
Aim: To investigate the effects of EPA- and DHA-enriched omega-3 polyunsaturated fatty acid dietary supplements on overnight **verbal and visual memory** consolidation as well as morning alertness before and after 26 weeks of supplementation.

Working

Working memory deficits are a transdiagnostic feature of adolescent psychopathology that substantially contribute to poor clinical and functional outcomes.

[R] Individualized Closed Loop TMS for Working Memory Enhancement
ID NCT04402294 - Last update posted: 2023-05-12
Sponsor: University of Pennsylvania, USA
Aim: To investigate **working memory** brain states by using transcranial magnetic stimulation (TMS) in combination with functional magnetic resonance imaging (fMRI).

[NYR] Modulation of Brain Oscillations Underlying Working Memory
ID NCT05923606 - Last update posted: 2023-09-05
Sponsor: Massachusetts General Hospital, Charlestown, Massachusetts, USA
Aim: To use novel transcranial alternating current stimulation (tACS) protocols and electroencephalography (EEG) to modulate and measure brain oscillations that underlie **working memory**. tACS is a noninvasive method used to modulate the timing and patterns of brain rhythms via weak electric currents passed through electrodes on the scalp.

[EBI] Electrophysiological Signatures of Distinct Working Memory Subprocesses That Predict Long-term Memory Success (WMLTM)

ID NCT05892419 - Last update posted: 2023-06-09

Sponsor: University of Chicago, Illinois, USA

Aim: To examine how measured electroencephalogram (EEG) brain activity relates to pictures of items viewed by healthy young adults.

[C] Influence of Fampridine on Working Memory in Healthy Young Subjects (FamH)

ID NCT04652557 - Last Update Posted 2023-02-06

Sponsor University of Basel, Switzerland

Aim: To investigate the hypothesis that Fampridine improves working memory performance by studying the acute effects on **working memory** of 10 mg Fampridine SR as well as the effects after repeated administration of 10 mg twice daily (3.5 days).

[C] Development of a Model-based Working Memory Training and Investigation of Its Comparative Efficacy

ID NCT04042779 - Last update posted: 2020-07-01

Sponsor: University Hospital, Basel, Switzerland

Aim: To investigate the efficacy of model-based **working memory** (WM) training using an appropriate control condition.

[C] Protocol Memory Deficit in Patients With Obstructive Sleep Apnea Syndrome

ID NCT00464659 - Last update posted: 2015-12-30

Sponsor: University Hospital, Grenoble, France

Aim: To evaluate the evolution of memory deficit (verbal **episodic memory, procedural memory, working memory, short-term memory**) in sleep apnea obstructive syndrome (SAOS) patients after treatment by continuous positive airway pressure treatment (CPAP).

[R] Traveling-wave Transcranial Electric Stimulation

ID NCT05399381 - Last update posted: 2022-10-06

Sponsor: University of Minnesota

Aim: To assess the impact of traveling wave transcranial alternating current stimulation (tACS) on **working memory** performance in adults.

[R] Non-Invasive Brain Stimulation to Control Large-Scale Brain Networks

ID NCT04680481 - Last update posted: 2023-02-08

Sponsor: University of Minnesota, Minneapolis, Minnesota, USA

Aim: To assess the feasibility of traveling wave transcranial alternating current stimulation (tACS) to modify **working memory** performance and large-scale brain connectivity in surgical epilepsy patients.

[NYR] Transcranial Direct Current Stimulation (tDCS) on Working Memory in College Going Students

ID NCT05737498 - Last update posted: 2023-02-21

Sponsor:Maharishi Markendeswar University (deemed to be University), India

Aim: To determine the effect of tDCS on **working memory** in college going students and improve their cognitive abilities.

[C] Galantamine Effects on Cognitive Function in Marijuana Users

ID NCT00969696 - Last update posted: 2012-07-25

Sponsor:Yale University, New Haven, Connecticut, USA

Aim: To evaluate galantamine's effects on cognitive performance in marijuana users who show impaired cognitive functioning, which predicts poor response to behavioral treatments, will improve **working memory**, **verbal learning/memory,** and response inhibition functions in marijuana users.

[R] NIMH K23: Modulation of Frontoparietal Dynamics in Adolescent Working Memory Deficits

ID NCT05662280 - Last update posted: 2023-01-05

Sponsor: National Institute of Mental Health, Bradley Hospital, East Providence, Rhodes Island, USA

Aim: To investigate whether non-invasive brain stimulation can modulate the neural mechanisms underlying adolescent **working memory** (WM) deficits and identify the contributing roles of prefrontal and parietal regions in WM processes, as well as identify optimal targets and parameters for novel brain-based treatments in adolescent psychopathology.

[C] Memory Rehabilitation by Means of Working Memory Training in Combination With a Recollection Training

ID NCT02790151 - Last update posted: 2016-10-18

Sponsor: University of Oldenburg, Oldenburg, Germany

Aim: To compare two therapeutic interventions and investigate whether therapy effects can be found on neuropsychological tests on a test measuring **memory** in everyday life and memory deficits after brain damage.

[C] Intrusive Re-experiencing: The Role of Working Memory Capacity and Thought Suppression

ID NCT01007682 - Last update posted: 2012-03-08

Sponsor: University Hospital, Basel, Switzerland

Aim: To identifying risk factors for the development of **intrusive** re-experiencing symptoms, in particular, the influence of **working memory** capacity and thought suppression on the occurrence of unpleasant memories of a negative experience.

Trials on memory aids and tools

[U] Smart-device Apps as Memory Aids

ID NCT02281617 - Last update posted: 2014-11-02

Sponsor: King's College, London, United Kingdom

Aim: To survey patients' use of memory aids and investigate the feasibility and efficacy of using smartphone and tablet apps as memory aids in a clinical setting.

[U] Examining the Effect of a Simple Memory Tool

ID NCT03244111 - Last update posted: 2017-08-09

Sponsor: University of Manitoba, Manitoba, Canada

Aim: To examine whether an intervention that involves a simple memory tool assists with daily life **memory performance** and goal attainment of older adults and whether the intervention has a different effect for individuals with healthy cognition versus individuals with mild cognitive impairment (MCI).

[C] Brain Fitness APP for Aging With a Healthy Brain
ID NCT03600545 - Last update posted: 2021-02-24

Sponsor: University of Manitoba, Winnipeg, Canada

Aim: To offer a novel approach to prevent dementia and age-related cognitive disorders by creating a brain fitness APP for the aging population, based on the premise of brain plasticity and targeting the brain functions that are declining with normal aging and dementia.

[C] Trial to Evaluate the Effectiveness of Memory Training Workshops in People From 65 to 80 Years
ID NCT02431182 - Last update posted{2015-04-30

Sponsor: Fundació Institut de Recerca de l'Hospital de la Santa Creu i Santa Pau, Spain

Aim: To assess the effectiveness of a memory training workshop in cognitive function, in terms of **self-perceived memory, everyday memory** and executive control abilities.

[U] Memory Intervention for Older Adults
ID NCT02499991 - Last update posted: 2016-05-10

Sponsor: University of Manitoba, Canada

Aim: To test a memory intervention that is potentially useful in everyday life.

[U] A Comparison of the Effectiveness of Two Types of Memory Training Programs in People With a Diagnosis of Mental Illness.
ID NCT01708200 - Last Update Posted 2012-10-16

Sponsor: St. Joseph's Healthcare, Hamilton, Canada

Aim: To compare the effectiveness of a psychoeducational memory program versus a computerized memory program in individuals with mental illness.

Trial for the virtual reality helmet

[C] Virtual Reality Helmet to Test for Problems With Memory (DETECT)
ID NCT00454454 - Last update posted: 2013-07-30

Sponsor: Emory University, USA

Aim: To compare a virtual reality display device with the standard neuropsychological evaluation for detecting mild cognitive impairment (problems with **memory**, concentration, reaction time, etc.).

Sidebar 19.1 – A brief primer on clinical trials

Clinical trials (CTs) are prospective biomedical or biobehavioral research studies on human participants designed to answer specific questions about biomedical or biobehavioral interventions, including new treatments (such as novel vaccines, drugs, dietary choices, dietary supplements, and medical devices) and known interventions that warrant further study and comparison. They are part of clinical research at the heart of all medical advances. They look at new ways to prevent, detect, or treat diseases by new drugs or new combinations of drugs, new surgical procedures or devices, or new ways to use existing treatments. They can also look at other aspects of care, such as improving the quality of life for people with chronic illnesses Their goal is to determine if a new test or treatment is safe and effective.. Some CTs involve healthy subjects with no pre-existing medical conditions, others pertain to people with specific health conditions who are willing to try an experimental treatment. Pilot experiments are conducted to gain insights for design of the CTs to follow.

Except for small, single-location trials, the design and objectives are specified in a document called a clinical trial protocol (CTP). This is the trial's "operating manual" to ensure that all researchers perform the trial in the same way on similar subjects, and that the data is comparable across all subjects. As a trial is designed to test hypotheses and rigorously monitor and assess outcomes, it can be seen as an application of the scientific method, specifically the experimental step.

CTs generate data on dosage, safety, and efficacy. They are conducted only after they have received regulatory approval (ethics committee approval and health authority), which vet the risk/benefit ratio of the trial and allow or deny it.

Depending on product type and development stage, investigators initially enroll volunteers or patients into small pilot studies, and subsequently conduct progressively larger-scale comparative studies.

CTs can vary in size and cost, and can involve a single research center or multiple centers, in one or in multiple countries. The clinical study design aims to ensure the scientific validity and reproducibility of the results. Costs for clinical trials can range into the billions of dollars per approved drug. The sponsor may be a governmental organization or a pharmaceutical, biotechnology, or medical device company. Certain functions necessary to the trial, such as monitoring and laboratory work, may be managed by an outsourced partner, such as a contract research organization (CRO) or a central laboratory. Only 10% of all drugs started in human clinical trials become approved drugs.

Overall goals

There are two goals to testing medical treatments: to learn whether they work well enough, called "efficacy" or "effectiveness"; and to learn whether they are safe enough, called "safety". Neither is an absolute criterion and both safety and efficacy are evaluated relative to how the treatment is intended to be used, what other treatments are available, and the severity of the disease or condition. The benefits must outweigh the risks.

The sponsor designs the trial in coordination with a panel of expert clinical investigators who also consider what alternative or existing treatments exist to compare to the new drug and what type(s) of patients might benefit.

Categories of trials

There are three trial categories:

Drugs

They are the most common to evaluate new pharmaceutical products, biologics, diagnostic assays, psychological therapies, or other interventions.

Devices

Similarly to drugs, manufacturers of medical devices may compare a new device to an established therapy, or may compare similar devices to each other. They are required for pre-market approval.

Procedures

Similarly to drugs, medical or surgical procedures may be subjected to clinical trials, They compare different surgical approaches in treatment.

Types of trials

CTs are classified by the research objective(s) or purpose(s) of the investigators:

By research objectives

This will depend on the kind of study. Thus, in an:

- **Observational study:** The investigators observe the subjects and measure their outcomes. They do not actively manage the study.
- **Interventional study:** The investigators give the research subjects an experimental drug, use of a medical device, a surgical procedure, diagnostic or other intervention to compare the treated subjects with those receiving no treatment or the standard treatment. Then, the researchers assess how the subjects' health changes.

By research purposes

There are ten such types:

- ➢ **Prevention trials:** They look for ways to prevent disease in people who have never had the disease or to prevent a disease from returning. These approaches may include drugs, vitamins or other micronutrients, vaccines, or lifestyle changes.
- ➢ **Screening trials:** They test for ways to identify certain diseases or health conditions.
- ➢ Di**agnostic trials:** They are conducted to find better tests or procedures for diagnosing a particular disease or condition.

- ➢ **Treatment trials:** They test experimental drugs, new combinations of drugs, or new approaches to surgery or radiation therapy.
- ➢ **Quality of life trials** or **supportive care trials:** They evaluate how to improve comfort and quality of care for people with a chronic illness.
- ➢ **Genetic trials:** They are conducted to assess the prediction accuracy of genetic disorders making a person more or less likely to develop a disease.
- ➢ **Epidemiological trials:** They have the goal of identifying the general causes, patterns or control(s) of diseases in large numbers of people.
- ➢ **Compassionate use trials** or **expanded access trials:** They provide partially tested, unapproved therapeutics to a small number of patients who have no other realistic options. Usually, this involves a disease for which no effective therapy has been approved, or a patient who has already failed all standard treatments and whose health is too compromised to qualify for participation in randomized clinical trials (RCTs). Usually in the U.S., case-by-case approval must be granted by both the FDA and the pharmaceutical company for such exceptions.
- ➢ **Fixed trials:** They consider existing data only during the trial's design, do not modify the trial after it begins, and do not assess the results until the study is completed.
- ➢ **Adaptive trials:** They use existing data to design the trial, and then use interim results to modify the trial as it proceeds. Modifications include dosage, sample size, drug undergoing trial, patient selection criteria, and "cocktail" mix.

Trial phases

CTs are conducted typically in four phases (Phases I to IV), with each phase using different numbers of subjects and having a different purpose to construct focus on identifying a specific effect. However, for new drugs, there are five phases (Phases 0 and I to IV), each phase being treated as a separate CT.

Table 19.1 recapitulates the aims of these phases:

Table 19.1 – Phases of clinical trials

Phase	Aim	Notes
0	**Pharmacodynamics** (what the drug does to the body) and **pharmacokinetics** (what the body does to the drug) in humans	o Optional o Sub-therapeutic doses o Small number of subjects (10-15) for preliminary data o Trial documents the absorption, distribution, metabolization, and clearance (excretion) of the drug, and the drug's interactions within the body, to confirm that these appear to be as expected
I	**Safety**	o Small number of subjects (20-30) o Determines safe dosage ranges o Identifies side effects
II	**IIa. Dosing** **IIb. Efficacy**	o IIa: Dosing requirements o IIb: Efficacy to establish therapeutic dose range
III	**Confirmation of safety and efficacy**	o Large group of subjects (1,000-3,000) o Monitors side effects o Compares to commonly-used treatments
IV	**Post-marketing safety**	o Delineates benefits, risks, optimal use o Ongoing during the drug's lifetime of active medical use

Reference: Wikipedia

Take-aways

➤ Clinical trials are prospective biomedical or biobehavioral research studies on human participants designed to answer specific questions about biomedical or biobehavioral interventions, including new treatments (such as novel vaccines, drugs, dietary choices, dietary supplements, and medical devices) and known interventions that warrant further study and comparison. Their overriding goal is to determine if a new test or treatment works and is safe.

➤ People with memory problems may be able to take part in clinical trials. Healthy people with no memory problems and no family history of such conditions may also be able to participate. Joining a clinical trial or other research study is also a way to help fight such issues.

➤ Typical questions asked by potential memory participants include: Can a memory patient participate in a clinical trial? Is the list of clinical trials available? Does it cost anything to participate in a clinical trial? What are the currently recruiting clinical trials.

➤ The particulars of the following categories of trials have been provided: Memory functions and physiological processes; memory processes; memory lapse /consolidation /reactivation; memory delays, deficits, impairments, and disorders; memory and mental health; various types of memory (autobiographical, declarative, emotional, episodic, intrusive, motor, prospective, spatial, subjective, verbal and visual, working); memory aids and tools; and the virtual realty helmet.

➤ A sidebar provides a brief primer on clinical trials: Nature; overall goal(s), design and objective(s); use of the data generated; categorization (drugs, devices, procedures); types by research objectives or research purposes (prevention, screening, diagnostic, treatment, quality of life or supportive care, genetic, epidemiological, compassionate use or expanded access, fixed, or adaptive). It also describes the various trial phases.

20

Treatment portfolio: V. Complementary and alternative treatments

Contents

20

Treatment portfolio: V. Complementary and alternative treatments

Tweaking memories

Can replacing bad memories with good ones or even erasing certain memories improve mental health? Researchers are exploring ways to manipulate memories to discover novel methods to treat post-traumatic stress disorder (PTSD), depression, and Alzheimer's. National Geographic is actually conducting public events that feature thought-provoking presentations by today's leading explorers, scientists, photographers, and performing artists.

Digital puzzle gaming

Since aging has a negative impact on **working memory**, are certain types of games connected with improvements in memory among younger and older adults? Certain experiments showed that adults who play *strategy* games show a greater working memory capacity compared to younger adults who play *action* games. This may be surprising because other experiments showed that action games have been associated with superior performance in various measures of attention, perception, and executive function.

For older people, puzzle games have the surprising ability to support mental capabilities to the extent that memory and concentration levels are the same as for 20 year-olds who had not played puzzle games. Older adults who play digital puzzle games may have a higher working memory capacity than older adults who play either other game types or do not play games at all. In addition, older adults who play digital puzzle games can ignore distractions better than other older adults. It seems that the strategy elements of the games (planning, problem solving, etc.) stimulate better memory and attention in younger rather than older people.

Alternative therapies

Aromatherapy and massage: Unclear benefits.

Cannabinoids: Can relieve behavioral and psychological symptoms of dementia.

Omega-3 fatty acid supplements from plants or fish sources: Do not appear to benefit or harm people with mild to moderate AD, or improve other types of dementia.

Dental hygiene: There is limited evidence linking poor oral health to cognitive decline. Poor oral hygiene can have an adverse effect on speech and nutrition, causing general and **cognitive health** decline. Oral bacteria (*P. gingivalis, F. Nucleatum; P. intermedia, T. Forsythia;* trepomena spirochetes) and oral viruses have been observed in the brains of AD patients.

Note on spirochetes: These are neurotrophic in nature, meaning they act to destroy nerve tissue and create inflammation. Inflammatory pathogens are an indicator of AD. Bacteria related to gum disease have been found in the brains of AD individuals. They invade nerve tissue in the brain, increasing the permeability of the blood brain barrier (BBB) and promoting the onset of AD among the elderly population (Fymat, 2018b).

Note on Herpes simplex virus (HSV): Found in over 70% of the 50 and older population, it persists in the peripheral nervous system (PNS) and can be triggered by stress, illness or fatigue. High proportions of viral-associated proteins in amyloid-containing plaques or neurofibrillary tangles (NFTs) highly confirm the involvement of HSV-1 in AD pathology. HSV-1 produces the main components of NFTs, the primary marker of AD.

Sleep therapies

Various medications can help people fall asleep, stay asleep, or both, such as Doxepin (Silenor®) and Ramelteon (Rozerem®). But, there may be some risks and side effects. Several are only for short-term use. This Section reviews 10 of the best prescribed medications to help a person sleep. It also explores some non-medical solutions for sleep issues.

Overview

Sleep disturbances are common. An estimated 50–70 million people in the U.S. experience chronic sleep or wakefulness conditions, which are more common in females and older individuals. A range of medications can help people fall asleep, stay asleep, or both. Prescription sleep aids can often relieve insomnia for short periods. However, many of these medications carry risks of side effects, misuse, and dependency. In addition, some sleep medications interact with other substances, including other medications, alcohol, and vitamin supplements.

1. Doxepin (Silenor®)

Doxepin is an immediate-release sleep aid tablet (dose: 3 and 6 [mg]), which may help a person fall asleep and stay asleep. People with insomnia use it for up to 3 months. It is not recommended for those taking monoamine oxidase inhibitors (MOI), a type of antidepressant, or people with glaucoma or urinary retention. It may cause side effects in some people, including: central nervous system (CNS) depression, where brain activity slows; worsening depression or suicidal thoughts; and unusual thinking patterns and behavior changes. If symptoms do not clear within 7–10 days, a doctor may need to rule out other possible causes of insomnia.

(Note: Pregnant or nursing mothers should consult a doctor before using Silenor. Parents or caregivers should only give it to children or adolescents if directed by a medical professional.)

2. Temazepam (Restoril®)

Temazepam (doses: 7.5 to 30 [mg]) is a benzodiazepine, which may cause dependency and addiction if a person misuses it. It is available by prescription for the short-term treatment of insomnia (typically, 7–10 days). It can cause a variety of side effects, which may include one or more of the following: Anxiety, confusion, depression, diarrhea, dizziness, drowsiness, dry mouth, fatigue, headache, nausea, nightmares, and vertigo.

(Note: Pregnant or nursing mothers should not take Restoril).

3. Eszopiclone (Lunesta®)

Lunesta (dose: 1 up to 3 [mg]) may help a person fall and stay asleep. It is a controlled substance with a tendency to lead to misuse and dependency. A person may also experience diminishing effects or increased tolerance to the medication over time. Though generally safe, its reported side effects include: Anxiety, dizziness, dry mouth, hallucinations, headache, rash, unpleasant mouth taste, and viral infections. In addition, it may cause a person to engage in complex sleep behaviors, such as sleep-walking or driving while asleep. Precautions before taking Lunesta include: Age: (older people should avoid taking higher doses); allergies (an allergic reaction can be caused in some people); liver function (people with reduced liver function should avoid taking Lunesta); mental health (Lunesta may worsen depression or suicidal thoughts); and safety (higher doses can impair a person's CNS even when awake, making driving and other complex tasks more dangerous).

(Note: Pregnant or nursing mothers should consult a doctor before taking Lunesta.)

4. Ramelteon (Rozerem®)

Unlike other medications, Rozerem (one size single dose not to be exceeded: 8 [mg]) may be prescribed for longer-term use to help a person fall asleep. It is not a controlled substance, has a low likelihood of misuse or dependency.

However, it can still cause side effects such as: Allergic reactions in some people, dizziness, drowsiness, fatigue, and worsening insomnia.

(Note: Use caution in taking this medication. Other groups may include people who may have had a past allergic reaction to the medication; have severe liver impairment; are taking the medication fluvoxamine; are pregnant.)

5. Suvorexant (Belsomra®)

This medication (dose: 5-20 [mg]; higher doses could lead to more adverse reactions) may help a person fall asleep and maintain sleep. However, there is a risk of misusing it and developing dependency. Like other controlled substances, it can cause CNS impairments that can lead to trouble with driving and other activities. It can also cause: Complex sleep behaviors; sleep paralysis; worsening suicidal thoughts or depression. Other potential side effects reported in clinical trials include: Cough, diarrhea, dizziness, unusual dreams, headache, dry mouth, or upper respiratory tract infection.

6. Triazolam (Halcion®)

Because the medication (dose: 0.25 and 0.50 [mg]) has the potential for dependency and misuse, it is not recommend as a long-term treatment for insomnia, typically for 7-10 days. Common side effects may include: Ataxia (or lack of muscle coordination), dizziness, drowsiness, lightheadedness. In some people. It can cause: CNS issues (anxiety, behavioral changes, and unusual thinking), dependency, worsening depression, worsening insomnia, complex sleep behaviors, issues with performing activities such as driving, or withdrawal symptoms when suddenly stopping taking it.

7. Trazodone (Desyrel®)

This medication (dose: typical starting 150 [mg] with a maximum [400 [mg] daily; typically 25-100 [mg] for sleep disturbances) modulates the neurotransmitter serotonin. It is typically used to treat major depressive disorder; however, it may be prescribed off-label to help a person fall asleep since one of its effects is drowsiness. Possible side effects include: Diarrhea, drowsiness, edema (body tissues contain too much fluid), fainting, fatigue, nasal congestion, increased suicide thoughts, blurred vision, or weight loss.

(Note: Alcohol consumption can increase the effects.)

8. Estazolam (Prosomc®)

Prescribed for the short-term treatment of insomnia (dose: 1-2 [mg]), it may help with falling and staying asleep. It has a risk of misuse and dependency and can cause some of the following reactions: Loss of coordination, dizziness, drowsiness, or hypokinesia (reduced range of movements).

9. Zaleplon (Sonata®)

This medicine (dose: 5-10 [mg]) may be useful for the short-term treatment of insomnia but, while it may help a person fall asleep, it does not help maintain sleep. It has some risk of dependency and a high likelihood of misuse. Side effects include: Diarrhea, difficulty concentrating, dizziness, drowsiness, and less commonly: hallucinations, memory loss, and mood changes.

10. Zolpidem (Ambien®, Intermezzo®, and Zolpimist®)

This sleep medication (dose: not exceeding 12.5 [mg]) may help with falling asleep and maintaining sleep maintenance. It may be prescribed for short-term insomnia relief but may cause complex sleep behaviors. It can also lead to anaphylactic reactions, CNS depression, worsening depression, and withdrawal effects. Common side effects may include: Dizziness, headache, next-day sleepiness.

(Note: It is not recommend during pregnancy.)

Table 20.1 compares the benefits and risks of these sleep medications.

Table 20.1 – Benefits and risks of various sleep medications

Medication	Pros	Cons	Helps fall asleep?	Helps maintain sleep?	Risk of dependence or misuse	Side effects
Silenor	May help fall and stay asleep	o May interact with other medications o May not be suitable for pregnant women	Yes	Yes	Unlikely	o CNS depression o Mood or behavior changes o Suicidal thoughts
Restoril	Strong sedative effect may help with insomnia	Risk of dependency, withdrawal, and misuse	Yes	Yes	Yes	o Anxiety o Depression o Headache o Fatigue o Nausea o Mouth dryness o Vertigo
Lunesta	o May help a person fall and stay asleep o Is generally safe	o Can cause complex sleep behaviors (such as sleep-walking)	Yes	Yes	Yes	o Anxiety o Dizziness o Headache o Taste unpleasantness o Viral infections
Rozerem	o Not a controlled substance o Little chance of causing dependency	Has the potential for adverse and allergic reactions	Yes	No	Unlikely	o Dizziness o Drowsiness o Fatigue o Insomnia worsening
Belsomra	May help fall and stay asleep	Risk of dependency or misuse	Yes	Yes	Yes	o Diarrhea o Dry mouth o Headache Upper respiratory tract infection
Halcion	May help fall asleep	Only for short term use	Yes	No	Yes	o Lack of coordination o Dizziness o Drowsiness o Lightheadedness
Desyrel	o Low dose anti-depressant o May cause fewer side effects than traditional sleep medications	o Can cause mental health side effects (suicidal ideation)	Yes	Yes	Unlikely	o Drowsiness o Edema o Suicidal thoughts o Vision blurs o Weight loss

Promos	May help fall and stay asleep	Risk of dependency or misuse	Yes	Yes	Yes	o Coordination lack o Dizziness o Drowsiness o Movements reduced
Sonata	May help fall asleep	o Risk of dependency and adverse effects o Does not help maintain sleep	Yes	No	Yes	o Abdominal pain o Headache o Weakness
Ambient/ Intermezzo/ Optimist	May help fall and stay asleep	o May cause complex sleep behaviors o Other adverse reactions	Yes	Yes	Yes	o Dizziness o Headache o Sleepiness (next day)

Lifestyle changes

Such alternative treatments and lifestyle changes include:

- Cognitive behavioral therapy (CBT).
- Herbal remedies (including supplements or teas).
- Relaxation techniques.
- Engaging in healthy sleep habits (sleeping in a cool, dark room, and avoiding distractions and large meals before bed).
- Increased exercise.

Take-aways

> Researchers are exploring ways to manipulate memories to discover novel methods to treat post-traumatic stress disorder (PTSD), depression, and Alzheimer's.

> Certain experiments showed that young adults who play strategy games show a greater working memory capacity compared to younger adults who play action games. For older people, puzzle games have the surprising ability to support mental capabilities to the extent that memory and concentration levels are the same as for 20 year-olds who had not played puzzle games.

- Older adults who play digital puzzle games may have a higher working memory capacity than older adults who play either other game types or do not play games at all. Further, older adults who play digital puzzle games can ignore distractions better than other older adults.
- The strategy elements of digital games (planning, problem solving, etc.) stimulate better memory and attention in younger rather than older people.
- Alternative therapies include: Aromatherapy and massage; cannabinoids; omega-3 fatty acid supplements from plants or fish sources; and dental hygiene.
- Various medications can help people fall asleep, stay asleep, or both but there may be some risks and side effects. Several are only for short-term use. Ten of the best prescribed medications have been reviewed including for their risk of dependency or misuse and their side effects.
- Alternative treatments and lifestyle changes for sleep include: Cognitive behavioral therapy, herbal remedies (including supplements or teas), relaxation techniques, engaging in healthy sleep habits, and increased exercise.

PART G
HOPE FOR THE FUTURE

21

Frequently asked questions

Contents

21

Frequently asked questions

On mild forgetfulness

What is mild forgetfulness?

Changes like taking longer to learn new things, remembering certain words, or finding glasses are often signs of mild forgetfulness, not serious memory problems.

Normal aging	Alzheimer's disease or a related dementia
Making an occasional bad judgment or decision	Making many poor judgments and decisions
Missing a regular financial obligation	Problems taking care of ordinary financial affairs
Forgetting which day it is and remembering later	Losing track of the date or time of year
Forgetting at times which words to use	Trouble having a conversation
Losing or misplacing things from time to time	Often misplacing things and unable to find them

What can be done about mind forgetfulness?

To help one's memory, one can take any or a number of the following steps:

- Get enough sleep, generally 7-8 hours each night.
- Exercise and eat well.
- Do not drink a lot of alcohol.
- Follow a daily routine.
- Every day, put regularly needed objects (wallet or purse, keys, phone, and glasses) in the same place each day.
- Use memory aids (calendars, to-do lists, notes, etc.).
- Get help if depressed for weeks at a time, etc.
- Learn a new skill.
- Volunteer in the community, at school, or at place of worship.

On serious memory problems

What are serious memory problems?

Serious memory problems make it hard to do everyday things such as to drive, shop, or even talk with a friend. Signs of serious memory problems may include:

- ➢ Asking the same questions over and over again.
- ➢ Getting lost in well-known places.
- ➢ Being unable to follow recipes or directions.
- ➢ Becoming more confused about time, people, and places.
- ➢ Not taking care of oneself (eating poorly, not bathing, or behaving unsafely).

What medical and other conditions cause serious memory problems?

Certain medical conditions can cause serious memory problems but can be managed. These problems should go away with treatment. Some conditions that may cause memory problems are:

- Head injury, such as a concussion from a fall or accident.
- Thyroid, kidney, or liver problems.
- Blood clots or tumors in the brain.
- Depression.
- Bad reaction to certain medicines.
- Having Alzheimer's disease or related dementias.
- Poor lifestyle habits (not eating enough healthy foods, or too few vitamins and minerals in the body; drinking too much alcohol, etc.).

What can be done about serious memory problems?

Seeing a doctor is important to find out what might be causing the serious memory problem and getting the right treatment. This may include a complete health check-up, medicines for blood and urine, and tests that check memory, problem solving, counting, and language skills. In addition, a brain scan may be ordered to show normal and problem areas in the brain. A referral to a neurologist who specializes in treating diseases of the brain and nervous system may also be obtained.

On emotional problems

What are the causes of emotional problems?

Some emotional problems in older adults (feeling sad, lonely, worried, or bored) can cause serious memory problems.

What treatments are available for emotional problems?

- See a doctor or counselor for treatment if these feelings last for more than two weeks.
- Being active, spending more time with family and friends, and learning new skills also can help one feel better and improve memory.

On mild cognitive impairment (MCI)

What are the signs and symptoms of MCI?

MCI is a medical condition that causes people to have more memory problems than other people of their age. The signs are not as severe as those of Alzheimer's disease. They include:

- Losing things often.
- Forgetting to go to events or appointments.
- Having more trouble coming up with words than other people of the same age.

How is MCI diagnosed?

➢ Your doctor can do thinking, memory, and language tests and eventually suggest a specialist for more tests. Because MCI may be an early sign of more serious memory problems, it is important to see the doctor or specialist regularly, say, every 6-12 months to see if any changes in memory or thinking skills have occurred over time.

How is MCI managed?

➢ People with MCI can take care of themselves and do their normal activities.

Can MCI be treated?

➢ At this time, there is no proven treatment for MCI.
➢ Even though there is no treatment for MCI, things can be done to help stay healthy and deal with changes in memory or thinking skills.

On dementia

What is dementia?

Dementia is the loss of the ability to think, remember, and reason to such a level that it interferes with activities of daily living (ADL).

What are the symptoms of dementia?

Dementia symptoms may include problems with language, vision (trouble reading or recognizing colors) or paying attention. Some people also experience changes in their personality and behavior.

What are the causes of dementia?

Many conditions can cause dementia or dementia-like symptoms. See below for the two most common forms of dementia (Alzheimer's disease and vascular disease).

What are the different forms of dementia?

There are different forms of dementia, characterized by symptoms and brain changes, including principally:

- ➤ Alzheimer's disease (AD).
- ➤ Vascular disease dementia (VDD).
- ➤ Lewy body dementia (LBD).
- ➤ Frontotemporal dementia (FTD).
- ➤ Mixed dementia (MD), and others.

On Alzheimer's disease (AD)

What are the signs and symptoms of AD?

AD causes serious memory problems. Its signs begin slowly and get worse over time because changes in the brain cause large numbers of brain cells to die. It may look like simple forgetfulness at first, but over time, people have trouble thinking clearly. They find it hard to do everyday things (shopping, driving, cooking, etc.). As the illness gets worse, they may need someone to take care of all their needs at home or in a nursing home, including feeding, bathing, and dressing.

In some people, the signs of AD can begin early, in their 40s, for example. However, most people do not begin to have symptoms until they are much older.

What treatments are available for AD?

> ➤ Taking certain medicines can help slow down some symptoms, such as memory loss, for a time. However, the medicines can have side effects and may not work for everyone.
> ➤ Other medicines can help against worriness, depression, or having problems sleeping.

On vascular dementia (VD)

What is VD?

Like AD, VD is caused by changes in the blood supply to the brain, often after a stroke. Signs can appear suddenly. These signs include changes in memory, language, thinking skills, and mood. However, unlike AD, it may appear suddenly because the memory loss and confusion are caused by changes in the blood supply to the brain, often after a stroke. If the stroke stops, a person may get better or stay the same for a long time. If more strokes occur, VD may get worse.

What is the treatment for VD?

The following steps can help reduce the risk of having more strokes:

> ➤ Control high blood pressure.
> ➤ Treat high cholesterol.

- ➢ Manage diabetes.
- ➢ Stop smoking.

On Lewy body dementia (LBD)

What is LBD?

LBD is a medical condition caused by changes in the brain from abnormal protein clusters, called 'Lewy bodies'.

What are the signs and symptoms of LBD?

Signs include problems with thinking, movement, behavior, and mood. Early on, the signs of LBD may be very mild but increase over time.

On mixed dementia (MD)

What is MD?

MD is a condition in which a person has two or more types of dementia. For example, someone may have both AD and VD at the same time.

On sleep-related myths

How much sleep does the average person need?

Sleep is not simply a lack of consciousness, but a rhythmic cycle of distinct neural patterns. For healthy young adults and adults with normal sleep, 7–9 hours is an appropriate amount but older adults need 7–8 hours. It is a myth that people can train their body to need fewer hours and it is more likely that they are used to the negative effects of sleep deprivation, but this does not mean that their body needs any less sleep. However, due to a rare genetic mutation, some rare individuals do seem to function fine with fewer than 6.5 hours' sleep each night.

Is daytime napping unhealthy?

Generally, daytime napping should be avoided to ensure a better night's sleep. However, if missing some sleep during previous nights, a tactical nap (around 20 minutes) can be helpful. This can help the body ample time to 'recharge'. Naturally, our bodies tend to dip in energy during the early afternoon, so perhaps napping around that time is more natural than avoiding sleep until nighttime. Some authors explain that afternoon naps in people who are not sleep deprived can lead to "*subjective and behavioral improvements*" and "*improvements in mood and subjective levels of sleepiness and fatigue*". Not all naps are equal, however. There is a great deal of variation, such as the time of day, duration, and frequency of naps. Another author suggested "*...a decrease in the risk of cardiovascular and cognitive dysfunction by the practice of taking short naps several times a week*". However, if an individual experiences severe tiredness during the day, this might be a sign of a sleep disorder, such as sleep apnea. More research is obviously needed to understand how factors associated with napping influence health outcomes.

Is more sleep always better?

Contrary to common belief, regularly sleeping longer than needed does not endow with superpowers. Actually, this was linked to poorer health, including developing obesity. Sleep duration might also impact mortality. According to a published meta-analysis "*both short- and long-sleep duration are significant predictors of death in prospective population studies*".

Can sleep deprivation be lethal?

In theory, it may be possible, but as far as scientists can ascertain, it is improbable. There is no record of anyone dying from sleep deprivation.

On medication approval

How is a medicine approved by FDA?

Drug companies seeking approval to sell a drug in the United States must test it. First, the drug company or sponsor performs laboratory and animal tests to discover how the drug works and whether it is likely to be safe and work well in humans. Next, a series of tests in humans is begun to determine whether the drug is safe when used to treat a disease and whether it provides a real health benefit. The company then sends the FDA's Center for Drug Evaluation and Research (CDER) the data from these tests to prove the drug is safe and effective for its intended use. A team of CDER physicians, statisticians, chemists, pharmacologists, and other scientists reviews the company's data and proposed labeling. If this review establishes that a drug's health benefits outweigh its known risks, the drug is approved for sale.

Over-the-counter (OTC) drugs are regulated by the FDA through OTC Drug monographs. OTC drug monographs are a kind of "recipe book" covering acceptable ingredients, doses, formulations, and labeling. Monographs will continually be updated adding additional ingredients and labeling as needed. Products conforming to a monograph may be marketed without further FDA clearance, while those that do not, must undergo separate review and approval through the "New Drug Approval System".

How can I find out if my medicine is FDA-approved?

To find out if your drug has been approved by the FDA, use Drugs@FDA, a catalog of FDA-approved drug products, as well as drug labeling. Drugs@ FDA contains most of the drug products approved since 1998.

Why are drugs evaluated by the FDA?

Drugs intended for human use are evaluated by the FDA's Center for Drug Evaluation and Research (CDER) to ensure that drugs marketed in the U.S.

are safe and effective. Biological products are evaluated by the FDA's Center for Biologics Evaluation and Research (CBER).

Does the FDA test drugs?

No. It is the responsibility of the company seeking approval to market a drug to conduct laboratory and animal tests on the safety and effectiveness of a proposed new drug and then to submit that information to the FDA for review by CDER physicians, statisticians, chemists, pharmacologists, and other scientists.

How long does the drug approval process take?

The 1992 Prescription Drug User Fee Act (PDUFA) established a two-tiered system – *Standard Review* and *Priority Review*. *Standard Review* is applied to a drug that offers at most, only minor improvement over existing marketed therapies. The 2002 amendments to PDUFA set a 10-month goal for a standard review. *Priority Review* designation is given to drugs that offer major advances in treatment, or provide a treatment where none existed. The goal for completing a Priority Review is six months.

What are the different types of drug applications that can be submitted to the FDA?

Four types of drug applications can be submitted o the FDA. These are:

> **Investigational New Drug (IND)** -- Federal law requires that a drug be the subject of an approved marketing application before it is transported or distributed across state lines.

> **New Drug Application (NDA)** -- When the sponsor of a new drug believes that enough evidence on the drug's safety and effectiveness has been obtained to meet FDA's requirements for marketing approval, the sponsor submits a new drug application (NDA) to the FDA. The application must contain data from specific technical viewpoints for review, including chemistry, pharmacology, medical, biopharmaceutics,

and statistics. If the NDA is approved, the product may be marketed in the United States.

➢ **Abbreviated New Drug Application (ANDA)** – An ANDA contains data that provides for the review and ultimate approval of a generic drug product. Generic drug applications are called "abbreviated" because they are generally not required to include preclinical (animal) and clinical (human) data to establish safety and effectiveness. Instead, a generic drug applicant must scientifically demonstrate that its product is bioequivalent (performs in the same manner as the innovator drug). Once approved, an applicant may manufacture and market the generic drug product.

➢ **Biologic License Application (BLA)** -- Biological products are approved for marketing under the provisions of the Public Health Service Act (PHSA). The Act requires a firm who manufactures a biologic for sale in interstate commerce to hold a license for the product. A biologics license application is a submission that contains specific information on the manufacturing processes, chemistry, pharmacology, clinical pharmacology, and the medical effects of the biologic product. If the information provided meets the FDA requirements, the application is approved and a license is issued allowing the firm to market the product.

Do over-the-counter (OTC) medications go through the same approval process as prescription drugs?

No. Because there are over 300,000 marketed OTC drug products, instead of individual drug products, the FDA reviews the active ingredients and the labeling of over 80 therapeutic classes of drugs, for example analgesics or antacids. For each class, an OTC drug monograph is developed and published in the *Federal Register*. OTC drug monographs are a kind of "recipe book" covering acceptable ingredients, doses, formulations, and labeling. Once a final monograph is implemented, companies can make and market an OTC product without the need for FDA pre-approval. These monographs define the safety, effectiveness, and labeling of all marketing OTC active ingredients. New products that conform to a final monograph may be marketed without further FDA review. Those that do not conform must be reviewed by the NDA process. A drug company may also petition to change a final monograph to include additional ingredients or to modify labeling.

On clinical trials and research studies

(See also Chapter 19.) People with memory problems, including AD, MCI, a family history of AD or a related dementia may be able to take part in clinical trials. Healthy people with no memory problems and no family history of such conditions may also be able to participate. Joining a clinical trial or other research study is also a way to help fight MCI, and AD and related dementias. To find out more about clinical trials:

➢ Check out www.ClinicalTrials.gov.
➢ See "NIH Clinical Research Trials and You" at www.nih.gov/health/ clinicaltrials.
➢ Visit the ADEAR Center website at www.alzheimers.gov.
➢ Call the Alzheimer's and related Dementias Education and Referral (ADEAR) Center.
Tel: 800-438-4380.

What are clinical trials and how do they relate to drug approval?

Clinical trials are studies that use human subjects (people) to see whether a drug is effective and what side effects it may cause. The trials are for gathering information about a drug that has not yet been proven to treat patients with a specific condition. A drug being studied in a clinical trial is called an 'investigational drug'. Clinical trials of drugs provide information about:

➢ Whether the drug has the effect it is supposed to have.
➢ How much of the drug to give to a patient and how often.
➢ What side effects are associated with the drug and how they can best be managed.
➢ How a drug is broken down in the body, and how long it stays in the body.

> Which foods, drinks, or other drugs can be used at the same time or should be avoided.

> Clinical trial results allow the FDA to make decisions about whether or not a drug should be approved for marketing.

How can I find a clinical trial for brain stimulation therapy?

The (U.S.) National Institute on Mental Health (NIMH) supports a wide range of research, including clinical trials that look at new ways to prevent, detect, or treat diseases and conditions. The goal of a clinical trial is again to determine if a new test or treatment works and is safe. Although people may benefit from being part of a clinical trial, they should know that the primary purpose is not necessarily to benefit them directly but to gain new scientific knowledge so that others can be better helped in the future. Researchers at NIMH and around the country conduct many studies with people experiencing mental disorders and healthy volunteers. Because of clinical trials, there are new and better treatment options today.

On help from family members

What can family members do to help?

If a family member or friend has a serious memory problem, other family members can help that person live as normal a life as possible, stay active, and keep up everyday routines. They can remind him/her of the time of day, where he/she lives, and what is happening at home and in the world. The following things could be done to help with memory problems:

> Keep large calendars to highlight important dates and events.

> Keep lists of the plans for each day.

> Keep notes about safety in the home.

> Provide written directions for using common household items.

> Have medication reminders using an alarm on mobile technology (smart watch, smart phone).

> Have maps and location services on mobile technologies to provide directions or help family members know a person's location.

How to communicate with someone with serious memory problems?

Some of the following tips can help make communication easier:

- ➤ Make eye contact and call the person by name.
- ➤ Be aware of how you look at the person, your body language, your tone, and how loud your voice is.
- ➤ Use other methods besides speaking, such as gentle touching.
- ➤ Try distracting the person if communication leads to a conflict or makes the person agitated or stressed (for example, look through a photo album together).
- ➤ Aim to be direct, specific, and positive.
- ➤ To encourage the person to communicate with you: Show a warm, loving, matter-of-fact manner; hold the person's hand while you talk; be open to the person's concerns, even if he/she is hard to understand; let him/her make some decisions and stay involved; be patient with angry outbursts, etc. And, remember, it's the illness "talking".

Take-aways

- ➤ This Chapter answered most of the frequently asked questions. For convenience, the questions have been grouped under the following categories as they would concern: Mild forgetfulness, serious memory problems, emotional problems, mild cognitive impairment, dementia and its various types (Alzheimer's, vascular, Lewy body, and mixed), sleep-related myths, medication approval, clinical trials and research studies, and help from family members.
- ➤ Mild forgetfulness has been contrasted between normal aging and Alzheimer's or a related dementia. Suggestions have been made as to what can be done about mild forgetfulness.
- ➤ Serious memory problems, as well as medical and other conditions that can cause them have been listed as well as what can be done about them.
- ➤ The causes of emotional problems and the available treatments have been discussed.

- The signs and symptoms of mild cognitive impairment, how the condition is diagnosed, managed, and treated have been presented.
- Dementia, its symptoms, causes, and treatments as well as the different forms in which it can present has been reviewed. The discussion also encompassed the various forms of dementia including Alzheimer's, vascular, Lewy body, and mixed dementia.
- Sleep- related myths have been dispelled.
- The various steps involved in the FDA drug approval process, **the different types of drug applications that can be submitted to that federal agency, as well as over-the-counter drugs, have been reviewed.**
- Clinical trials and research studies and how they relate to drug approval have been explained.
- Help from family members is too important to neglect and suggestions have been made as to how they can do so, and how they ought to communicate with someone with serious memory problems.

22

Support and resources

Contents

22

Support and resources

Federal resources

U.S. National Library of Medicine: "Memory".

Behavioral Brain Research: "Skill-memory consolidation".

Current Biology: "Memory reconsolidation".

Drugs@FDA database: Everything to know about approved medicines (approved brand name and generic drugs; therapeutic biological products) and almost every drug approved by the FDA since 1998. The database has drug labels, patient information, approval letters, and other information for most drug products approved. Drugs@FDA can be used to find:

➢ Labels for drug products, including: name; active ingredient; dosage form (such as tablet, capsule or injection), route of administration (oral, nasal, or intramuscular), strength, and whether it is a prescription, over-the-counter, discontinued product, or tentatively approved.

➢ If there are generic drug products for an innovator ("brand name") drug product.

➢ Therapeutically equivalent drug products. Drug products that are therapeutically equivalent and control a symptom or condition in the exact same way as another drug product.

- Consumer information for drugs.
- All drugs with a specific active ingredient.
- The approval history of a drug, including approval letters and review documents.

Journal of Clinical and Experimental Neuropsychology: "Digit-span assessments".

MedlinePlus.

General resources:

- Brain Stimulation Therapies for Epilepsy: National Institute of Neurological Disorders and Stroke.
- Deep Brain Stimulation (DBS): MedlinePlus Medical Encyclopedia.
- Deep Brain Stimulation for the Treatment of Parkinson's Disease and Other Movement Disorders: National Institute of Neurological Disorders and Stroke.
- Electroconvulsive Therapy: MedlinePlus Medical Encyclopedia.

Information about memory loss and forgetfulness

The following organizations can provide information about memory loss, brain health, Alzheimer's disease and related dementias, and support groups and services. They can also share information about research centers and clinical trials and studies.

(U.S.) National Institute of Mental Health
866-615-6464
866-415-8051 (TTY)
nimhinfo@nih.gov
www.nimh.nih.gov
1-866-615-6464

(U.S.) National Institute of Neurological Disorders and Stroke (NINDS)
The National Institute of Neurological Disorders and Stroke aims to increase knowledge about the brain and nervous system and to use that knowledge to reduce the burden of related diseases.
800-352-9424 (toll-free)
www.ninds.nih.gov
braininfo@ninds.nih.gov

(U.S.) National Institute on Aging (NIA) -
Alzheimer's and related Dementias Education and Referral (ADEAR) Center
"Instruments to Detect Cognitive Impairment in Older Adults".
The National Institute on Aging's ADEAR Center offers information and free print publications about Alzheimer's and related dementias for families, caregivers, and health professionals on Alzheimer's disease and related dementias, including information on clinical trials, and research. ADEAR Center staff answer inquiries by telephone, email, and written requests and make referrals to local and national resources. Visit the ADEAR website to learn more about Alzheimer's and related dementias, find clinical trials, and sign up for email updates.

P.O. Box 8250
Silver Spring, MD 20907-8250
800-438-4380 (toll-free)
adear@nia.nih.gov
www.nia.nih.gov/alzheimers

(U.S.) National Library of Medicine
This service of the National Library of Medicine, a part of the National Institutes of Health, provides consumer-friendly information and videos on various health topics and medical tests.
www.medlineplus.gov

Eldercare Locator
The Eldercare Locator is a service of the Administration on Aging that provides information about community resources, such as home

care, adult day services, and nursing homes. Contact the Eldercare Locator to find these resources in your area.
800-677-1116 (toll-free)
eldercarelocator@n4a.org
https://eldercare.acl.gov

Alzheimers.gov
Explore the Alzheimers.gov website for information and resources on Alzheimer's and related dementias from across the federal government.
www.alzheimers.gov

Alzheimer's Association
The Alzheimer's Association is a nonprofit organization offering information and support services to people with Alzheimer's and their caregivers and families. This association provides a toll-free hotline with the federal government's Administration for Community Living.
225 N. Michigan Avenue, Suite 1700
Chicago, IL 60611-7633
800-272-3900 (toll-free)
866-403-3073 (TTY/toll-free)
info@alz.org
www.alz.org

Alzheimer's Foundation of America
This foundation serves people with dementia and their caregivers and families. Services include a toll-free hotline, publications, and online resources.
866-232-8484 (toll-free)
info@alzfdn.org
www.alzfdn.org

Association for Frontotemporal Degeneration
This nonprofit organization provides information and support to people living with frontotemporal dementia and their care partners. Services include a toll-free hotline and support groups.

866-507-7222 (toll-free)
info@theaftd.org
www.theaftd.org

Lewy Body Dementia Association
This nonprofit organization sponsors research and provides support to people living with Lewy body dementia, their families, and caregivers.
404-935-6444
800-539-9767 (toll-free LBD Caregiver Link)
www.lbda.org

McKnight Brain Research Foundation
This foundation, dedicated to discovering the mysteries of the aging brain, provides information about brain health, age-related cognitive decline, and memory loss.
407-237-4485
https://mcknightbrain.org

Information about agnosia

The following organizations and resources help people living with agnosia and their families, friends, and caregivers:

Merck Manuals Online Medical Library
203-744-0100
800-999-6673 (toll-free)
844-259-7178

Spanish National Organization for Rare Disorders (NORD)

Information about palliative care

Palliative care is recommended before the late stages of dementia. Given the progressive and terminal nature of the disease, palliative care can be helpful to patients and their caregivers by helping both people with the disorder and their caregivers understand what to expect, deal with loss of physical and mental abilities, plan out a patient's wishes and goals including surrogate decision-making, and discuss wishes for or against cardiopulmonary resuscitation (CPR) and life support.

Information about caregiving

To help, caregivers should learn different ways to communicate and to deescalate possibly aggressive situations. Because decision-making skills can be impaired, it can be beneficial to give simple commands instead of asking multiple questions. By keeping the patient active, focusing on their positive abilities, and avoiding stress, these tasks can easily be accomplished. Routines for bathing and dressing must be organized in a way so that the individual still feels a sense of independence. Simple approaches such as finding clothes with large buttons, elastic waist bands, or Velcro straps can ease the struggles of getting dressed in the morning.

When household chores begin to pile up, find ways to break down large tasks into small, manageable steps that can be rewarded. Finally, talking with and visiting a family member or friend with memory issues is very important. Using a respectful and simple approach, talking one-on-one can ease the pain of social isolation and bring much mental stimulation. Many people who experience memory loss and other cognitive impairments can have changes in behaviors that are challenging to deal with for care givers.

Further, finances should be managed or have a trusted individual appointed to manage them. Changing passwords to prevent over-use and involving a trusted family member or friend in managing accounts can prevent financial issues.

Caregiving can be a physically, mentally, and emotionally taxing job to take on. Caregivers also need to remember to care for themselves, taking breaks, finding time to themselves, and possibly joining a support group in the search for a few ways to avoid burnout.

Take-aways

➢ The available (U.S.) federal resources have been listed along with their particulars.

➢ Information about memory loss and forgetfulness has been provided including several U.S. institutions (**National Institute of Mental Health, National Institute of Neurological Disorders and Stroke, National Institute on Aging with its Alzheimer's and related Dementias Education and Referral,** National Library of Medicine, **Eldercare Locator, Alzheimers.gov) and private organizations (Alzheimer's Association, Alzheimer's Foundation of America,** Association for Frontotemporal Degeneration, Lewy Body Dementia Association, and the McKnight Brain Research Foundation).

➢ Information was also provided concerning agnosia, palliative care, and caregiving.

23

Research and latest developments

Contents

23

Research and latest developments

The following is a synopsis of a few selected research and latest developments.

From the (U.S.) National Institutes of Health (NIH)

The *Brain Research Through Advancing Innovative Neurotechnologies*® Initiative, or The BRAIN Initiative®

Under the leadership of the NIH, this Initiative is a partnership between 10 Federal and non-Federal Institutes and Centers whose missions and current research portfolios complement the goals of the Initiative, including the:

> - National Center for Complementary and Integrative Health (NCCIH).
> - National Eye Institute (NEI).
> - National Institute on Aging (NIA).
> - National Institute on Alcohol Abuse and Alcoholism (NIAAA).
> - National Institute of Biomedical Imaging and Bioengineering (NIBIB).
> - Eunice Kennedy Shriver National Institute of Child Health and Human Development (NICHD).
> - National Institute on Drug Abuse (NIDA).

- ➢ National Institute on Deafness and Other Communication Disorders (NIDCD).
- ➢ National Institute of Mental Health (NIMH).
- ➢ National Institute of Neurological Disorders and Stroke (NINDS).

This transformative BRAIN Initiative, initiated in 2014, seeks to revolutionize our understanding of the human brain by advancing innovative neurotechnologies. Through the application and dissemination of these scientific advancements, it is hoped that researchers will be able to produce a revolutionary new dynamic picture of the brain that, for the first time, will show how individual cells and complex neural circuits interact in both time and space.

Investigative human neuroscience program

The NIH BRAIN Initiative funds research on investigative human neuroscience through the Research Opportunities in Humans (ROH) program. While fundamental basic research often provides insights relevant to disorders of the nervous system, this program is not intended to generate research that is explicitly disease therapeutic. Rather, it provides support for research projects focused on investigative neuroscience with intracranial access to recording and manipulating the brain directly. Such investigations offer revolutionary, but challenging, opportunities for experimental investigation in how the human brain senses, thinks, perceives, remembers, plans, registers emotions, activates movements, engages language, and makes decisions. By leveraging surgical procedures with direct access to the brain, there is the opportunity to design experiments specifically about human neuroscience in ways that are both uniquely human and otherwise impossible.

Neural recording and modulation

The NIH BRAIN Initiative supports the development and optimization of new tools and technologies for modulation and recording of cellular or near-cellular resolution signals of the central nervous system and the biology and biophysics underlying those technologies. These technologies include electrodes, micro/miniscopes, molecular probes for neurotransmitters, magnetothermal tools, bioluminescent recorders, and voltage indicators, as well as supplemental components for these base technologies like custom application-specific integrated circuits (ASICs), adaptive optics, and signal processing techniques. The primary goal of this research is to develop new tools that enable new capabilities for *in vivo* experiments, at or near cellular resolution, in animal models.

Neural activity is defined broadly to include electrical activity, neurotransmitter and neuropeptide signaling, as well as plasticity and intracellular signaling events. The technologies employed represent diverse modalities including optical, electrical, magnetic, acoustic, and genetic recording/ manipulation.

The brain and memory: Understanding how the brain thinks

In a groundbreaking finding that could affect how we treat brain conditions such as Alzheimer's disease (AD) and dementia, and as part of the NIH's *Brain Research through Advancing Innovative Neurotechnologies®* (**BRAIN**) ***Initiative***, transcontinental researchers discovered "boundary" and "event" cells that are involved in making and marking memories, and are activated at memory starting and stopping points, respectively. They were operating under the existing memory framework of "boundaries"—the idea that memories can have *hard* and *soft* starting and ending points (think of hard boundaries as a file folder and soft boundaries as the files inside it). It is unclear how exactly the brain sets these boundaries. For 20 consenting patients across the country undergoing intracranial recordings for epilepsy treatment, the researchers looked at their brain activity while they were shown clips mimicking hard and soft boundaries. They found that "boundary" cells were activated by both hard and soft boundaries whereas "event" cells were activated only by hard boundaries. The team believes that, activating both boundary and event cells, hard boundaries are what trigger the brain to create a new memory. Knowing what cells are involved with memory production, the next step is to figure out what activates the cells, which could have a huge effect on treating memory-related issues like AD and dementia.

Brain ripples of activity could hold clues to memory

As it turns out, a split second before a person calls up a memory, fast waves of activity ripple across key parts of the brain that help store memories. Recording brain activity of epilepsy patients, researchers found out what was causing the seizures related to their disorder. The recordings also provided a chance to study how the brain stores memories. The ripples could help better understand how the brain processes and retrieves memories: Coordinated ripple activity may play a critical role in replaying the neural codes behind memories. How we remember may come down to unique firing patterns in our brains.

Brain circuits susceptible to aging, Alzheimer's disease

This University of California, Irvine study aims to create maps of the brain that identify specific brain cells and circuits related to aging and AD. These findings can hopefully lead to earlier diagnoses and help create new treatments.

Brain cells' Atlas Project

The Seattle Alzheimer's Disease Brain Cell Atlas consortium, led by the Allen Institute, is attempting to create a cellular- and molecular-level atlas of the human brain to determine the causes and effects of AD. The project relies heavily on brain-mapping technology developed by researchers funded by the NIH BRAIN Initiative.

The human brain is not uniform in nature, comprising an incredibly intricate system of neurons and non-neuronal cells, each with distinct roles. Each brain cell possesses an identical DNA sequence, but various cell types utilize distinct genes in varying quantities. This diversity results in the creation of numerous brain cell types, adding to the intricacy of neural networks. Creating a comprehensive map of these diverse brain cell types and deciphering their collaborative functions will ultimately lead to a greater understanding of the brain and its functioning.

Gaining insights into the molecular distinctions among these cell types is crucial for comprehending brain functionality and devising innovative approaches to address neuropsychiatric disorders. This will further **advance our understanding of the genetic foundations of neuropsychiatric disorders, potentially paving the way for more targeted treatments and precision medicine in neuropsychiatry.**

In a collaborative study led by the University of California at San Diego, scientists have examined over 1 million human brain cells to craft intricate maps of gene regulators specific to different brain cell types. This research not only demonstrated the intricate links between distinct cell categories and prevalent neuropsychiatric disorders but also pioneers the use of artificial intelligence (AI) to predict the impact of high-risk gene variations within these cells, potentially unlocking insights into disease development.

Subsequently, the researchers constructed machine learning models aimed at forecasting how specific DNA sequence variations can impact gene regulation and contribute to the development of diseases. Researchers are still in the process of comprehensively mapping the brain. If the technology becomes effective, this will not only play a role in treating the conditions but, even more exciting, preventing them.

Different firing patterns in epileptic brains could help in future dementia and other memory loss

To study how brains make and find memories, researchers tracked the electrical activity of thousands of individual neurons of epileptic subjects. They found that there are distinct "firing" patterns that happen when they tried to remember. These unique patterns could help better understand how brains stop working properly in various memory and thinking disorders, like dementia and Alzheimer's. The lead investigator of the study describes the finding as follows: *"Just as musical notes are recorded as grooves on a record, it appears that our brains store memories in neural firing patterns that can be replayed over and over again"*.

Reading the brain's map: Coordinated brain activation supports spatial learning and decision-making

Specialized internal brain activation "replay" processes have revealed that animals (here, rodents) learn from past experiences to form memories of paths leading toward goals, and subsequently to recall these paths for planning future decisions. These results help better understand how coordinated activation at the level of neurons can contribute to the complex processes involved in learning and decision-making. The hippocampus, a structure critical to learning and **memory,** contains specialized "place" cells that relay information about location and orientation in space. These place cells show specific patterns of activity during navigation that can be "replayed" later in forward or reverse order, almost as if the brain were fast-forwarding or rewinding through routes the animals had taken. These replay events, marked by bursts of neural activity (called "sharp-wave ripples") lead to coordinated activity in certain brain areas (the hippocampus and the prefrontal cortex) and helped show how neural representations changed as the animals were learning. The findings suggest that coordinated replay across the hippocampus and prefrontal cortex serves an important function in spatial learning and memory-guided decision-making. Specifically, the results suggest that reverse replay is likely to support the ability to reflect on and evaluate paths that have led to goals in the past, whereas forward replay seems to support the ability to think ahead and plan choices that will lead to goals in the future.

Workshop on the definition of working memory

Working memory (WM) is the active maintenance and flexible updating of goal/task relevant information (items, goals, strategies, etc.) in a form that has limited capacity and resists interference. These representations may:

- ➢ **Involve flexible binding of representations;**
- ➢ **Be characterized by the absence of external support for the internally maintained representations; and**
- ➢ **Are frequently temporary, though this may be due to ongoing interference.**

This 2010 workshop was the first in a series with goals to:

> Arrive at an agreed-upon definition of WM, incorporating how the field views WM currently, and how it is distinguished from other similar constructs in cognition.

> Provide an annotated listing (based on current knowledge) of the elements that would populate the research domain criteria (RDoC) matrix with respect to the genes, molecules, cells, and circuits sub-serving WM.

> Identifying promising behavioral tasks to reliably assess disruptions in WM functioning.

For the above purposes, the participants agreed to the following pre-requisites:

- WM is distinct from short-term memory (STM), long-term memory (LTM), cognitive control, attentional processes, and perception.

- WM and STM represent different processes, even in the absence of a clear agreement regarding how they differed from each other.

- WM and LTM have distinct features: Compared to WM, LTM has a longer time frame, less accessible representations, and may be reactivated/accessed more automatically.

- LTM is associated with at least partially distinct circuits within the brain (medial temporal lobe versus dorsal frontal parietal in WM).

- Cognitive control processes are distinguishable from WM in that they involve processes that are not present in WM: Motivation, goal selection, motor inhibition, and error conflict monitoring.

- WM differs from attentional processes in that they operate on or involve perceptual processes/ representations and "bottom-up inputs" that are not formally part of WM.

- The circuitries associated with WM and attentional processes may be different in that the former appear to be more "frontal." whereas the latter are generally considered more "parietal".

- Perception is different from WM in that it depends on external versus internal support for the representations.

- Integrity of perceptual processes and representations may influence the integrity of derived WM representations.

From the (U.S.) National Institute of Mental Health (NIMH)

Understanding the brain, mood, memory, and thinking

This research study seeks to learn about the brain, moods, memory, thinking, and concentration in healthy adults and compares them to those who have HIV infections. For this purpose, researchers will evaluate the relationship among brain inflammation, protein function, and motor neuron diseases (MND); and how HIV infection may cause problems with blood vessel function and contribute to thinking and mood disorders, such as early dementia and depression.

Brain processes underlying the extinction and reactivation of fear memories

Exposure therapy is a technique often used to reduce or eliminate learned fear by repeatedly exposing to a fear-provoking stimulus in the absence of a negative or aversive outcome. Over time, this exposure helps reduce emotional and physiological responses associated with the learned-fear. Although exposure therapy and fear extinction have shown effectiveness, fear memories can sometimes relapse over time — an event called "spontaneous recovery", which may occur because extinction training does not erase fear memories but instead creates a new memory that either suppresses the fear memory or competes with it for expression. Neurons called "engram cells" and their reactivation are necessary for memory recall; they are genetically tagged (a technique called optogenetics) and manipulated to evidence their activity changes during the formation, extinction, and spontaneous recovery of a fear memory. Researchers found that during extinction training, the engram cells associated with the fear memory are suppressed and a second set of engram cells associated with the extinction memory are activated. During the spontaneous recovery of fear, the engram cells associated with the fear memory become more active than the engram cells associated with the extinction memory.

Daily multivitamins may enhance memory in older adults

Memory and thinking skills tend to decline as one gets older. Certain lifestyle factors — such as a healthy diet, physical activity, and social interactions — might help to protect cognitive health as one ages. Some studies have suggested that taking multivitamins or other dietary supplements may help protect thinking and **memory**. But few large-scale studies have directly examined how dietary supplements affect cognitive health in older adults. Clinical trials to date have shown mixed results (see Chapter 19). In a random clinical trial, people taking multivitamins had significantly higher scores on a test of immediate recall compared to the placebo group, the scores having improved from an average of about 7.1 recalled words to 7.8 words after the first year. For comparison, scores changed from about 7.2 words to about 7.6 words in the placebo group. The improved scores in the multivitamin group continued but did not significantly increase over that of the placebo group into the second and third years of the study. Other types of cognitive tests showed no significant differences between the groups. Notably, participants with a history of cardiovascular disease had lower immediate-recall scores at the start of the study compared to those without such history. But after one year of taking multivitamins, the scores of those with cardiovascular disease improved significantly, becoming comparable to those without the disease.

These results refine the findings of a related NIH-supported study that found that the use of a daily multivitamins improved a broad measure of cognitive function. Improvements were likewise more prominent in those with a history of cardiovascular disease.

Daily multivitamins may improve cognition in older adults

Safe and affordable treatments to prevent **cognitive** decline in older adults are urgently needed. In response to this need, certain dietary supplements have been touted as having protective effects on cognition. Normal brain function requires various vitamins, minerals, and other nutrients. Deficiencies in these nutrients may increase the risk for cognitive decline and dementia with age. Yet clinical trials of individual nutrients' effects on cognition have yielded mixed results. Prior research suggests that Flavanols in particular — compounds found in high levels in unprocessed cocoa — might benefit cognition. Much of the research on Flavanols was based on observational studies, rather than clinical trials. And previously, the effects of a multivitamin on cognition in older adults had been studied only in a few short clinical trials (less than 12 months) and a single longer trial that included older male physicians. There is no difference in global cognition between people who take cocoa extract and those who do not. But participants taking the multivitamin had higher **global cognition** scores than those who did not. The improvement was most pronounced in those with a history of cardiovascular disease. Significant improvements with daily multivitamins use were also seen in **memory** and **executive function**. Cocoa extract had no effect on either.

Higher levels of education may help preserve memory in the face of accumulating age-related brain pathology

Several research studies have shown that higher educational attainment is associated with better late-life cognitive functioning and reduced risk for dementia. Although the relationship between education and cognition, especially **memory**, has been known for some time, exactly how and why cognition is preserved in the brains of people with higher education levels is still unknown. While many factors could be involved, scientists have proposed two theories to explain how factors like higher educational attainment may support cognitive function in older adults. The first, called "brain maintenance", suggests that higher education levels act as a shield to protect the brain from age-related pathology and that older adults with higher educational attainment have less age-related brain pathology, such as white matter damage, which accumulates in all older adults. An alternative theory, called "cognitive reserve", suggests that people who attain higher levels of education process and store information in the brain in a way that allows them to maintain normal cognitive performance even in the face of white matter damage or brain pathology. Basically, higher education levels somehow equip the brain to navigate around the effects of age-related brain pathology. A (U.S.) National Institute on Aging (NIA)-funded study used data from a large, racially and ethnically diverse sample of older adults to support the latter hypothesis — that more education predicts better **memory** later in life **through better cognitive reserve.**

To attempt to tease apart these two hypotheses, researchers evaluated how education affects a well-studied pathway that occurs during aging: 'white matter hyperintensities", which are a sign of cardiovascular-related brain damage linked to high blood pressure in older adults. Increased volume of white matter hyperintensities are linked to decreased memory performance in older adults, and are a predictor of Alzheimer's disease. The researchers did not find evidence supporting the brain maintenance hypothesis for education—education level did not affect blood pressure or white matter hyperintensity volume—they did find evidence to support the cognitive reserve pathway. Specifically, education was shown to affect the relationship between white matter hyperintensity volume and memory scores; the memory scores of individuals with higher educational attainment were less affected by increases in white matter hyperintensity volume compared to those with less education. This is consistent with the theory that **education may only be able to buffer the effects of age-related brain pathology at earlier stages**. The pattern supporting the cognitive reserve hypothesis held up across Hispanic, non-Hispanic black, and non-Hispanic white subgroups.

While this study does not address how cognitive reserve supports memory function in the face of brain pathology, future research could shed light on the hypothesis that education may improve the efficiency or ability of brain networks involved in **memory**, or enhance the brain's ability to flexibly use non-damaged areas to support memory. This study suggests that education could play an important role in protecting the brain from age-related cognitive decline and dementia.

Positive mood in older adults suggests better brain function

Research findings support links between a positive mental outlook and physical health benefits such as lower blood pressure, less heart disease, and healthier blood sugar levels. Healthy brain function may also result in maintaining a positive outlook. There appears to be a potential neurobiological connection between an older adult's mood with changes, over a period of time, in white brain matter and cognitive ability. White matter is where information is transmitted from one brain region to another. As one ages, changes can occur in the white matter that may lead to thinking, walking, and balance problems. The integrity of the white matter and stable executive function appear to be important for maintaining healthy mood states in late life. Observations showed that mood improved with increasing age until around the early 70s, at which point the positive effect of age on mood plateaued, and eventually reversed. Stable white matter integrity, along with stable executive function and processing speed, appeared to protect against this reversal of positive mood. However, because the underlying study was observational, the above findings cannot be interpreted to show causation. Further research is needed to determine whether the brain-mood relationships are bidirectional. Further, observed relationships between mood, age, white matter integrity, and cognition need to be evaluated in racially and educationally diverse groups. In addition, they should be large-scale, longitudinal, and use methods to allow capture of the full range of neurodevelopment to inform interventions across a variety of neurodegenerative and neuropsychiatric conditions.

From the (U.S.) National Library of Medicine (NLM)

Memory loss

Memory loss is unusual forgetfulness; it may be transient (last a short time and then resolve) or be semi-permanent (not go away and, depending on the cause, get worse over time). In severe cases, such memory impairment may interfere with daily living activities. Normal aging can cause some forgetfulness but does not lead to dramatic memory loss. Such memory loss is due to other diseases.

Memory loss can be caused by many things. Because many brain areas help one create and retrieve memories, a problem in any of these areas can lead to memory loss. This may result from a new injury to the brain, which is caused by or is present after:

- Brain tumor.
- Cancer treatment, such as brain radiation, bone marrow transplant, or chemotherapy.
- Concussion or head trauma.
- Not enough oxygen getting to the brain when one's heart or breathing is stopped for too long.
- Severe brain infection or infection around the brain.
- Major surgery or severe illness, including brain surgery.
- Transient global amnesia (TGA) – a sudden, temporary loss of memory of unclear cause.
- Transient ischemic attack (TIA) or stroke.
- Hydrocephalus (fluid collection in the brain).
- Multiple sclerosis (MS).
- Dementia.

Sometimes, memory loss occurs with mental health problems, such as:

- After a major, traumatic or stressful event.
- Bipolar disorder (BD).
- Depression or other mental health disorders, such as schizophrenia.

Memory loss may be a sign of dementia. Dementia also affects thinking, language, judgment, and behavior. Common types of dementia associated with memory loss are:

- Alzheimer disease (AD).
- Vascular dementia (VD).
- Lewy body dementia (LBD).
- Fronto-temporal dementia (FTD).
- Progressive supranuclear palsy (PSP).
- Normal pressure hydrocephalus (NPH).
- Creutzfeldt-Jakob disease (CJD).

Other causes of memory loss include:

- Alcohol or use of prescription or illegal drugs.
- Brain infections such as Lyme disease (LD), syphilis, or HIV/AIDS.
- Overuse of medicines, such as barbiturates or (hypnotics).

- ECT (electroconvulsive therapy) (most often short-term memory loss).
- Epilepsy that is not well controlled.
- Illness that results in the loss of, or damage to brain tissue or nerve cells, such as Parkinson's disease (PD), Huntington's disease (HD), or multiple sclerosis (MS).
- Low levels of important nutrients or vitamins, such as low vitamin B1 or B12.

From the Alzheimer's Association (AA)

Medications for memory, cognition, and dementia-related behaviors

Although current medications cannot cure Alzheimer's, two U.S. Food and Drug Administration (FDA)-approved treatments address the underlying biology. Other medications may help lessen symptoms, such as memory loss and confusion. The FDA has approved medications that fall into the following two categories (see also Chapter 17, Table 17.1):

Drugs that change disease progression

Drugs in this category slow disease progression by going after the underlying biology of the disease process. They aim to slow the decline of memory and thinking, as well as function, in people living with Alzheimer's disease (AD).

Amyloid-targeting approaches

Anti-amyloid treatments work by attaching to and removing beta-amyloid, a protein that accumulates into plaques, from the brain. Each works differently and targets beta-amyloid at a different stage of plaque formation. These treatments change the course of the disease in a meaningful way for people in the early stages, giving them more time to participate in daily life and live independently. Clinical trial participants who received anti-amyloid treatments experienced reduction in cognitive decline observed through measures of cognition and function. Anti-amyloid treatments do have side effects and can cause serious allergic reactions, amyloid-related imaging abnormalities (ARIA), infusion-related reactions, headaches, and falls. ARIA is typically a temporary swelling in areas of the brain that usually resolves over time. Some people may also have small spots of bleeding in or on the surface of the brain with the swelling, although most people with swelling in areas of the brain do not have symptoms. Some may have symptoms of ARIA such as headache, dizziness, nausea, confusion, and vision changes. Some people have a genetic risk factor (ApoE ε4 gene carriers) that may cause an increased risk for ARIA.

- ○ **Aducanumab (Aduhelm®): A**n anti-amyloid antibody intravenous (IV) infusion therapy that is delivered every month. It has received accelerated approval from the FDA to treat early AD, including people living with mild cognitive impairment (MCI) or mild dementia due to AD who have confirmation of elevated beta-amyloid in the brain. Aducanumab was the first therapy to demonstrate that removing beta-amyloid from the brain reduces cognitive and functional decline in people living with early AD. The drug was later discontinued and removed from the market by its manufacturer.
- ○ **Lecanemab (Leqembi®): A**n anti-amyloid antibody intravenous (IV) infusion therapy that is delivered every two weeks. It has received traditional approval from the FDA to treat early AD, including people living with mild cognitive impairment (MCI) or mild dementia due to AD who have confirmation of elevated beta-amyloid in the brain. There is no safety or effectiveness data on initiating treatment at earlier or later stages of the disease than were studied. Lecanemab was the second therapy to demonstrate that removing beta-amyloid from the brain reduces cognitive and functional decline in people living with early AD.

Drugs that treat cognitive symptoms (memory and thinking)

As AD progresses, brain cells die and connections among cells are lost, causing cognitive symptoms to worsen. While the following medications do not stop the damage AD causes to brain cells, they may help lessen or stabilize symptoms for a limited time by affecting certain chemicals involved in carrying messages among and between the brain's nerve cells.

- ➢ **Cholinesterase inhibitors: They** are prescribed to treat symptoms related to **memory**, thinking, language, judgment, and other thought processes. Further, they prevent the breakdown of acetylcholine, a chemical messenger important for memory and learning. Still further, they support communication between nerve cells. Though generally well-tolerated, if side effects occur, they commonly include nausea, vomiting, loss of appetite and increased frequency of bowel movements. The cholinesterase inhibitors most commonly prescribed are:
  - ○ **Donepezil (Aricept®)**: To treat all stages of AD.
  - ○ **Rivastigmine (Exelon®)**: For mild-to-moderate AD as well as mild-to-moderate dementia associated with Parkinson's disease (PD).
  - ○ **Galantamine (Razadyne®)**: For mild-to-moderate stages of AD.

- ➢ **Glutamate regulators: They** are prescribed to improve **memory**, attention, reason, language and the ability to perform simple tasks. This type of drug works by regulating the activity of glutamate, a different chemical messenger that helps the brain process information. This drug is known as:
  - ○ **Memantine (Namenda®):** Approved for moderate-to-severe AD. It can cause side effects, including headache, constipation, confusion, and dizziness.

- ➢ **Cholinesterase inhibitor + glutamate regulator:** This type of drug is a combination of a cholinesterase inhibitor and a glutamate regulator:
  - ○ Donepezil and Memantine (Namzaric®): Approved for moderate-to-severe AD. Possible side effects include nausea, vomiting, loss of appetite, increased frequency of bowel movements, headache, constipation, confusion, and dizziness.

Drugs that treat non-cognitive symptoms (behavioral and psychological symptoms)

AD affects more than just memory and thinking. A person's quality of life may be impacted by a variety of behavioral and psychological symptoms that accompany dementia, such as sleep disturbances, agitation, hallucinations, and delusions. Some medications focus on treating these non-cognitive symptoms for a time, though it is important to try non-drug strategies to manage behaviors before adding medications. The FDA has approved one drug to address symptoms of insomnia that has been tested in people living with dementia and one that treats agitation.

> **Orexin receptor antagonist (ORA):** Prescribed to treat insomnia, this drug inhibits the activity of orexin, a type of neurotransmitter involved in the sleep-wake cycle.

> **Suvorexant (Belsomra®):** Approved for treatment of insomnia, it has been shown in clinical trials to be effective for people living with mild to moderate AD. Possible side effects include, but are not limited to: risk of impaired alertness and motor coordination (including impaired driving), worsening of depression or suicidal thinking, complex sleep behaviors (such as sleep-walking and sleep-driving), sleep paralysis, and compromised respiratory function.

> **Atypical antipsychotics: A** group of antipsychotic drugs that target the serotonin and dopamine chemical pathways in the brain. These drugs are largely used to treat schizophrenia and bipolar disorder and as add-on therapies for major depressive disorder. The FDA requires that all atypical antipsychotics carry a safety warning that the medication has been associated with an increased risk of death in older patients with dementia-related psychosis.

> Many atypical antipsychotic medications are used "off-label" to treat dementia-related behaviors, and there is currently only one FDA-approved atypical antipsychotic to treat agitation associated with dementia due to AD. It is important to try non-drug strategies to manage non-cognitive symptoms — like agitation — before adding medications.

> **Brexpiprazole (Rexulti®):** Approved for the treatment of agitation associated with dementia due to AD. Possible side effects include, but are not limited to: weight gain, sleepiness, dizziness, common cold symptoms, and restlessness or feeling like you need to move. Warning for serious side effects: increased risk of death in older adults with dementia-related psychosis. Rexulti is not approved for the treatment

of people with dementia-related psychosis without agitation that may happen with dementia due to AD.

Pharmacologically reinstating the hippocampal theta frequency may lead to early AD treatment

The "hippocampal theta rhythm" is a specific type of electrical activity (the theta rhythm at 4-7 [Hz]) that can be observed in the hippocampus and other brain structures in numerous species of mammals. In rats, hippocampal theta is seen mainly when an animal is running, walking or in some other way actively interacting with its surroundings, or else during REM sleep. Its presence in the EEG can be predicted on the basis of what an animal is doing, rather than why the animal is doing it. Theta-frequency EEG activity is also manifested during some short-term **memory** tasks. Theta rhythms are very strong in rodent hippocampi during learning and **memory** retrieval, and are believed to be vital to the induction of long-term potentiation, a cellular mechanism of learning and **memory**. Amyloid-ß dampens the electrical theta oscillations of the rat hippocampus, and this modulation correlates with a decline in learning ability. This decline in theta is not due to cell death, but instead reflects a change in firing patterns. The findings point to another mechanism by which AD may disrupt normal cognitive functions, such as learning and memory. Further, in Aß-treated rats, the theta frequency stayed constant at 7.6 Hz, correlating with a lack of learning. Thus, beta-amyloid appears to negatively impact **memory** function even when the brain is still structurally intact (that is, no hippocampal atrophy has taken place). It may also be causing trouble before it has even deposited into plaques. More importantly, reinstating the theta frequency pharmacologically might possibly open a new avenue to consider for early AD treatment.

A hormonal connection between stress and AD

People who are susceptible to stress are at more risk of developing AD. Physical activity, which reduces stress levels, may reduce the chances of developing the disease. It is widely believed that the stress hormone corticotrophin-releasing factor (CRF) may have a protective effect on the brain, including the **memory** changes brought on by AD, It is associated with the production of stress and is found in high levels in people experiencing various forms of anxiety. Normal CRF levels are beneficial to the brain, keeping cognitive abilities sharp and aiding the survival of nerve cells. People with AD have a reduced level of CRF. An experimental drug to prevent CRF from binding to the brain receptor called CRFR1 in mice with AD showed that the animals were free from **memory** impairments. Further, moderate exercise restored the normal function of the CRF system allowing its **memory** enhancing effects.

Brain atrophy and B vitamins

Brain atrophy involves the loss of neurons. Some degree of atrophy and subsequent brain shrinkage is common with old age, even in people who are cognitively healthy. However, this atrophy is accelerated in people with mild cognitive impairment (MCI) and even faster in those who ultimately progress from MCI to AD. Many factors have been implicated in affecting the rate of brain atrophy, one of which is high levels of an amino acid in the blood called homocysteine. Raised levels of homocysteine increase the risk of AD. Researchers have investigated the role of vitamin B in regulating levels of homocysteine, specifically whether lowering it through giving high doses of vitamin B for two years could reduce the rate of brain atrophy in people with pre-existing MCI. Even accounting for such other factors as age, blood pressure, initial brain volume, and concentration of homocysteine, treatment with vitamin B tablets has notable effects on the levels of homocysteine in the blood, reducing it by 22.5 percent. Overall, treatment with B vitamins for a period of 24 months can lead to a reduction in the rate of brain atrophy. Overall, the safety of vitamins is good with no adverse events. This "simple and safe treatment" can slow down the accelerated rate of brain atrophy in people with MCI. mild cognitive impairment. Other studies have also found that the rate of brain atrophy is linked to cognitive decline. Based on the evidence gathered so far, it is too early to claim that vitamin B can prevent clinical disease, but the results so far are promising.

From the European Human Brain Project

The European Human Brain Project (HBP) was a 10-year project that was initiated on 1 October 2013 and terminated on its anniversary date. It was a multinational and uniquely interdisciplinary project that drew together 500+ researchers from 155 institutions from 19 countries. It pioneered digital neuroscience, a new approach to studying the brain based on multidisciplinary collaborations and high-performance computing. The researchers came from diverse disciplines, including neuroscience, philosophy, and computer science to take advantage of the loop of experimental data, modelling theories, and simulations.

The primary objective of the HBP was to create an ICT-based research infrastructure for brain research, cognitive neuroscience, and brain-inspired computing, which can be used by researchers world-wide.

The Project was divided into the following 12 Subprojects (SP):

> **SP1 Mouse Brain Organization:** To understand the structure of the mouse brain, and its electrical and chemical functions.
> **SP2 Human Brain Organization:** To understand the structure of the human brain, and its electrical and chemical functions.
> **SP3 Systems and Cognitive Neuroscience:** To understanding how the brain performs its systems-level and cognitive functional activities.
> **SP4 Theoretical Neuroscience:** To derive high-level mathematical models to synthesize conclusions from research data.
> **SP5 Neuroinformatics Platform:** To gather, organize, and make available brain data.
> **SP6 Brain Simulation Platform:** To develop data-driven reconstructions of brain tissue and simulation capabilities to explore these reconstructions.
> **SP7 High-performance Analytics and Computing Platform:** To provide the ICT capability to map the brain in unprecedented detail, construct complex models, run large simulations, and analyze large volumes of data.
> **SP8 Medical Informatics Platform:** To develop the infrastructure to share hospital and medical research data for the purpose of understanding disease clusters and their respective disease signatures.
> **SP9 Neuromorphic Computing Platform:** To develop and apply brain-inspired computing technology.
> **SP10 Neurorobotics Platform:** To develop virtual and real robots and environments for testing brain simulations.

- ➢ **SP11 Management and Coordination:** To generally coordinate the project.
- ➢ **SP12 Ethics and Society:** To explore the ethical and societal impact of HBP's work.

The HBP produced more than 3000 academic publications and more than 160 digital tools, medical and technological applications, and an open digital research infrastructure called EBRAINS, offering access to digital tools, models, data and services, and facilitating the integration of brain science across disciplines and national borders. It drove outstanding advances in brain research, the 3D atlases of the brain, breakthroughs in personalized brain medicine, and the development of new brain-inspired technologies (e.g., in artificial intelligence and neuromorphic computing).

The brain model provided by the HBP can be used to investigate signatures of disease in the brain and the impact of certain drugs, enabling the development of better diagnosis and treatment methods. Ultimately, these technologies will likely lead to more advanced medical options available to patients at a lower cost.

Take-aways

- ➢ Several research programs of interest have been summarized in the case of (U.S.) federal and private research entities.
- ➢ The (U.S.) National Institutes of Health (NIH)'s BRAIN Initiative aims to revolutionize our understanding of the human brain with the common goal to accelerate the development of innovative neurotechnologies.
- ➢ The BRAIN Initiative is focused on investigative neuroscience with intracranial access to recording and manipulating the brain directly. Such investigations offer opportunities for investigating how the human brain senses, thinks, perceives, remembers, plans, registers emotions, activates movements, engages language, and makes decisions.
- ➢ The BRAIN Initiative also supports the development and optimization of new tools and technologies for modulation and recording of cellular or near-cellular resolution signals of the central nervous system. The primary goal is to develop new tools that enable new capabilities for *in vivo* experiments, at or near cellular resolution, in animal models.

- As part of the BRAIN Initiative, researchers discovered "boundary" and "event" cells that are involved in making and marking memories and are activated at memory starting and stopping points, respectively. This finding will help treat memory-related issues like Alzheimer's and dementia.

- Brain maps have been created to identify specific brain cells and circuits related to aging and Alzheimer's disease, hopefully leading to earlier diagnoses and new treatments.

- A cellular- and molecular-level atlas of the human brain was created to determine the causes and effects of Alzheimer's disease.

- Before a person calls up a memory, fast waves of activity ripple across key parts of the brain, showing how the brain stores memories. The ripples could help better understand how the brain processes and retrieves memories.

- To study how brains make and find memories, researchers tracking the brain electrical activity in epileptic subjects found that there are distinct "firing" patterns that happen when they tried to remember. These unique patterns could help better understand how brains stop working properly in various memory and thinking disorders, like dementia and Alzheimer's.

- Coordinated replay across the hippocampus and prefrontal cortex serves an important function in spatial learning and memory-guided decision-making. Reverse replay is likely to support the ability to reflect on and evaluate paths that have led to goals in the past, whereas forward replay seems to support the ability to think ahead and plan choices that will lead to goals in the future.

- Researchers at the (U.S.) National Institute of Mental Health (NIMH) evaluated the relationship among brain inflammation, protein function, motor neuron diseases, and how HIV infection may cause problems with blood vessel function and contribute to thinking and mood disorders, such as early dementia and depression.

- Neurons called "engram cells" and their reactivation are necessary for memory recall. They are genetically tagged and manipulated to evidence their activity changes during the formation, extinction, and spontaneous recovery of a fear memory.

- Certain lifestyle factors (healthy diet, physical activity, and social interactions) might help to protect cognitive health as one ages. Some studies have suggested that use of a daily multivitamin or other dietary supplements improved a broad measure of cognitive function. There is no difference in global cognition between people who take cocoa extract and those who do not.

- Higher levels of education may help preserve memory, better late-life cognitive functioning, and reduced risk for dementia in the face of accumulating age-related brain pathology. More education predicts better memory later in life through better cognitive reserve.

- There appears to be a potential neurobiological connection between an older adult's mood with changes, over a period of time, in white brain matter and cognitive ability. Maintaining a positive outlook suggests better brain function, physical health benefits such as lower blood pressure, less heart disease, and healthier blood sugar levels.

- Memory loss may be transient or semi-permanent and may interfere with daily living activities. It may result from a number of diseases or mental health problems.

- Medications for memory loss and confusion, cognition, and dementia-related behaviors can be categorized as d**rugs that change disease progression, target amyloid-targeting, or treat c**ognitive and non-cognitive symptoms (behavioral and psychological symptoms).

- **Pharmacologically reinstating the hippocampal theta frequency may lead to early Alzheimer treatment.**

- A hormonal connection exists between stress and Alzheimer. It is widely believed that the stress hormone corticotrophin-releasing factor (CRF) may have a protective effect on the brain, including the **memory** changes brought on by Alzheimer's. Further, moderate exercise may restore normal function of the CRF system, allowing its memory enhancing effects.

- Some degree of atrophy and subsequent brain shrinkage is common with old age, even in people who are cognitively healthy. However, this atrophy is accelerated in people with mild cognitive impairment and even faster in those who ultimately progress to Alzheimer's. Overall, treatment with B vitamins can lead to a reduction in the rate of brain atrophy.

24

Conclusions

Contents

24

Conclusions

We have seen in Chapter 6 that several pathologies of the central nervous system may lead to memory issues. These include those pathologies due to *inflammation* or/and *encephalopathies* including memory reduction problems or alteration in consciousness.

The five categories of diseases

We must here distinguish between five categories of diseases (a) degenerative, (b) neurodegenerative, (c) demyelinating, (d) episodic paroxysmal, and (e) other related diseases.

Degenerative diseases

Degenerative diseases of concern include extrapyramidal & movement disorders, particularly Alzheimer's disease, Creutzfeldt-Jakob disease, Huntington's disease, panthotenate kinase-associated degeneration, Parkinson's disease and parkinsonism, and progressive supranuclear palsy. They also involve dementias of various forms (Alzheimer's disease, early onset, frontotemporal lobar degeneration, HIV, juvenile, Lewy bodies, late onset; Parkinson's disease and parkinsonism, pugilistica, vascular, etc.) as well as posterior cortical atrophy, primary progressive aphasia, synucleinopathies, tauopathies, and seizures (epileptic and others), including Dravet's and Lennox-Gastaud syndrome.

Non-degenerative diseases

On the other hand, neurodegenerative diseases encompass motor neuron diseases such as, in particular, amyotrophic lateral sclerosis.

Demyelinating diseases

Demyelinating diseases include multiple sclerosis and Canavan's disease.

Episodic paroxysmal diseases

Episodic paroxysmal diseases include epileptic and other seizures, cerebrovascular diseases such as acute aphasia, stroke, transcranial global and anteretrograde amnesia, and sleep disorders, especially sleep apnea.

Other related diseases

The other related diseases include the encephalopathies of Nicker, anti-MDS receptor, and HIV.

The above multiple possible contributors to memory impairments would theoretically need to be differentiated against, as appropriate, for a correct diagnosis and associated treatment.

The twenty(+) types of memory

The various types of memory (twenty in number, perhaps more) were identified in Chapter 12 and include (in alphabetical order); Active (see also short term), autobiographical, declarative (see also explicit), emotional and nostalgia, episodic, explicit, implicit, *kinesthetic, l*ong term (see also semantic), motor, objective, photographic, prospective, semantic, sensory (*verbal, auditory or echoic, olfactory,* short-term, spatial, subjective, and working.

The three classes of possible causes of memory issues

Because many brain areas help one create and retrieve memories, a problem in any one of them can lead to memory loss. There are three classes of possible **causes of memory** issues that include (a) clinical, (b) psychological, and (c) lifestyle issues.

Clinical issues

Clinical issues may result from a new injury to the brain, which is caused by - or is present after - a brain tumor; brain infections such as Lyme disease, syphilis, or HIV/AIDS; a cancer treatment such as brain radiation, bone marrow transplant, or chemotherapy; a concussion or head trauma; epilepsy that is not well controlled; insufficient oxygen getting to the brain when one's heart or breathing is stopped for too long; a severe brain infection or infection around the brain; a major surgery or severe illness including brain surgery, electroconvulsive therapy; a transient global amnesia' an illness that results in the loss of, or damage to brain tissue or nerve cells such as Parkinson's disease, Huntington's disease, or multiple sclerosis; a transient ischemic attack or stroke; hydrocephalus (a fluid collection in the brain); multiple sclerosis; or dementia.

Psychological issues

Sometimes, memory loss occurs with mental health problems such as after a major, traumatic or stressful event, bipolar disorder, depression or other mental health disorders such as schizophrenia. Memory loss may be a sign of dementia from any one or a combination of several forms of the disease, including dementia associated with Alzheimer's disease, vascular problems, Lewy bodies, fronto-temporal issues, progressive supranuclear palsy, normal pressure hydrocephalus, or Creutzfeldt-Jakob disease.

Lifestyle issues

Other causes of memory loss relate to lifestyle choices such as excess use of alcohol, use of prescription or illegal drugs, overuse of medicines such as barbiturates or (hypnotics), or low levels of important nutrients or vitamins such as low vitamin B1 or B12.

The six theories advanced to explain memory issues

In attempts to explain memory loss, **six** theories or effects have been advanced (mnemonic <u>ACIAP) covering a</u>ssociative deficit, contiguity, inhibition and inhibitory control, working memory decline, attentional resources limitation, and processing speed effects.

The four categories of medications for memory and cognition

Medications for memory, cognition, and dementia-related behaviors have been discussed in Chapter 23. In particular, for Alzheimer's, although current medications cannot cure it, two (U.S.) FDA-approved treatments address the underlying biology. Other medications may help lessen symptoms, such as memory loss and confusion. The FDA-approved medications fall into categories (a) d**rugs that change disease progression, (b) drugs that target the amyloid-beta plaques, (c) drugs that treat cognitive symptoms (memory and thinking), and (d) drugs that treat non-cognitive (behavioral and psychological symptoms).**

Drugs to slow disease progression

The drugs that slow disease progression go after the underlying biology of the disease process and aim to slow the decline of memory and thinking, as well as function, in people living with the disease.

Anti-amyloid drugs

The anti-amyloid drugs, specifically, **Aducanumab (Aduhelm®) and Lecanemab (Leqembi®)** work by attaching to and removing the beta-amyloid plaques from the brain.

Drugs to treat cognitive symptoms

The drugs that treat cognitive symptoms may help lessen or stabilize symptoms for a limited time by affecting certain chemicals involved in carrying messages among and between the brain's nerve cells. They include **cholinesterase inhibitors Donepezil (Aricept®), Rivastigmine (Exelon®), and Galantamine (Razadyne®); glutamate receptors such as Memantine (Namenda®), or the combination (cholinesterase inhibitor + glutamate regulator).**

Drugs to treat non-cognitive symptoms

In addition to treating memory and thinking, drugs that treat non-cognitive symptoms address quality of life such as, for example, insomnia and agitation. Such drugs include **Orexin receptor antagonist, Suvorexant (Belsomra®), atypical antipsychotics, and Brexpiprazole (Rexulti®).**

An overview of memory loss issues and cognitive impairment is provided in Table 24.1 and further illustrated in the synoptic flow chart of Figure 24.1

Table 24.1 – Memory loss issues and cognitive impairment overview

	Categories	**Diseases**
Diseases (5)	**1. Degenerative**	o Alzheimer's disease o Creutzfeldt-Jakob disease o Dementias of various forms o Dravet's syndrome o Huntington's disease o Lennox-Gastaud syndrome o Panthotenate kinase-associated degeneration o Parkinson's disease and parkinsonism o Posterior cortical atrophy o Primary progressive aphasia o Progressive supranuclear palsy o Seizures (epileptic and others) o Synucleinopathies o Tauopathies
	2. Neurodegenerative	o Amyotrophic lateral sclerosis
	3. Demyelinating	o Canavan's disease o Multiple sclerosis

	4. Episodic paroxysmal	o Acute aphasia o Amnesia (transcranial global and anteretrograde) o Cerebrovascular diseases: such o Epileptic and other seizures o Sleep disorders (sleep apnea) o Stroke
	5. Other related diseases	o Wernicke encephalopathy o Anti-MDS receptor o HIV encephalopathy
Memory types (21)	**1. Active**	
	2.Autobiographical	
	3.Declarative	
	4. Emotional and nostalgia	
	5.Episodic	
	6. Explicit	
	7. Implicit	
	8. *Kinesthetic*	
	9. *Long-term*	
	10. Motor	
	11. Objective.	
	12. Photographic	
	13. Prospective	
	14. Semantic	
	15. Sensory *verbal*	
	16. *Sensory auditory (or echoic)*	
	17. *Sensory olfactory*	
	18. *Short-term*	
	19. Spatial	
	20. Subjective	
	21. Working	

Causes of memory issues (3)	1. Clinical	o Bone marrow transplant o Brain tumor o Brain infection: - Lyme disease - Syphilis - HIV/AIDS o Brain oxygen insufficient o Brain surgery: o Brain radiation o Cancer treatment: o Chemotherapy o Concussion or head trauma o Dementia. o Epilepsy not well controlled o Hydrocephalus o Multiple sclerosis o Severe illness o Stroke o Transient ischemic attack
	2. Psychological	o Bipolar disorder o Creutzfeldt-Jakob disease. o Dementia o Depression or other mental health disorder o Major, traumatic or stressful event o Normal pressure hydrocephalus o Progressive supranuclear palsy o Schizophrenia
	3. Lifestyle	o Alcohol use excessive o Illegal drugs use o Medicines overuse: - Barbiturates - Hypnotics - Important nutrients or vitamins low levels: vitamin B1 or B12.
Theories (6)	1. Associative deficit	
	2. Attentional resources limitation	
	3. Contiguity	
	4. Inhibition and inhibitory control	
	5. Processing speed effects	
	6. Working memory decline	
Drugs (4)	1. To change disease progression	
	2. To target the amyloid-beta plaques	o Aducanumab (Aduhelm®) o Lecanemab (Leqembi®)

| | 3. To treat cognitive symptoms | o Cholinesterase inhibitors:
- Donepezil (Aricept®)
- Rivastigmine (Exelon®)
- Galantamine (Razadyne®)
o Glutamate receptors:
- Memantine (Namenda®)
o Combination (cholinesterase
   inhibitor + glutamate regulator). |
| | 4. To treat non-cognitive
symptoms (agitation, insomnia) | o Atypical antipsychotics
o Brexpiprazole (Rexulti®)
o Orexin receptor antagonist
o Suvorexant (Belsomra®) |

Figure 24.1 – Synoptic flow chart of memory
loss issues and cognitive impairment

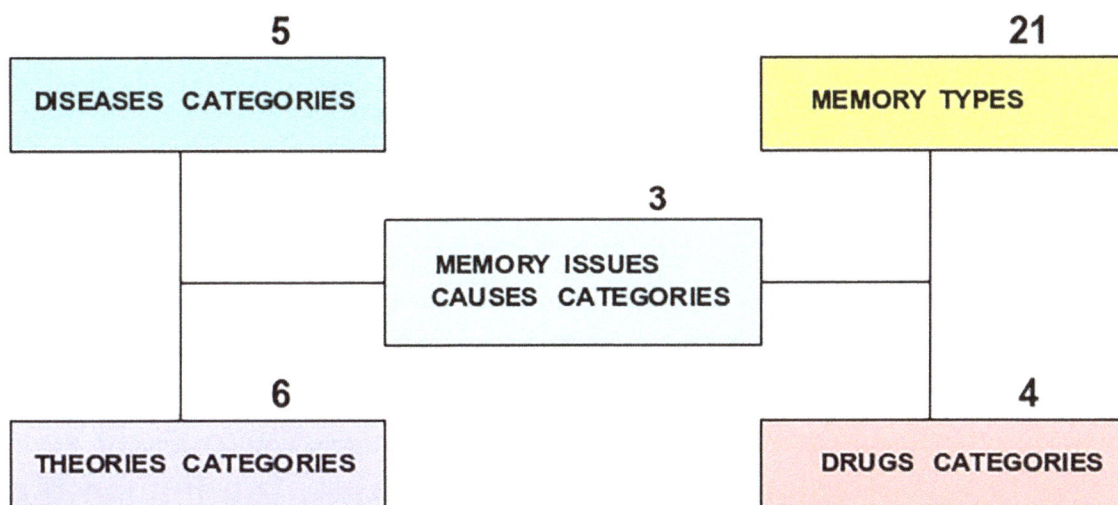

For the practicing medical professional, Table 24.1 and the flow chart of Figure 24.1 provide a roadmap for tackling, diagnosing, and treating the memory issues presented by their patient. S/he would begin by understanding the memory issues presented (center box of the flow chart), identifying the memory types involved (upper right box), conducting a differential diagnosis to eliminate as many confounding diseases as possible (upper left box), determining the applicable causal theory(ies) (lower left box), and prescribing the appropriate medication(s) (lower right box), as applicable.

Artificial intelligence (AI) experts have traditionally aimed to use their techniques and technologies to better understand the human brain and its functions. Such tools comprise neural networks, machine learning systems, brain modeling and mapping, the connectome and transcriptome projects, the European Human Brain Project, the (U.S.) BRAIN Initiative (see Chapter 23), etc.

Recently, however, researchers at the University of Massachusetts Amherst and the Baylor College of Medicine, Texas have adopted the contrarian approach in which it is rather human brain mechanisms that are employed to improve on AI. In this manner, they have confronted a "*major, long-standing obstacle to increasing AI capabilities*" by drawing inspiration from the human brain memory "replay" mechanism.

They pointed out that deep neural networks are the main drivers behind recent AI advances but, upon learning new lessons, progress had been held back by the networks forgetting what they had learned before. They pointed out that one solution would be, upon learning something new, to revisit previously stored encountered examples. Unfortunately, such an approach would quickly result in unmanageable amounts of data. By contrast, the human brain accumulates information throughout its lifetime and builds upon earlier lessons. Here, an important protecting mechanism against forgetting is the replay of the neuronal activity patterns representing those memories. Rather than storing data, the brain generates "*representations of memories at a high, more abstract level with no need to generate detailed memories*". The researchers then created an "*abstract generative brain replay*" and demonstrated that replaying just a few generated representations sufficed to remember older memories while learning new ones. Generative replay not only prevents catastrophic forgetting but also "*enables the system to generalize learning from one situation to another*".

References

On Santiago *Ramón* y Cajal

Cajal, Santiago Ramón y (1905)."*Manual de Anatomia Patológica General*" (Handbook of General Anatomical Pathology) (in Spanish) (4th ed.).

Cajal, Santiago Ramón y and Greeff R (1894). "*Die Retina der Wirbelthiere: Untersuchungen mit der Golgi-cajal'schen Chromsilbermethode und der ehrlich'schen Methylenblaufärbung*" (Retina of vertebrates) (in German). Bergmann.

Cajal, Santiago Ramón y and Azoulay L (1894). "*Les Nouvelles Idées sur la Structure du Système Nerveux chez l'Homme et chez les Vertébrés*" ('New Ideas on the Fine anatomy of the Nerve Centers in Man and in Vertebrates) (in French). C. Reinwald.

Cajal, Santiago Ramón y, Bresler J, and Mendel E (1896). "*Beitrag zum Studium der Medulla Oblongata: Des Kleinhirns und des Ursprungs der Gehirnnerven*" (in German). Verlag von Johann Ambrosius Barth.

Cajal, Santiago Ramón y (1898). "*Estructura del Quiasma Optico y Teoría General de los Entrecruzamientos de las Vías Nerviosas*" (Structure of the Chiasma Opticum and General Theory of the Crossing of Nerve Tracks)" [Die Structur des Chiasma opticum nebst einer allgemeine Theorie der Kreuzung der Nervenbahnen (German, 1899, Verlag Joh. A. Barth)]. Rev. Trim. Micrográfica (in Spanish) **3**:15–65.

Cajal, Santiago Ramón y (1899). "Comparative Study of the Sensory Areas of the Human Cortex". Clark University. p. 85.

Cajal, Santiago Ramón y (1899–1904). "*Textura del Sistema Nervioso del Hombre y los Vertebrados*" (Texture of the Nervous System of Man aand

Vertebrates) (in Spanish). Madrid. ISBN 978-84- 340-1723-8.; ISBN 978-3-211-83202-8.

Cajal, Santiago Ramón y (1909). "*Histologie du Système Nerveux de l'Homme et des Vertébrés*" (Histology of the Nervous Syste of Man and Vertebrates) (in French) – via Internet Archive.

Cajal, Santiago Ramón y (1906). "*Studien über die Hirnrinde des Menschen v.5*" (Studies about the Meninges of Man) (in German). Johann Ambrosius Barth.

Cajal, Santiago Ramón y, Sánchez, Domingo y Sánchez (1915). "*Contribución al Conocimiento de los Centros Nerviosos de los Insectos*" (Contribution to the Knowledge of the Central Nervous System of Insects) (in Spanish). Madrid: Imprenta de Hijos de Nicolas Moya.

Carlos de Juan A and Borrell J (2007). "A historical reflection of the contributions of Cajal and Golgi to the foundations of neuroscience". *Brain Research Reviews***55**(1):8–16. doi:10.1016/j.brainresrev.2007.03.010. hdl:10261/62299.

On brain anatomy and physiology

Ackerman S (1992). "Discovering the Brain". National Academy Press. Washington, D.C, pp. 22–5. ISBN 978-0-309-04529-2.

Adelman G (2010). "The neurosciences research program at MIT and the beginning of the modern field of Nnuroscience". *Journal of the History of the Neurosciences* **19**(1):15–23. doi:10.1080/09647040902720651.

Arsava EY, Arsava EM, Oguz KK, and Topcuoglu MA (2019). "Occipital petalia as a predictive imaging sign for transverse sinus dominance". *Neurological Research* **41**(4):306–11. doi:10.1080/01616412.2018.1560643.

Azevedo F *et al.* (2009). "Equal numbers of neuronal and non-neuronal cells make the human brain an isometrically scaled-up primate brain". *The Journal of Comparative Neurology* **513**(5):532–41. doi:10.1002/cne.21974. (Note: Despite the widespread quotes that the human brain contains 100 billion neurons and ten times more glial cells, the absolute number of neurons and glial cells in the human brain remains unknown. Actually, the adult male human brain contains on average 86.1 ± 8.1 billion NeuN-positive cells ("neurons") and 84.6 ± 9.8 billion NeuN-negative ("nonneuronal") cells.)

Bacyinski A, Xu M, Wang W, and Hu J (2017). "The paravascular pathway for brain waste clearance: Current understanding, significance and controversy". *Frontiers in Neuroanatomy* **11**:101. doi:10.3389/fnana.2017.00101. (Note: The paravascular pathway, also known as the "glymphatic" pathway, is a recently described system for waste clearance in the brain. According to this model, cerebrospinal fluid (CSF) enters the paravascular spaces surrounding penetrating arteries of the brain, mixes with interstitial fluid (ISF) and solutes in the parenchyma, and exits along paravascular spaces of draining veins. ...In addition to Aβ clearance, the glymphatic system may be involved in the removal of other interstitial solutes and metabolites.)

Bear MF, Connors MA, and Paradiso (2001). "Neuroscience: Exploring the Brain". Baltimore: Lippincott. ISBN 978-0-7817-3944-3.

Berntson G and Cacioppo J.(2009). "Handbook of Neuroscience for the Behavioral Sciences", Volume 1. John Wiley & Sons. p. 145. ISBN 978-0-470-08355-0.

Bigos KL, Hariri A, and Weinberger D (2015). "Neuroimaging Genetics: Principles and Practices". Oxford University Press. p. 157. ISBN 978-0-19-992022-8.

Bliss M (2005). "Harvey Cushing: A Life in Surgery:", USA: Oxford University Press. pp. ix–x. ISBN 978-0-19-534695-4.

Bogart BI and Ort V(2007). "Integrated Anatomy and Embryology". Philadelphia, PA: Elsevier Saunders. ISBN 978-1-4160-3165-9.

Boraud T, Bezard E *et al.* (2002). "From single extracellular unit recording in experimental and human Parkinsonism to the development of a functional concept of the role played by the basal ganglia in motor control". *Progress in Neurobiol* **66**(4):265–83. doi:10.1016/s0301-0082(01)00033-8.

Bornstein MH and Lamb ME (2015). "Developmental Science: An Advanced Textbook". Psychology Press. p. 220. ISBN 978-1-136-28220-1.

Borrell V (2018). "How cells fold the cerebral cortex". *The Journal of Neuroscience* **38**(4):776–83. doi:10.1523/JNEUROSCI.1106-17.2017.

Budzyński J and Kłopocka M (2014). "Brain-gut axis in the pathogenesis of *Helicobacter pylori* infection". *World J. Gastroenterol.* **20**(18):5212–25. doi:10.3748/wjg.v20.i18.5212.

Burke RE (2007). "Sir Charles Sherrington's The integrative action of the nervous system: A centenary appreciation". *Brain* **130**(Pt 4):887–94. doi:10.1093/brain/awm022.

Buxton R, Uludag K, and Liu T (2004). "Modeling the hemodynamic response to brain activation". *NeuroImage* **23**:S220–3. doi:10.1016/j.neuroimage.

Carabotti M, Scirocco A, Maselli MA, and Severi C (2015). "The gut-brain axis: Interactions between enteric microbiota, central and enteric nervous systems". *Ann Gastroenterol.* **28**(2):203–9.

Clark BD, Goldberg EM, and Rudy B (2009). "Electrogenic tuning of the axon initial segment". *The Neuroscientist* **15**(6):651–68. doi:10.1177/1073858409341973.

Clark DD and Sokoloff. L (1999). In Siegel GJ, Agranoff BW, Albers RW, Fisher SK, and Uhler MD (eds.). "Basic Neurochemistry: Molecular, Cellular, and Medical Aspects". Philadelphia: Lippincott. pp. 637–670. ISBN 978-0-397-51820-3.

Cobb M (2020). "The Idea of the Brain: The Past and Future of Neuroscience". New York: Hachette UK. ISBN 9781541646865.

Cosgrove KP, Mazure CM, and Staley JK (2007). "Evolving knowledge of sex differences in brain structure, function, and chemistry". *Biol Psychiatry* **62**(8):847–55. doi:10.1016/j.biopsych.2007.03.001.

Cowan WM, Harter DH, and Kandel ER (2000). "The emergence of modern neuroscience: Some implications for neurology and psychiatry". *Annual Review of Neuroscience* **23**:345–6. doi:10.1146/annurev.neuro.23.1.343.

Cowin SC and Doty SB (2007). "Tissue Mechanics". Springer Science & Business Media. p. 4. ISBN 978-0-387-49985-7.

Damasio (2001). "Neural basis of language disorders". In Chapey, Roberta (ed.). "Language Intervention Strategies in Aphasia and Related Neurogenic Communication Disorders" (4th ed.). Lippincott Williams & Wilkins. pp. 18–36. ISBN 978-0-7817-2133-2. OCLC 45952164.

Daneman R, Zhou L, Kebede AA, and Barres BA (2010). "Pericytes are required for blood-brain barrier integrity during embryogenesis". *Nature* **468**(7323):562–6. Natur.468..562D. doi:10.1038/nature09513.

Dawodu ST (2017). "Traumatic brain injury (TBI) – Definition and pathophysiology: Overview, epidemiology, primary injury". *Medscape.*

Dhanwate AD (2014). "Brainstem death: A comprehensive review in Indian perspective". *Indian Journal of Critical Care Medicine* **18**(9):596–605. doi:10.4103/0972-5229.140151.

Diamond A (2013). "Executive functions". *Annual Review of Psychology* **64**:135–68. doi:10.1146/annurev-psych-113011-143750.

Dissing-Olesen L, Hong S, and Stevens B (2015). "New brain lymphatic vessels drain old concepts". *EBioMedicine* **2**(8):776–7. doi:10.1016/j.ebiom.2015.08.019.

Domínguez JF, Lewis ED, Turner R, and Egan GF (2009). In Chiao JY (ed.)." The Brain in Culture and Culture in the Brain: A Review of Core Issues in Neuroanthropology". **178**:43–6. doi:10.1016/S0079-6123(09)17804-4. ISBN 978-0-444-53361-6.

Emery A (2000). "A Short History of Neurology: The British Contribution 1660–1910". Edited by F. Clifford Rose pp. 282. ISBN 07506 4165 7. Oxford: Butterworth-Heinemann and *Journal of Anatomy* **197**(3):513–8. doi:10.1046/j.1469-7580.2000.197305131.x.

Eagleman D (2015). "The Brain", Pantheon Books, p. 28-9.

Fan X and Markram H (2019). "A brief history of simulation neuroscience". *Frontiers in Neuroinformatics* **13:** 32. doi:10.3389/fninf.2019.00032.

Farris SP *et al.* (2015). "Applying the new genomics to alcohol dependence". *Alcohol* **49**(8):825–36. doi:10.1016/j.alcohol.2015.03.001.

Fedorenko E and Kanwisher N (2009). "Neuroimaging of language: Why hasn't a clearer picture emerged?". *Language and Linguistics Compass* **3**(4):839–65. doi:10.1111/j.1749- 818x.2009.00143.x. S2CID 2833893.

Finkelstein GW (2013). "Emil du Bois-Reymond: Neuroscience, Self, and Society in Nineteenth- Century Germany". Cambridge, Massachusetts. ISBN 978-1-4619-5032-5.

Flores CE and Méndez P (2014). "Shaping inhibition: Activity dependent structural plasticity of GABAergic synapses". *Frontiers in Cellular Neuroscience* **8:**327. doi:10.3389/fncel.2014.00327.

Frigeri, T, Paglioli E, De Oliveira E, and Rhoton Jr. AL (2015). "Microsurgical anatomy of the central lobe". *Journal of Neurosurgery* **122**(3):483–98. doi:10.3171/2014.11.JNS14315.

Fymat AL (2021). "The Human Brain: Wonders and Disorders", Tellwell Talent Publishers, pp 500,29. ISBN: 978-0-2288-4885-1 (Hardcover); 978-0-2288-4884-4 (Paperback).

Gaillard F (2017). "Glymphatic pathway". *Radiopaedia.org.*

Gianaros PJ, Gray MA, Onyewuenyi I and Critchley HD (2010). "Chapter 50. Neuroimaging methods in behavioral medicine". In Steptoe A (ed.). "Handbook of Behavioral Medicine: Methods and Applications". Springer Science & Business Media. p. 770.

Glees P (2005). "The Human Brain". Cambridge University Press. p.1. ISBN 978-0-521-01781-7. doi:10.1007/978-0-387-09488-5_50. ISBN 978-0-387-09488-5.

Goard M and Dan Y (2009). "Basal forebrain activation enhances cortical coding of natural scenes". *Nature Neuroscience* **12**(11):1444–9. doi:10.1038/nn.2402.

Goila AK and Pawar M (2009). "The diagnosis of brain death". *Indian Journal of Critical Care Medicine* **13**(1):7–11. doi:10.4103/0972-5229.53108.

Goll Y, Atlan G, and Citri A (2015). "Attention: The claustrum". *Trends in Neurosciences* **38**(8):486– 95. doi:10.1016/j.tins.2015.05.006.

Gray's Anatomy (2008), pp. 227–9, 242–244, 247, 248, 250-2, 254-6, 275, 297, 325-6, 335–7.

Gross CG (1987). In Adelman G (ed.). "Encyclopedia of Neuroscience" (2. ed.). Boston: Birkhäeuser pp. 843–7. ISBN 978-0-8176-3335-6.

Gross CG (1999). "Brain, Vision, Memory: Tales in the History of Neuroscience" (1st MIT Press pbk. ed.). Cambridge, Mass.: MIT. pp. 37–51. ISBN 978-0-262-57135-7.

Guyton and Hall (2011). "Principles of Anatomy and Physiology" (12th Edition), Tortora, p. 519, 574, and 667.

Hall J (2011). "Guyton and Hall Textbook of Medical Physiology" (12th ed.). Philadelphia, PA: Saunders/Elsevier. ISBN 978-1-4160-4574-8.

Hellier J (2014). "The Brain, the Nervous System, and their Diseases" (3 volumes). ABC-CLIO. pp. 300–303. ISBN 978-1-61069-338-7.

Hickok G (2009). "The functional neuroanatomy of language". *Physics of Life Reviews* **6**(3):121–43. doi:10.1016/j.plrev.2009.06.001.

Hofman MA (2014). "Evolution of the human brain: When bigger is better". *Frontiers in Neuroanatomy* **8**:15. doi:10.3389/fnana.2014.00015.

Hyun JC, Weyandt LL, and Swentosky A (2014). "Chapter 2: The physiology of Eeecutive functioning". In Goldstein S and Naglieri J. (eds.). "Handbook of Executive Functioning". New York: Springer. pp. 13–23. ISBN 978-1-4614-8106-5.

Iliff JJ and Nedergaard M (2013). "Is there a cerebral lymphatic system?" *Stroke* **44**(6 Suppl 1):S93-5. doi:10.1161/STROKEAHA.112.678698.

Jarrett C (2014). "Great Myths of the Brain". John Wiley & Sons. ISBN 978-1-118-31271-1.

Jones EG and Mendell LM (1999). "Assessing the Decade of the Brain". *Science* **284**(5415):739. doi:10.1126/science.284.5415.739.

Jones R (2012). "Neurogenetics: What makes a human brain?". *Nature Reviews Neuroscience* **13**(10): 655. doi:10.1038/nrn3355.

Kandel ER, Schwartz JH, and Jessel TM (2000) (eds.). "Principles of Neural Science", 4th ed. McGraw-Hill Professional:New York, NY. p. 324. ISBN 978-0-8385-7701-1.

Karbowski K (2008). "Sixty years of Ccinical Eeectroencephalography". *European Neurology* **30**(3):170–5. doi:10.1159/000117338.

Kretzer RM, Coon AL, and Tamargo RJ (2010). "Walter E. Dandy's contributions to vascular neurosurgery". *Journal of Neurosurgery* 112(6): 1182–91. doi:10.3171/2009.7.JNS09737.

Kuzawa CW, Chugani HT, Grossman LI, Lipovich L, Muzik O, Hof PR, Wildman DE, Sherwood C C, Leonard WR, and Lange N (2014). "Metabolic costs and evolutionary implications of human brain development". *Proceedings of the O.S. National Academy of Sciences* **111**(36):13010–5. doi:10.1073/pnas.1323099111.

Lambert KG (2003). "The life and career of Paul MacLean". *Physiology & Behavior* **79**(3):343–9. doi:10.1016/S0031-9384(03)00147-1.

Lancaster MA, Renner M, Martin CA, Wenzel D, Bicknell LS, Hurles ME, Homfray T, Penninger JM, Jackson AP, and Knoblich JA (2013). "Cerebral organoids model human brain development and microcephaly". *Nature* **501**(7467):373–9. doi:10.1038/nature12517.

Larsen WJ (2001). "Human Embryology" (3rd ed.). Philadelphia, PA: Churchill Livingstone. ISBN 978-0-443-06583-5.

Laterra J, Keep R, Betz LA, *et al.* (1999). "Blood–Cerebrospinal Fluid Barrier". Basic Neurochemistry: Molecular, Cellular, and Medical Aspects (6th ed.). Philadelphia: Lippincott-Raven.

Lee CT, Bendriem RM, Wu WW, and Shen RF (2017). "3D brain organoids derived from pluripotent stem cells: Promising experimental models for brain development and neurodegenerative disorders". *Journal of Biomedical Science* **24**(1):59. doi:10.1186/s12929-017-0362-8.

Llewellyn DJ (2018). "Stroke and dementia risk: A systematic review and meta-analysis". *Alzheimer's & Dementia* **14**(11):1416–26. doi:10.1016/j.jalz.2018.06.3061.

Malenka RC, Nestler EJ, and Hyman SE (2009). "Preface". In Sydor A and Brown, RY (eds.). "Molecular Neuropharmacology: A Foundation for Clinical Neuroscience" (2nd ed.). New York: McGraw-Hill Medical. p. xiii. ISBN 978-0-07-148127-4.

Malenka RC, Nestler EJ, Hyman SE, and Holtzman DM (2015). "Chapter 14: Higher cognitive function and behavioral control". In "Molecular Neuropharmacology: A Foundation for Clinical Neuroscience" (3rd ed.). New York: McGraw-Hill Medical. ISBN 978-0-07-182770-6.

(Note: ADHD can be conceptualized as a disorder of executive function; specifically, ADHD is characterized by reduced ability to exert and maintain cognitive control of behavior. Compared with healthy individuals, those with ADHD have diminished ability to suppress inappropriate prepotent responses to stimuli (impaired response inhibition) and diminished ability to inhibit responses to irrelevant stimuli (impaired interference suppression). ...Functional neuroimaging in humans demonstrates activation of the prefrontal cortex and caudate nucleus (part of the dorsal striatum) in tasks that demand inhibitory control of behavior. ...Early results with structural MRI show a thinner cerebral cortex, across much of the cerebrum, in ADHD subjects compared with age-matched control, including areas of [the] prefrontal cortex involved in working memory and attention.)

Marin-Valencia I *et al.* (2013). "Heptanoate as a neural fuel: Energetic and neurotransmitter precursors in normal and glucose transporter I-deficient (G1D) brain". *Journal of Cerebral Blood Flow and Metabolism* **33**(2):175–82. doi:10.1038/jcbfm.2012.151.

Marshall LH and Magoun HW (2013). "Discoveries in the Human Brain: Neuroscience Prehistory, Brain Structure, and Function". Springer Science & Business Media. p. 44. ISBN 978-1- 475-74997-7.

McDaniel M (2005). "Big-brained people are smarter". *Intelligence* **33**(4):337–46. doi:10.1016/j.intell.2004.11.005.

Molina DK and DiMaio JM (2012). "Normal organ weights in men". *The American Journal of Forensic Medicine and Pathology* **33**(4):368–72. doi:10.1097/PAF.0b013e31823d29ad.

Molina DK and DiMaio JM (2015). "Normal organ weights in women". *The American Journal of Forensic Medicine and Pathology* **36**(3):182–7. doi:10.1097/PAF.0000000000000175.

Møllgård K, Beinlich FRM, Kusk P Miyakoshi LM, Delle C, Plá V, Hauglund NL, Esmail T, Rasmussen MK, Gomolka RS, Mori Y, and Nedergaard M (2023). "A mesothelium divides the subarachnoid space into functional compartments". *Science* **379**(627):84–8. doi:10.1126/science.adc8810.

Moore SP (2005). "The Definitive Neurological Surgery Board Review". Lippincott Williams & Wilkins. p. 112. ISBN 978-1-4051-0459-3.

Mrsulja BB (2012). "Pathophysiology of Cerebral Energy Metabolism". Springer Science & Business Media. pp. 2–3. ISBN 978-1-4684-3348-7.
(U.S.) National Institutes of Health (2013). "Brain may flush out toxins during sleep".

(U.S.) National Institute of Neurological Disorders and Stroke (2017). "Brain Basics: Understanding Sleep". www.ninds.nih.gov.

Netter F (2014). "Atlas of Human Anatomy Including Student Consult Interactive Ancillaries and Guides" (6th ed.). Philadelphia, Penn.: W B Saunders Co. p. 114. ISBN 978-1-4557-0418-7.

Nieuwenhuys R, Donkelaar ten HJ, and Nicholson C (2014). "The Central Nervous System of Vertebrates". Springer. p. 2127. ISBN 978-3-642-18262-4.

NPR (2017). "A Surgeon's-Eye View of the Brain". NPR.org.

Obel LF, Müller MS, Walls AB, Sickmann HM, Bak LK, Waagepetersen HS, and Schousboe A (2012). "Brain glycogen-new perspectives on its metabolic function and regulation at the subcellular level". *Frontiers in Neuroenergetics* **4**:3. doi:10.3389/fnene.2012.00003.

O'Connor J (2003). "Thomas Willis and the background to *Cerebri Anatome*". *Journal of the Royal Society of Medicine* **96**(3):139–143. doi:10.1177/014107680309600311.

Olesko KM, Holmes FL (1994). In Cahan D (ed.). "Experiment, Quantification, and Discovery: Helmholtz's Early Physiological Researches, 1843-50". Hermann von Helmholtz and the Foundations of Nineteenth Century

Science. Berkeley; Los Angeles; London: University of California Press: 50–108.

Parent A and Carpenter MB (1995). "Carpenter's Human Neuroanatomy", Chapter 1, Williams & Wilkins. ISBN 978-0-683-06752-1.

Pavel F and Jiří V (2013). "Central Nervous System". Karolinum Press p.79. ISBN 978-80-246-2067.1.

Pearce JMS (2009). "Marie-Jean-Pierre Flourens (1794–1867) and Cortical Localization". *European Neurology* **61**(5):311–14. doi:10.1159/000206858.

Pennington BF (2008). "Diagnosing Learning Disorders", 2nd Edition: "A Neuropsychological Framework'. Guilford Press. pp. 3–10. ISBN 978-1-60623-786-1.

Pocock G and Richards C (2006). "Human Physiology: The Basis of Medicine" (3rd ed.). Oxford: Oxford University Press. ISBN 978-0-19-856878-0.

Poeppel D, Emmorey K, Hickok G, and Pylkkänen L (2012). "Towards a new neurobiology of language". *The Journal of Neuroscience* **32**(41):14125–31. doi:10.1523/JNEUROSCI.3244- 12.2012.

Polyzoidis S, Koletsa T, Panagiotidou S, Ashkan K, and Theoharides TC (2015). "Mast cells in meningiomas and brain inflammation". *Journal of Neuroinflammation* **12**(1):170. doi:10.1186/s12974-015-0388-3.

Popova M (2011). "'Brain culture': How neuroscience became a pop culture fixation". *The Atlantic.*

Psych Central News (2017). "Cultural Environment Influences Brain Function". *Psych Central News.*

Purves D (2012). "Neuroscience" (5th ed.). Sunderland, MA: Sinauer associates. ISBN 978-0- 87893- 695-3.

Purves D, Augustine GJ, Fitzpatrick D, Katz LC, LaMantia AS, McNamara JO, Williams SM, eds. (2001). "Rhombomeres". *Neuroscience* (2nd ed.). ISBN 978-0-87893-742-4.

Quistorff B, Secher N, and Van Lieshout J (2008). "Lactate fuels the human brain during exercise". *The FASEB Journal* **22**(10):3443–9. doi:10.1096/fj.08-106104.

Raichle M and Gusnard DA (2002). "Appraising the brain's energy budget". *Proc. (U.S.) Natl. Acad. Sci. U.S.A.* **99**(16):10237–9. doi:10.1073/pnas.172399499.

Ribas GC (2010). "The cerebral sulci and gyri". *Neurosurgical Focus* **28**(2):7. doi:10.3171/2009.11. FOCUS09245.

Rozycka A and Liguz-Lecznar M (2017). "The space where aging acts: Focus on the GABAergic synapse". *Aging Cell* **16**(4):634–43. doi:10.1111/acel.12605.

Sabbatini RME "Sabbatini RME: The Discovery of Bioelectricity. Nerve Conduction". www.cerebromente.org.br.

Sadler T (2010). "Langman's Medical Embryology" (11th ed.). Philadelphia: Lippincott Williams & Wilkins. p. 293. ISBN 978-0-7817-9069-7.

Sampaio-Baptista C and Johansen-Berg H (2017). "White matter plasticity in the adult brain". *Neuron.* **96**(6):1239–51. doi:10.1016/j.neuron.2017.11.026.

Saver J. (2005). "Time is brain—quantified". *Stroke* **37**(1):263–6. doi:10.1161/01.STR.0000196957.55928.ab.

Schwartz JH (2000). "Appendix D: Consciousness and the neurobiology of the twenty-first century". In Kandel ER, Schwartz, JH, and Jessell TM (2000). "Principles of Neural Science", 4th Edition.

Science (2017). "A $4.5 Billion Price Tag for the BRAIN Initiative?" *Science* | AAAS. June 5, 2014.

Selimbeyoglu A and Parvizi J (2010). "Electrical stimulation of the human brain: Perceptual and behavioral phenomena reported in the old and new literature". *Frontiers in Human Neuroscience* **4**:46. doi:10.3389/fnhum.2010.00046.

Sherwood L (2012). "Human Physiology: From Cells to Systems". Cengage Learning. p. 181. ISBN 978-1-133-70853-7.

Sharwood S and Mike (2017). "Introducing Language and Cognition". Cambridge University Press. p. 206. ISBN 978-1-107-15289-2.

Silverstein J (2012). "Mapping the motor and sensory cortices: A historical look and a current case study in sensorimotor localization and direct cortical motor stimulation". *The Neurodiagnostic Journal* **52**(1):54–68.

Simpkins CA and Simpkins AM (2012). "Neuroscience for Clinicians: Evidence, Models, and Practice". Springer Science & Business Media. p. 143. ISBN 978-1-4614-4842-6

Sjöstedt E, Fagerberg L, Hallström BM, Häggmark A, Mitsios N, Nilsson P, Pontén F, Hökfelt T, and Uhlén M (2015). "Defining the human brain proteome using transcriptomics and antibody- based profiling with a focus on the cerebral cortex". PLOS ONE **10** (6):e0130028. doi:10.1371/journal.pone.0130028.

Squire LR ed. (1996). The History of Neuroscience: An Autobiography". Washington DC: Society for Neuroscience. pp. 475–97. ISBN 978-0-12-660305-7.

Squire L (2013). "Fundamental Neuroscience". Waltham, MA: Elsevier. ISBN 978-0-12-385870-2

Standring S (ed.) (2008). "Gray's Anatomy: The Anatomical Basis of Clinical Practice" (40th ed.). London: Churchill Livingstone. ISBN 978-0-8089-2371-8.

Sun BL, Wang LH, Yang T, Sun JY, Mao LL, Yang MF, Yuan H, Colvin RA, and Yang XY (2018). "Lymphatic drainage system of the brain: A novel target for intervention of neurological diseases". *Progress in Neurobiology* **163–4:** 118–43. doi:10.1016/j.pneurobio.2017.08.007.

Swaminathan N (2008). "Why does the brain need so much power?" *Scientific American.*

Swanson LW (2014). "Neuroanatomical Terminology: A Lexicon of Classical Origins and Historical Foundations". Oxford University Press. ISBN 978-0-19-534062-4.

Tessman PA and Suarez JI (2002). "Influence of early printmaking on the development of neuroanatomy and neurology". *Archives of Neurology* **59**(12):1964–9. doi:10.1001/archneur.59.12.1964.

Thornton DJ (2011). "Brain Culture: Neuroscience and Popular Media". Rutgers University Press. ISBN 978-0-8135-5013-8.

Tsuji A (2005). "Small molecular drug transfer across the blood-brain barrier via carrier-mediated transport systems". *NeuroRx* **2**(1):54–62. doi:10.1602/neurorx.2.1.54.

Uhlén M, Fagerberg L, Hallström BM, Lindskog Ce Oksvold P, Mardinoglu A, Sivertsson A, Kampf C, and Sjöstedt E (2015). "The human proteome in brain – The Human Protein Atlas" (2017). "Tissue-based map of the human proteome". *Science* **347**(6220): 1260419. doi:10.1126/science.1260419. *www.proteinatlas.org.*

University of Rochester Medical Center via medicalxpress.com (2023). "University press release: Newly discovered anatomy shields and monitors brain", January 7, 2023.

Van Essen DC (1997). "A tension-based theory of morphogenesis and compact wiring in the central nervous system". *Nature* **385**(6614):313–8. doi:10.1038/385313a0.

Van Essen DC *et al.* (2012). "The Human Connectome Project: A data acquisition perspective". *NeuroImage* **62**(4):2222–31. doi:10.1016/j.neuroimage.2012.02.018.

Vijay N and Morris ME (2014). "Role of monocarboxylate transporters in drug delivery to the brain". *Curr. Pharm. Des.* **20**(10):1487–98. doi:10.2174/13816128113199990462.

Volkow ND, Koob GF, and McLellan AT (2016). "Neurobiologic advances from the brain disease model of addiction". *The New England Journal of Medicine* **374**(4):363–71. doi:10.1056/NEJMra1511480.

Warden A (2017). "Gene expression profiling in the human alcoholic brain". *Neuropharmacology* **122:** 161–74. doi:10.1016/j.neuropharm.2017.02.017.

Wijdicks EFM (2002). "Brain death worldwide: Accepted fact but no global consensus in diagnostic criteria". *Neurology* **58**(1):20–5. doi:10.1212/wnl.58.1.20.

Wingo AP, Fan W, Duong DM, Gerasimov ES, Dammer EB, Liu Y, Harerimana NV, White B, Thambisetty M, Troncoso JC, Kim N, Schneider JA, Hajjar IM, Lah JJ, Bennett DA, Seyfried NT, Levey AI, and Wingo TS (2020). "Shared proteomic effects of cerebral atherosclerosis and Alzheimer's disease on the human brain". *Nat Neurosci* **23**(6):696–700. doi:10.1038/s41593- 020-0635-5.

Xie L, Kang H, Xu Q, Chen MJ, Liao Y, Thiyagarajan M, O'Donnell J, Christensen DJ, Nicholson C, Iliff JJ, Takano T, Deane R, and Nedergaard M (2013). "Sleep drives metabolite clearance from the adult brain". *Science* **342**(6156): 373–7. doi:10.1126/science.1241224. (Note: The restorative function of sleep may be a consequence of the enhanced removal of potentially neurotoxic waste products that accumulate in the awake central nervous system.)

Zhong-Lin L and Dosher B (2013). "Visual Psychophysics: From Laboratory to Theory". MIT Press. p. 3. ISBN 978-0-262-01945-3.

On neuropsychology/psychiatry

Andrews DG (2001). "Neuropsychology". Psychology Press. ISBN 978-1-84169-103-9.

Barker P (2003). Psychiatric and mental health nursing: the craft of caring. *London: Arnold.* ISBN 0-340-81026-2. OCLC 53373798.

Benton AL, Eslinger P, and Damasio A (1981). "Normative observations on neuropsychological test performances in old age". *Journal of Clinical Neuropsychology* **3**(1):33–42. doi:10.1080/01688638108403111.

Bernstein D (2010). "Essentials of Psychology". Cengage Learning. p. 64. ISBN 978-0-495-90693-3.

Brady JV and Nauta WJH (2013). "Principles, Practices, and Positions in Neuropsychiatric Research", Proceedings of a Conference Held in June 1970 at the Walter Reed Army Institute of Research, Washington, D.C., in Tribute to Dr. David Mckenzie Rioch upon His Retirement as Director of the Neuropsychiatry Division of That Institute. Elsevier. p. vii. ISBN 978-1- 4831-5453-4.

Carrier M and Mittelstrass J (1991). "Mind, Brain, Behavior: The Mind-Body Problem and the Philosophy of Psychology" [Geist, Gehirn, Verhalten]. Translated by Lindberg, Steven. Berlin: Walter de Gruyter. p. 11. ISBN 9783110128765.

Chatterjee A and Branch CH (2013). "The Roots of Cognitive Neuroscience: Behavioral Neurology and Neuropsychology". OUP USA. pp. 337–8. ISBN 978-0-19-539554-9.

Churchland PS (1989). "Ch. 8 - Neurophilosophy". MIT Press. ISBN 978-0-262-53085-9.

Davey G (2011). "Applied Psychology". John Wiley & Sons. p. 153. ISBN 978-1-4443-3121-9.

Freberg L (2009). "Discovering Biological Psychology". *Cengage Learning* pp. 44–46. ISBN 978-0- 547-17779-3.

Geddes J, Gelder MG, and Mayou R (2005). Psychiatry. Oxford [Oxfordshire]: Oxford University Press. p. 141. ISBN 0-19-852863-9.

Gray P (2002). "Psychology" (4th ed.). Worth Publishers. ISBN 978-0-7167-5162-5.

Hart WD (1996). Guttenplan S (ed.). "A Companion to the Philosophy of Mind". Blackwell pp. 265–7.

Hoppe C and Stojanovic J (2008). "High-aptitude minds". *Scientific American Mind* **19**(4):60–7. doi:10.1038/scientificamericanmind0808-60.

Kalat J (2015). "Biological Psychology. Cengage Learning". p. 425. ISBN 978-1-305-46529-9.

Kane RL and Parsons TD (2017). "The Role of Technology in Clinical Neuropsychology". Oxford University Press. p. 399. ISBN 978-0-19-023473-7.

Kearney C and Trull TJ (2016). "Abnormal Psychology and Life: A Dimensional Approach". Cengage Learning. p. 395. ISBN 978-1-337-09810-6.

Kolb B.and Whishaw IQ (2009). "Fundamentals of Human Neuropsychology". Macmillan. pp. 73–75. ISBN 978-0-7167-9586-5.

Kolb B and Whishaw IQ. (2013). "Introduction to Brain and Behavior". Macmillan Higher Education. p. 21. ISBN 978-1-4641-3960-4.

Lezak MD, Howieson DB, and Loring DW (2004). Neuropsychological Assessment" (4th ed.). Oxford: Oxford University Press. ISBN 978-0-19-511121-7.

Lilienfeld SO, Lynn SJ., Ruscio J, and Beyerstein BL (2011). "50 Great Myths of Popular Psychology: Shattering Widespread Misconceptions about Human Behavior". John Wiley & Sons. p. 89. ISBN 978-1-4443-6074-5.

Lindquist KA, Wager TD, Kober H, Bliss-Moreau E, and Barrett LF (2012). "The brain basis of emotion: A meta-analytic review". *Behavioral and Brain Science* **35**(3):121–43. doi:10.1017/S0140525X11000446.

Lokhorst GJ (2016). "Descartes and the Pineal Gland". The Stanford Encyclopedia of Philosophy. Metaphysics Research Lab, Stanford University.

Luders E *et al.* (2008). "Mapping the relationship between cortical convolution and intelligence: Effects of gender". *Cerebral Cortex* **18**(9):2019–26. doi:10.1093/cercor/bhm227.

Morris CG and Maisto AA (2011). "Understanding Psychology". Prentice Hall. p. 56. ISBN 978-0- 205-76906-3.

Papez JW (1995). "A proposed mechanism of emotion. 1937". *The Journal of Neuropsychiatry and Clinical Neurosciences* **7**(1):103–12. doi:10.1176/jnp.7.1.103.

Phan KL, Wager,T, Taylor SF, and Liberzon I (2002). "Functional neuroanatomy of emotion: A meta-analysis of emotion activation studies in PET and fMRI". *NeuroImage* 16(2):331–48. doi:10.1006/nimg.2002.1087.

Sander D (2013) in Armony J, and Vuilleumier P (eds.). "The Cambridge Handbook of Human Affective Neuroscience". Cambridge: Cambridge Univ. Press. p. 16. ISBN 978-0-521-17155-7.

Schacter DL, Gilbert DT, and Wegner DM (2009). "Introducing Psychology". Macmillan. p. 80. ISBN 978-1-4292-1821-4.

Simpson JM and Moriarty GL (2013). "Multimodal Treatment of Acute Psychiatric Illness: A Guide for Hospital Diversion". Columbia University Press. pp. 22–24. ISBN 978-0-231-53609-7.

On what the eyes can tell us about the brain

Dhana K, James BD, Agarwal P, Agarwal NT, Cherian LJ, Leurgans SE, Barnes LL, Bennett DA, and Schneider JA. (2021). "MIND Diet, common brain pathologies, and cognition in community-dwelling older adults". *Journal of Alzheimer's Disease* **83**(2):683-92.

Fassier P, Kang JH, Lee IM, Grodstein F, and Vercambre MN. (2022). "Vigorous physical activity and cognitive trajectory later in life: Prospective association and interaction by Apolipoprotein E e4 in the Nurses' Health Study". *Journals of Gerontology Series A: Biological Sciences and Medical Science* 1;**77**(4):817-25.

Han SB, Yang HK, and Hyon JY. (2018). "Influence of diabetes mellitus on anterior segment of the eye". *Clinical Interventions of Aging* 27;14:53-63.

Morris MC, Tangney CC, Wang Y, Sacks FM, Barnes LL, Bennett DA, and Aggarwal NT. (2015). "MIND diet slows cognitive decline with aging". *Alzheimer's & Dementia* **11**(9):1015-22.

(U.S.) National Institute on Aging (NIA). (2022). *"Vision impairment is associated with as many as 100,000 U.S. dementia cases" (10 NOVEMBER 2022)*. https://www.nia.nih.gov/news/vision- impairment-associated-many-100000-u-s-dementia-cases.

(U.S.) National Institute of Diabetes and Digestive and Kidney Diseases (NIDDKD). *"Diabetic eye disease"*.https://www.niddk.nih.gov/health-information/diabetes/overview/preventing-problems/diabetic-eye-disease

Varadaraj V, Munoz B, Deal JA, *et al.* (2021). "Association of vision impairment with cognitive decline across multiple domains in older adults". *JAMA Network Open* 4(7):e2117416.

On the healthy aging brain

Alverzo JP (2006). "A review of the literature on orientation as an indicator of level of consciousness". *Journal of Nursing Scholarship* **38**(2):159–64. doi:10.1111/j.1547-5069.2006.00094.x.

Anderton BH (2002). "Aging of the brain". *Mechanisms of Aging and Development* **123**(7):811–7. doi:10.1016/S0047-6374(01)00426-2.

Audet JN and Lefebvre L (2017). "What's flexible in behavioral flexibility?". *Behavioral Ecology* **28**(4):943–7. doi:10.1093/beheco/arx007.

Baker LD, Frank LL, Foster-Schubert K, Green PS, Wilinson CW, McTiernan A *et al.* (2010). "Effects of aerobic exercise on mild cognitive impairment: A controlled trial". *Archives of Neurology* 67(1):71–9. doi:10.1001/archneurol.2009.307.

Banich M T and Compton RJ (2011). Cognitive neuroscience". Belmont, CA: Wadsworth. p. 334.

Barnes C and Burke S (2006). "Neural plasticity in the aging brain". *Nature Reviews Neuroscience* **7**(1):30–40. doi:10.1038/nrn1809.

Barnes LL, Mendes de Leon CF, Wilson RS, Bienias JL, and Evans DA (2004). "Social resources and cognitive decline in a population of older African-Americans and whites". *Neurology* **63**(12):2322–6. doi:10.1212/01.wnl.0000147473.04043.b3.

Benveniste H, Liu X, Koundal S, Sanggaard S, Lee H, and Wardlaw J (2019). "The glymphatic system and waste clearance with brain aging: A review". *Gerontology* **65**(2):106–19. doi:10.1159/000490349.

Boehme M, Guzzetta KE, Bastiaanssen TFS, van de Wouw M, Moloney GM, Gual-Grau, Spichak S, Olavarría-Ramírez L, Fitzgerald P, Morillas E, Ritz NL, Jaggar M, Cowan CSM, Crispie F, Donoso F, Halitzki E, Neto MC, Sichetti M, Golubeva AV, Fitzgerald RS, Claesson MJ, Cotter PD, O'Leary OF, Dinan TG, and Cryan JF (2021). "Microbiota from young mice counteracts selective age-associated behavioral deficits". *Nature Aging* **1**(8):666–76. doi:10.1038/s43587- 021-00093-9.

Braidy N and Liu Y (2020). "Can nicotinamide riboside protect against cognitive impairment?". *Current Opinion in Clinical Nutrition & Metabolic Care* **23**(6):413–20. doi:10.1097/MCO.0000000000000691.

Breton YA, Seeland KD, and Redish AD (2015). "Aging impairs deliberation and behavioral flexibility in inter-temporal choice". *Frontiers in Aging Neuroscience* **7**:41. doi:10.3389/fnagi.2015.00041.

Brotchie J, Brennan J, and Wyke M (1985). "Temporal orientation in the presenium and old age". *British Journal of Psychiatry* **147**(6):692–5. doi:10.1192/bjp.147.6.692.

Carrier JSA, Cheyne A, Solman GJF, and Smilek D (2010). "Age trends for failures of sustained attention". *Psychology and Aging* **25**(3):569–74. doi:10.1037/a0019363.

Chang L, Jiang CS, and Ernst T (2009). "Effects of age and sex on brain glutamate and other metabolites". *Magnetic Resonance Imaging* **27**(1):142–5. doi:10.1016/j.mri.2008.06.002.

Chappus-McCendie H, Chevalier L, Roberge C, and Plourde M (2019). "Omega-3 PUFA metabolism and brain modifications during aging". *Progress in Neuro- Psychopharmacology and Biological Psychiatry* **94**:109662. doi:10.1016/j.pnpbp.2019.109662.

Charuchandra S (2023). "Scientists discover a new protective layer in the brain". *Advanced Science News* (30 January 2023).

Craik F and Salthouse T (2000). "The Handbook of Aging and Cognition" (2nd ed.). Mahwah, NJ: Lawrence Erlbaum. ISBN 0-8058-2966-0. OCLC 44957002.

Crosson B, Garcia A, Mcgregor K, and Wierenga CE (2013). "The impact of aging on neural systems for language". In M. F. G. Sandra Koffler, Joel Morgan, Ida Sue Baron (Ed.) "Neuropsychology", Volume 1 (pp. 149–87). Oxford University Press. ISBN 9780199794317.

Denis I, Potier B, Heberden C, and Vancassel S (2015). "Omega-3 polyunsaturated fatty acids and brain aging". Current Opinion in Clinical Nutrition & Metabolic Care **18**(2):139–46. doi:10.1097/MCO.0000000000000141.

Ding XQ, Maudsley AA, Sabati M, Sheriff S, Schmitz B, Schütze MBP, Kahl KG, and Lanfermann H (2016). "Physiological neuronal decline in healthy aging human brain — An *in vivo* study with MRI and short echo-time whole-brain 1H MR spectroscopic imaging". *NeuroImage* **137**:45–51. doi:10.1016/j.neuroimage.2016.05.014.

Fymat AL (2021). "The Human Brain: Wonders and Disorders", Tellwell Talent Publishers, pp 500. ISBN: 978-0-2288-4885-1 (Hardcover); 978-0-2288-4884-4 (Paperback).

Gabrieli J and Hedden T (2004). "Insights into the aging mind: A view from cognitive neuroscience". *Nature Reviews Neuroscience* **5**(2):87–96. doi:10.1038/nrn1323.

Harris SE, Deary IJ, MacIntyre A, *et al.* (2006). "The association between telomere length, physical health, cognitive aging, and mortality in non-demented older people". *Neuroscience Letters* **406**(3): 260–4. doi:10.1016/j.neulet.2006.07.055.

Horvath S (2013). "DNA methylation age of human tissues and cell types". *Genome Biology* **14**(10): R115. doi:10.1186/gb-2013-14-10-r115.

Horvath S, Mah V, Lu AT, Woo JS, Choi OW, Jasinska AJ, Riancho JA, Tung S, Coles NS, Braun J, Vinters HV, and Coles LS (2015). "The cerebellum ages slowly according to the epigenetic clock". *Aging* **7**(5):294–306. doi:10.18632/aging.100742.

Langner R (2021). "The aging brain and executive functions revisited: Implications from meta- analytic and functional-connectivity evidence". *Journal of Cognitive Neuroscience* **33**(9):1716– 52. doi:10.1162/jocn_a_01616.

Hof PR and Morrison JH (2004). "The aging brain: Morphomolecular senescence of cortical circuits". *Trends in Neurosciences* **27**(10):607–13. doi:10.1016/j.tins.2004.07.013.

Hopp GA, Dixon RA, Grut M, and Bacekman L (1997). "Longitudinal and psychometric profiles of two cognitive status tests in very old adults". *Journal of Clinical Psychology* **53**(7):673–86. doi:10.1002/(sici)1097-4679(199711)53:7<673::aid-jclp5>3.0.co;2-j.

Iram T, Kern F, Kaur A, Myneni S, Morningstar AR, Shin H, Garcia MA, Yerra L, Palovics R, Yang AC, Hahn O, Lu N, Shuken SR, Haney MS, Lehallier B, Iyer M, Luo J, Zetterberg H, Keller A, Zuchero J, Bradley, and Wyss-Coray T (2022). "Young CSF restores oligodendrogenesis and memory in aged mice via Fgf17". **Nature** 605(7910):509–15. doi:10.1038/s41586-022-04722.0.

Ishizaki J, Meguro K, Ambo H, Shimada M, Yamaguchi S, and Harasaka C *et al.* (1998). "A normative community based study of mini-mental state in elderly adults: The effect of age and educational level". *The Journal of Gerontology:* Series B. **53**(6):359–63. doi:10.1093/geronb/53b.6.p359.

Iyo M and Yamasaki T (1993). "The detection of age-related decrease of dopamine, D1, D2 and serotonin 5-HT2 receptors in living human brain". *Progress in Neuro-Psychopharmacology and Biological Psychiatry* **17**(3):415–21. doi:10.1016/0278-5846(93)90075-4.

Kaasinen V, Vilkman H, Hietala J, Någren K, Helenius H, Olsson H, Farde L, and Rinne JO (2000). "Age-related dopamine D2/D3 receptor loss in extrastriatal regions of the human brain". *Neurobiology of Aging* **21**(5): 683–8. doi:10.1016/S0197-4580(00)00149-4.

Kadakkuzha BM and Akhmedov K (2013). "Age-associated bidirectional modulation of gene expression in single identified R15 neuron of Aplysia". *BMC Genomics* **14**(1):880. doi:10.1186/1471-2164-14-880.

Kaiser LG, Schuff N, Cashdollar N, and Weiner MW (2005). "Age-related glutamate and glutamine concentration changes in normal human brain: 1H MR spectroscopy study at 4 T". *Neurobiology of Aging* **26**(5):665–72. doi:10.1016/j.neurobiolaging.2004.07.001.

Keller JN, Schmitt FA, Scheff SW *et al.* (2005). "Evidence of increased oxidative damage in subjects with mild cognitive impairment". *Neurology* **64**(7):1152–6. doi:10.1212/01.WNL.0000156156.13641.BA.

Kensinger EA (2009). "Cognition in aging and age-related disease". In P. R. Hof & C. V. Mobbs (Eds.), *Handbook of the neuroscience of aging* (249-56). London: Elsevier Press.

Kolb B and Whishaw IQ (1998). "Brain plasticity and behavior". *Annual Review of Psychology* **49**(1):43–64. doi:10.1146/annurev.psych.49.1.43. hdl:2027.42/74427.

Kolb B, Gibb R, and Robinson TE (2003). "Brain plasticity and behavior". *Current Directions in Psychological Science* **12**(1):1–5.doi:10.1111/1467-8721.01210. hdl:2027.42/74427.

Light LL (1991). "Memory and aging: Four hypotheses in search of data". *Annual Review of Psychology* **42**:333–76. doi:10.1146/annurev. ps.42.020191.002001.

Liu T, Wei W, Wanlin Z, Kochan NA, Trollor JN, Reppermund S, Jin JS, Luo S, Brodaty H, and Sachdev PS (2011). "The relationship between cortical sulcal variability and cognitive performance in the elderly". *NeuroImage* **56**(3):865–73. doi:10.1016/j.neuroimage.2011.03.015.

Lu T, Pan Y, Kao SY, Li C, Kohane I, Chan J, and Yankner BA (2004). "Gene regulation and DNA damage in the aging human brain". *Nature* **429**(6994):883–91. doi:10.1038/nature02661.

Mandavilli BS and Rao KS (1996). "Accumulation of DNA damage in aging neurons occurs through a mechanism other than apoptosis". *J Neurochem.* **67**(4):1559–65. doi:10.1046/j.1471- 4159.1996.67041559.x.

Marcusson J, Oreland L, and Winblad B (1984). "Effect of age on human brain serotonin (S-1) binding sites". *Journal of Neurochemistry* **43**(6):1699–705. doi:10.1111/j.1471-4159.1984.tb06098.x.

Mattson MP and Arumugam TV (2018). "Hallmarks of brain aging: Adaptive and pathological modification by metabolic states". *Cell Metabolism* **27**(6):1176–99. doi:10.1016/j.cmet.2018.05.011.

Minhas PS, Latif-Hernandez A, McReynolds MR, Durairaj AS, Wang Q, Rubin A, Joshi AU, He JQ, Gauba E, Liu L, Wang C, Linde M, Sugiura Y, Moon PK, Majeti R, Suematsu M, Mochly- Rosen D, Weissman IL, Longo FM, Rabinowitz JD, and Andreasson KI (2021). "Restoring metabolism of myeloid cells **reverses cognitive decline in aging**". *Nature* **590**(7844):122–8. doi:10.1038/s41586-020-03160-0.

Mobbs CV and Hof PR (2009). "Handbook of the neuroscience of aging". Amsterdam: Elsevier/Academic Press. ISBN 978-0-12-374898-0.

Møllgård K, Beinlich FRM, Kusk P, Miyakoshi LM, Delle C, Plá V, Hauglund NL, Esmail T, Rasmussen MK, Gomolka RS, Mori Y, and Nedergaard M (2023). "A mesothelium divides the subarachnoid space into functional compartments". *Science* **379**(6627):84–8. doi:10.1126/science.adc8810.

Mou Y, Du Y, Zhou L, Yue Ji, Hu Xi, Liu Y, Chen S, Lin X, Zhang G Xiao H, and Dong B (2022). "Gut microbiota interact with the brain through systemic chronic inflammation: Implications on neuroinflammation, neurodegeneration, and aging". *Frontiers in Immunology* **13**:796288. doi:10.3389/fimmu.2022.796288.

(U.S.) National Institute on Aging. "Instruments to Detect Cognitive Impairment in Older Adults."

Ota M, Yasuno F, Ito H, Seki C, Kozaki S, Asada T, and Suhara T (2006). "Age-related decline of dopamine synthesis in the living human brain measured by positron emission tomography with L-[β-11C]DOPA". *Life Sciences* **79**(8):730–6. doi:10.1016/j.lfs.2006.02.017.

Raz N *et al.* (2005). "Regional brain changes in aging healthy adults: General trends, individual differences, and modifiers". *Cerebral Cortex* **15**(11):1676–89. doi:10.1093/cercor/bhi044.

Raz N and Rodrigue KM (2006). "Differential aging of the brain: Patterns, cognitive correlates and modifiers". *Neuroscience & Biobehavioral Reviews* **30**(6):730–48. doi:10.1016/j.neubiorev.2006.07.001.

Reuter-Lorenz PA and Park DC (2014). "How does it STAC Up? Revisiting the Scaffolding Theory of Aging and Cognition". *Neuropsychology Rev* **24**(3):355–70. doi:10.1007/s11065-014-9270-9.

Riley KP, Snowdon DA, Desrosiers MF, and Markesbery WR (2005). "Early life linguistic ability, late life cognitive function, and neuropathology: Findings from the Nun Study". *Neurobiology of Aging* **26** (3):341–7. doi:10.1016/j.neurobiolaging.2004.06.019.

Rinne Juha O, Lonnberg Pirkko, and Marjamaiki Paivi (1989). "Age-dependent decline in human brain dopamine D1 and D2 receptors". *Brain Research* **508**(2):349–52. doi:10.1016/0006- 8993(90)90423-9.

Sailasuta N, Ernst T, and Chang L (2008). "Regional variations and the effects of age and gender on glutamate concentrations in the human brain". *Magnetic Resonance Imaging* **26**(5):667–75. doi:10.1016/j.mri.2007.06.007.

Sanders A, Wang C, Katz M, Derby C, and Barzilai N (2011). "Association of a functional polymorphism in the cholesteryl ester transfer protein (CETP) gene with memory decline and incidence of dementia". *Journal of the American Medical Association* **303**(2):150–8. doi:10.1001/jama.2009.1988.

Scarmeas N and Stern Y (2003). "Cognitive reserve and lifestyle". *Journal of Clinical and Experimental Neuropsychology* **25**(5):625–33. doi:10.1076/jcen.25.5.625.14576.

Sowell ER, Peterson BS, Thompson PM, Welcome SE, Henkenius AL, and Toga AW (2003). "Mapping cortical change across the human life span". *Nature Neuroscience* **6**(3):309–15. doi:10.1038/nn1008.

"Study reveals immune driver of brain aging". medicalxpress.com (13 February 2021).

Sweet JJ, Such Y, Leahy B, Abramowitz C, and Nowinski CJ (1999). "Normative clinical relationships between orientation and memory: Age as an important moderator variable". T*he Clinical Neuropsychologist* **13**(4):495–508. doi:10.1076/1385-4046(199911)13:04;1-y;ft495.

Tao L, Wei W, Wanlin Z, Julian T, Reppermund S, Crawford J, Jin JS, Luo S, Brodaty H, and Sachdev P (2010). "The effects of age and sex on cortical sulci in the elderly". *NeuroImage* **51**(1):19–27. doi:10.1016/j.neuroimage.2010.02.016.

Uddin LQ (2021). "Cognitive and behavioral flexibility: neural mechanisms and clinical considerations". *Nature Reviews Neuroscience* **22**(3):167–79. doi:10.1038/s41583-021-00428-w

University of Rochester Medical Center (press release, 7 January 2023): "Newly discovered anatomy shields and monitors brain". *Medicalxpress. com*.

Wang E and Snyder SD (1998). "Handbook of the aging brain". San Diego, California: Academic Press. ISBN 0-12-734610-4. OCLC 636693117.

Wang Y, Chan GL, Holden JE *et al.* (1998). "Age-dependent decline of dopamine D1 receptors in human brain: A PET study". *Synapse* **30**(1):56–61. doi:10.1002/(SICI)1098- 2396(199809)30:1<56.

Whalley LJ, Deary IJ, Appleton CL, and Starr JM (2004). "Cognitive reserve and the neurobiology of cognitive aging". Aging *Research Reviews* **3**(4):369–82. doi:10.1016/j.arr.2004.05.001.

Winder NR, Reeve EH, and Walker AE (2021). "Large artery stiffness and brain health: Insights from animal models". *American Journal of Physiology. Heart and Circulatory Physiology* **320** (1):H424–31. doi:10.1152/ajpheart.00696.2020.

Wong DF *et al.* (1984). "Effects of age on dopamine and serotonin receptors measured by positron tomography in the living human brain". *Science* **226**(4681):1393–6. doi:10.1126/science.6334363.

Wyss-Coray T (2016). "Aging, neurodegeneration, and brain rejuvenation". *Nature* **539**(7628): 180–6. doi:10.1038/nature20411.

Yamamoto M, Suhara T, Okubo Y, Ichimiya T, Sudo Y, Inoue Y, Takano A, Yasuno F, Yoshikawa K, and Tanada S (2001). "Age-related decline of serotonin transporters in living human brain of healthy males". *Life Sciences* **71**(7):751–57. doi:10.1016/S0024-3205(02)01745-9.

Yang W, Zhou X, and Ma T (2019). "Memory decline and behavioral inflexibility in aged mice are correlated with dysregulation of protein synthesis capacity". *Frontiers in Aging Neuroscience* **11:**246. doi:10.3389/fnagi.2019.00246.

Yin C, Imms P, Cheng M,*et al.* (2023). "Anatomically interpretable deep learning of brain age captures domain-specific cognitive impairment". *Proceedings of the (U.S.) National Academy of Sciences* **120**(2):e2214634120. doi:10.1073/pnas.2214634120.

Yin F, Sancheti H, Patil I, and Cadenas E (2016). "Energy metabolism and inflammation in brain aging and Alzheimer's disease". *Free Radical Biology and Medicine* **100:**108–22. doi:10.1016/j.freeradbiomed.2016.04.200.

Yirka B (2022). "Giving an old mouse cerebrospinal fluid from a young mouse improves its memory". *Medicalxpress.com* (22 June 2022).

Zhang G, Li J, Purkayastha, Tang Y, Zhang H, Yin Y, Li B *et al.* (2013). "Hypothalamic programming of systemic aging involving IKK-[bgr], NF-[kgr]B and GnRH". *Nature* **497**(7448):211–6. doi:10.1038/nature12143.

Longitudinal studies

Bennett DA, Schneider JA, Arvanitakis WZ, and Wilson RS (2012). "Overview and findings from the Religious Orders Study". *Current Alzheimer Research* 9(6):628–45. doi:10.2174/156720512801322573.

Danner DD, Snowdon DA, and Friesen WV (2001). "Positive emotions in early life and longevity: Findings from the Nun Study", *Journal of Personality and Social Psychology* **80**(5):804–13. doi:10.1037/0022-3514.80.5.804.

Dunkel T (2006). "Offering an education in aging". *Baltimore Sun*.

Eisenstadt EE (2021). "20 years later, lessons on aging from the 'Nun Study' resonate today". *Global Sisters Report.* https://katoactonalz.org/

Iacono D, Markesbery WR, Gross M, Pletnikova O, Rudow G, Zandi P, and Troncoso JC (2009). "The Nun Study". *Neurology* **73**(9):665–73. doi:10.1212/WNL.0b013e3181b01077.

Patzwald GA and Wildt S (2004). "The use of convent archival records in medical research: The School Sisters of Notre Dame archives and the Nun Study". *The American Archivist* **67**(1):86– 106. doi:10.17723/aarc.67.1.d558520196w85573.

Riley KP, Snowdon DA, Desrosiers MF, and Markesbery WR (2005). "Early life linguistic ability, late life cognitive function, and neuropathology:

Findings from the Nun Study". *Neurobiology of Aging* **26**(3):341–7. doi:10.1016/j.neurobiolaging.2004.06.019.

Snowdon DA (2002). "Aging with grace: What the Nun Study teaches us about leading longer, healthier, and more meaningful lives". New York, New York: Bantam Books. ISBN 0-553- 38092-3.

Tyas SL, Snowdon DA, Desrosiers MF, Riley KP, and Markesbery WR (2007). "Healthy aging in the Nun Study: Definition and neuropathologic correlates". *Age and Aging* **36**(6):650–55. doi:10.1093/ageing/afm120.

Weinstein N, Legate N, Ryan WS, and Hemmy L (2019). "Autonomous orientation predicts longevity: New findings from the Nun Study". *Journal of Personality* 87(2):181–93. doi:10.1111/jopy.12379. ISSN 1467-6494.

On the pathogenic brain

Fymat AL (2019a). "The pathogenic brain". *Current Opinions in Neurological Science* **3**(2):669- 671.

Fymat AL (2019b). "On the pathogenic hypothesis of neurodegenerative diseases", *Journal of Clinical Research in Neurology* 2(1):1-7.

Fymat AL (2020). "On the symbiosis between our two interacting brains", Proceedings of the European Union Academy of Sciences *147-151, 2020 Newsletter.*

Fymat AL (2021). "The Human Brain: Wonders and Disorders", Tellwell Talent Publishers, pp 500. ISBN: 978-0-2288-4885-1 (Hardcover); 978-0-2288-4884-4 (Paperback).

Fymat AL (2023). "Pathogens in the brain and neurodegenerative diseases", Journal of Neurology and Psychology Research *5(1):1-14.*

On some neurological diseases of interest

> ### *In general:*

Bredesen DE, Rao RV, and Mehlen P (2006). "Cell death in the nervous system". Nature *443(7113): 796–802.* doi:10.1038/nature05293.

Brody DL and Holtzman DM (2008). "Active and passive immunotherapy for neurodegenerative disorders". Annual Review of Neuroscience *31:175– 93.* doi:10.1146/annurev.neuro.31.060407.125529.

Caccamo D, Currò M, Condello S, Ferlazzo N, and Ientile R (2010). "Critical role of transglutaminase and other stress proteins during neurodegenerative processes". Amino Acids **38** (2):653–8. doi:10.1007/s00726-009-0428-3.

Camandola S and Mattson MP (June 2017). "Brain metabolism in health, aging, and neurodegeneration". The EMBO Journal **36**(11):1474–92. do i:10.15252/embj.201695810.

Chung CG, Lee H, and Lee SB (2018). "Mechanisms of protein toxicity in neurodegenerative diseases". Cellular and Molecular Life Sciences **75**(17):3159–80. doi:10.1007/s00018-018- 2854-4.

De Vos KJ, Grierson AJ, Ackerley S, and Miller CC (2008). "Role of axonal transport in neurodegenerative diseases". Annual Review of Neuroscience **31**:151–73. doi:10.1146/annurev.neuro.31.061307.090711.

Erkkinen MG, Kim M-O, and Geschwind MD (2018). "Clinical neurology and epidemiology of the major neurodegenerative diseases". Cold Spring Harbor Perspectives in Biology **10**(4):20. doi:10.1101/cshperspect. a033118.

Fymat AL (2018a). "Regulating the brain's autoimmune system: The end of all neurological disorders?" Journal of Current Opinions in Neurological Science **2**(3):475-9.

Fymat AL (2018b). "Harnessing the immune system to treat cancers and neurodegenerative diseases", Journal of Clinical Research in Neurology **1**(1):1-14.

Fymat AL (2019). "From The Heart To The Brain: My Collected Works in Medical Science Research (2016- 2018), Tellwell Talent Publishers, pp 580, 1 February 2019. ISBN: 978-0-2288-0910-4 (Hardcover); 978-0-2288-0575-5 (Paperback).

Fymat AL (2020a). "The Odyssey of Humanity's Diseases: Epigenetic and Ecogenetic Modulations From Ancestry Through Inheritance, Environment, Culture, And Behavior", Volume 1, Tellwell Talent Publishers, pp 610. ISBN: 978-0-2288-2385-8 (Hardcover); 978-0-2288-2387-2 (Paperback).

Fymat AL (2020b). "The Odyssey of Humanity's Diseases: Epigenetic and Ecogenetic Modulations From Ancestry Through Inheritance, Environment, Culture, And Behavior" Volume 2, Tellwell Talent Publishers, pp 484. ISBN: 978-0-2288-2388-9 (Hardcover); 978-0-2288- 2386-5 (Paperback).

Fymat AL (2020c). "The Odyssey of Humanity's Diseases: Epigenetic and Ecogenetic Modulations From Ancestry Through Inheritance, Environment, Culture, And Behavior", Volume 3, Tellwell Talent Publishers, pp 388. ISBN: 978-0-2288-2390-2 (Hardcover); 978-0-2288- 2389-6 (Paperback).

Fymat AL (2021). "Nanomedicine". Tellwell Talent Publishers, pp 196. ISBN: 978-0-2288-6970-2 (Hardcover); 978-0-2288-6969-2 (Paperback).

Jeppesen DK, Bohr VA, and Stevnsner T (2011). "DNA repair deficiency in neurodegeneration". Progress in Neurobiology 94(2):166–200. doi:10.1016/j.pneurobio.2011.04.013.

Kanter I et al. (2023);. "Neuronal plasticity features are independent of neuronal holding membrane potential", Physica A.

Lin MT and Beal MF (2006). "Mitochondrial dysfunction and oxidative stress in neurodegenerative diseases". Nature 443 (7113):787–95. doi:10.1038/nature05292.

Liu Z, Zhou T, Ziegler AC, Dimitrion P, and Zuo L (2017). "Oxidative stress in neurodegenerative diseases: From molecular mechanisms to clinical applications". Oxidative Medicine and Cellular Longevity 2017: 2525967. doi:10.1155/2017/2525967.

Lobsiger CS and Cleveland DW (November 2007). "Glial cells as intrinsic components of non-cell- autonomous neurodegenerative disease". Nature Neuroscience 10(11):1355–60. doi:10.1038/nn1988.

Madabhushi R, Pan L, and Tsai LH (2014). "DNA damage and its links to neurodegeneration". Neuron 83(2):266–82. doi:10.1016/j.neuron.2014.06.034.

Maynard S, Fang EF, Scheibye-Knudsen M, Croteau DL, and Bohr VA (2015). "DNA damage, DNA repair, aging, and neurodegeneration". Cold Spring Harbor Perspectives in Medicine 5 (10):a025130. doi:10.1101/cshperspect.a025130.

Nabais MF, Laws SM, Lin T, Vallerga CL, Armstrong NJ, Blair IP, Kwok JB, Mather KA, Mellick GD, Sachdev PS, and Wallace L (2021)." Meta-analysis of genome-wide DNA methylation identifies shared associations across neurodegenerative disorders". Genome Biology 22(1):90. doi:10.1186/s13059-021-02275-5.

Pereira TMC, Côco LZ Ton AMM, Meyrelles SS, Campos-Toimil M, Campagnaro BP, and Vasquez EC (2021). "The emerging scenario of the gut-brain axis:

The therapeutic actions of the new actor Kefir against neurodegenerative diseases". Antioxidants **10**(11):1845. do i:10.3390/antiox10111845.

Rubinsztein DC (2006). "The roles of intracellular protein-degradation pathways in neurodegeneration" Nature **443**(7113):780–6. doi:10.1038/nature05291.

Singh A, Kukreti R, Saso L, and Kukreti S (2019). "Oxidative stress: A key modulator in neurodegenerative diseases". Molecules **24**(8):1583. d oi:10.3390/molecules24081583.

Stephenson J, Nutma E, van der Valk P, and Amor S (2018)." Inflammation in CNS neurodegenerative diseases". Immunology **154**(2):204–19. doi:10.1111/imm.12922.

Thompson LM (2008). "Neurodegeneration: A question of balance". Nature **452**(7188):707–8. d oi:10.1038/452707a.

Vila M and Przedborski S (2003). "Targeting programmed cell death in neurodegenerative diseases". Nature Reviews-Neuroscience **4**(5):365–75. doi:10.1038/nrn1100.

Wang H, Dharmalingam P, Vasquez V, Mitra J, Boldogh I, Rao KS et al. (2017). "Chronic oxidative damage together with genome repair deficiency in the neurons is a double whammy for neurodegeneration: Is damage response signaling a potential therapeutic target?". Mechanisms of Ageing and Development **161**(Pt A):163–76. doi:10.1016/j.mad.2016.09.005.

➤ Alzheimer's disease:

Alzheimer's Association (2022). "What Is Alzheimer's?". https://www.alz.org/alzheimers- dementia/what-is-alzheimers
(U.K.) Alzheimer's Society (2021). "Physical exercise and dementia".

Archer MC, Hall PH, and Morgan JC (2017). "Accuracy of clinical diagnosis of Alzheimer's disease in Alzheimer's disease centers". Alzheimer's & Dementia **13**(7S Part 16):P800–1. doi:10.1016/j.jalz.2017.06.1086.

Birks J (2006). "Cholinesterase inhibitors for Alzheimer's disease". The Cochrane Database of Systematic Reviews (1): CD005593. doi:10.1002/14651858.CD005593.

Brookmeyer R, Johnson E, Ziegler-Graham K, and Arrighi HM (2007). "Forecasting the global burden of Alzheimer's disease". Alzheimer's Dement **3:**186–91.

Chen Y, Zhou K, Wang R, Liu Y, Kwak YD, Ma T et al. (2009). "Antidiabetic drug metformin (Glucophage(R)) increases biogenesis of Alzheimer's amyloid peptides via up-regulating BACE1 transcription". Proc Natl Acad Sci USA **106:***3907–12.*

Commission de la transparence (2012). "Drugs for Alzheimer's disease: best avoided. No therapeutic advantage" Prescrire International. **21***(128):150.*

Cummings JL (2002). "Alzheimer's disease". *J. Amer. Med. Assoc.* **287**(18):2335-8. doi:10.1001/jama.287.18.2335.

Davis P, Morris J et al. (1991). "The distribution of tangles, plaques, and related immunohistochemical markers in healthy aging and Alzheimer's disease". Neurobiology of Aging **12***(4):295–312.* doi:10.1016/0197-4580(91)90006-6.

Delrieu J, Ousset PJ, Caillaud C, and Vellas B (2012). "'Clinical trials in Alzheimer's disease': immunotherapy approaches". Journal of Neurochemistry **120***(Suppl 1):186–93. doi:10.1111/j.1471-4159.2011.07458.x.*

Duthie A, Chew D, and Soiza RL (2011). "Non-psychiatric comorbidity associated with Alzheimer's disease". *Q J Med* **104:**913–20.

Fymat AL (2017a). "Alzheimer's disease: A review", *Journal of Current Opinions in Neurological Science* **2**(2);415-36.

Fymat AL (2018a). "Alzheimer's disease: Prevention, delay, minimization and reversal", *Journal of Clinical Research in Neurology* **1**(1):1-16.

Fymat AL (2018b). "Is Alzheimer's an autoimmune disease gone rogue?", *Journal of Clinical Research in Neurology* 2(1):1-4.

Fymat AL (2018c). "Is Alzheimer's a runaway autoimmune disease? And how to cure it?" *Proceedings of the European Union Academy of Sciences*, 2018 Newsletter, pages 379-83.

Fymat AL (2019). "Alzhei ... Who? Demystifying The Disease And What You Can Do About It", Tellwell Talent Publishers, pp 236. ISBN: 978-0-2288-2420-6 (Hardcover); 978-0-2288- 2419-0 (Paperback).

Fymat AL (2020a). "Is Alzheimer's an autoimmune disease gone rogue? The role of brain immunotherapy", *Journal of Clinical Research in Neurology* **3**(2):1-3.

Fymat AL (2020b). "Alzheimer's: What do we know about the disease and what can be done about it?" *EC Journal of Psychology & Psychiatry* **9**(11):69-74.

Fymat AL (2020c). "Alzheimer's: Will there ever be a cure?" *Journal of Clinical Psychiatry and Neuroscience* **3**(4):1-5.

Fymat AL (2022a). "Alzheimer's disease: A path to a cure", *Journal of Neurology and Psychology Research* **3**(1):1-15. https://researchnovelty. com/articles.php?journal_id=5.

Fymat AL (2022b). "Alzheimer's disease: A path to a cure", *Current Opinions in Neurological Science* **3**(1):1-16.

Gosche KM, Mortimer JA, Smith CD, Markesbery WR, and Snowdon DA(2002). "Hippocampal volume as an index of Alzheimer neuropathology: Findings from the Nun Study". Neurology ***58**(10): 1476–82. doi:10.1212/ WNL.58.10.1476.*

Graff BJ, Harrison SL, Payne SJ, and El-Bouri WK (2023). "Regional cerebral blood flow changes in healthy aging and Alzheimer's disease: A narrative review". Cerebrovascular Diseases ***52**(1):11–20. doi:10.1159/000524797.*

Habes M, Janowitz D, Erus G, Toledo JB, Resnick SM, Doshi J, Van der Auwera S, Wittfeld K, Hegenscheid K, Hosten N, Biffar R, Homuth G, Völzke H, Grabe HJ, Hoffmann W, and Davatzikos C (2016). "Advanced brain aging: Relationship with epidemiological and genetic risk factors, and overlap with Alzheimer's disease atrophy patterns". Translational Psychiatry ***6**(4):e775. doi:10.1038/tp.2016.39.*

Hyman BT, Phelps CH, Beach TG, Bigio EH, Cairns NJ, Carrillo MC, Dickson DW, Duyckaerts C, Frosch MP, Masliah E, Mirra SS, Nelson PT, Schneider JA, Thal DR, and Thies B (2012). "National Institute on Aging– Alzheimer's Association guidelines for the neuropathologic assessment of Alzheimer's disease". Alzheimer's & Dementia ***8**(1):1–13. doi:10.1016/j. jalz.2011.10.007.*

Karlawish JH, Klocinski JL, Merz J, Clark CM, and Asch DA (2000). "Caregivers' preferences for the treatment of patients with Alzheimer's disease". Neurology ***55**:1008–14.*

Keohane K and Balfe M (2019). "The Nun Study and Alzheimer's disease: Quality of vocation as a potential protective factor?". Dementia ***18**(5):1651–62. doi:10.1177/1471301217725186.*

Krivanek TJ, Gale SA, McFeeley BM, Nicastri CM, and Daffner KR (2021). "Promoting successful cognitive aging: A ten-year update". Journal of Alzheimer's Disease ***81**(3):871–920. doi:10.3233/JAD-201462.*

Larson EB, Shadlen MF, Wang L, McCormick WC, Bowen JD, Teri L et al. (2004). "Survival after initial diagnosis of Alzheimer's disease". Ann Intern Med **140:**501–9+I526.

Lock MM (2013). "The Alzheimer conundrum: Entanglements of dementia and aging". Princeton. ISBN 978-1-4008-4846-1.

McCormick WC, Kukull WA, van Belle G, Bowen JD, Teri L, and Larson EB (1994). "Symptom patterns and comorbidity in the early stages of Alzheimer's disease". J Am Geriatr Soc **42:**517– 21.

Montine TJ, Phelps CH, Beach TG, Bigio EH, Cairns NJ, Dickson DW, Duyckaerts C, Frosch MP, Masliah E, Mirra SS, Nelson PT, Schneider JA, Thal D, Trojanowski JQ, and Vinters HV (2012). "National Institute on Aging–Alzheimer's Association guidelines for the neuropathologic assessment of Alzheimer's disease: A practical approach". Acta Neuropathologica **123**(1):1–11. doi:10.1007/s00401-011-0910-3.

Moore BA (1995). "Study of Nuns turns up clues to brain aging and Alzheimer's disease". Public Health Reports **110**(4):508.
(U.S.) National Institute on Aging (NIA), U.S. Department of Health and Human Services (2022). "What Is Alzheimer's disease?" https://www.nia.nih.gov/health/what-alzheimers-disease.

Nicolazzo JA and Mehta DC (2010). "Transport of drugs across the blood-brain barrier in Alzheimer's disease". Ther Deliv **1:**595–611.

Pini L, Pievani M, Bocchetta M, Altomare D, Bosco P, Cavedo E, Galluzzi S, Marizzoni M, Frisoni GB (2016). "Brain atrophy in Alzheimer's Disease and aging". Ageing Research Reviews **30:**25–48. doi:10.1016/j.arr.2016.01.002.

Priller C, Bauer T, Mitteregger G, Krebs B, Kretzschmar HA, and Herms J (2006). "Synapse formation and function is modulated by the amyloid precursor protein". The Journal of Neuroscience **26**(27):7212–21. doi:10.1523/JNEUROSCI.1450-06.2006.

Reisberg B, Borenstein J, Salob SP, and Ferris SH (1987). "Behavioral symptoms in Alzheimer's disease: Phenomenology and treatment". J Clin Psychiatry **48:**9–15.

Sauer A (2017). "What Nuns are teaching us about Alzheimer's". Alzheimers.net.

Schenk D, Basi GS, and Pangalos MN (2012). "Treatment strategies targeting amyloid β-protein". Cold Spring Harbor Perspectives in Medicine *2(9): a006387*. doi:10.1101/cshperspect.a006387.

Sirts K, Piguet O, and, Johnson M (2017). "Idea density for predicting Alzheimer's disease from transcribed speech". *arXiv:1706.04473*.

Snowdon DA (1997). "Aging and Alzheimer's disease: Lessons from the Nun Study". The Gerontologist *37(2):150–6. doi:10.1093/geront/37.2.150.*

Snowdon DA, Kemper SJ, Mortimer JA, Greiner LH, Wekstein DR, and Markesbery WR (1996). "Linguistic ability in early life and cognitive function and Alzheimer's disease in late life: Findings from the Nun Study". JAMA *275(7):528–32.*

doi:10.1001/jama.1996.03530310034029.

Stewart WF, Kawas C, Corrada M, and Metter EJ (1997). "Risk of Alzheimer's disease and duration of NSAID use". Neurology *48:626–32.*

Svob S, Dubravka K, Konjevod M, Sagud M, Nikolac PM, Nedic EG, Vuic B, Simic G, Vukic V, Mimica N, and Pivac N (2021). "Personalizing the care and treatment of Alzheimer's disease: An overview". Pharmacogenomics and Personalized Medicine *14:631–53.* doi:10.2147/PGPM.S284615.

Tiraboschi P, Hansen LA, Thal LJ, and Corey-Bloom J (2004). "The importance of neuritic plaques and tangles to the development and evolution of AD". Neurology *62(11):1984–9.* doi:10.1212/01.WNL.0000129697.01779.0A.

Turner PR, O'Connor K, Tate WP, and Abraham WC (2003). "Roles of amyloid precursor protein and its fragments in regulating neural activity, plasticity and memory". Progress in Neurobiology *70(1):1–32.* doi:10.1016/S0301-0082(03)00089-3.

University of Southern California (2023). "How old is your brain, really? AI-powered analysis accurately reflects risk of cognitive decline and Alzheimer's disease". Press release: via medicalxpress.com.

Veld in t' BA, Ruitenberg A, Hofman A, Launer LJ, van Duijn CM, Stijnen T et al. (2001). "Nonsteroidal anti-inflammatory drugs and the risk of Alzheimer's disease". N Engl J Med *345:1515–21.*

Wenk GL (2003). "Neuropathologic changes in Alzheimer's disease". The Journal of Clinical Psychiatry 64(Suppl 9):7–10.

➢ **Creutzeldt-Jakob disease:**

(U.S.) National Institute of Neurological Disorders and Stroke (2022). "Creutzfeldt-Jakob Disease Fact Sheet ".

Mayo Clinic (2022). "Creutzfeldt-Jakob disease - Symptoms and causes".

➢ **Dementia:**

Alzheimer's Society (2015). *"Sight, perception and hallucinations in dementia".*

Alzheimer's Association (2022). "What Is dementia? https://www.alz.org/ alzheimers-dementia/what-is- dementia

American Psychiatric Association(2013). Diagnostic and statistical manual of mental disorders: DSM-5 *(5ᵗʰ ed.). Washington, D.C.: American Psychiatric Association. pp. 591– 603. I* SBN 978-0-89042-554-1.

American Speech Language Hearing Association. "Dementia-Signs and symptoms".

Annear MJ, Toye C, McInerney F, Eccleston C, Tranter B, Elliott KE, and Robinson A (2015). "What should we know about dementia in the 21ˢᵗ century? A Delphi consensus study".
*BMC Geriatr.***15:**5. doi: 10.1186/s12877-015-0008-1.

Australian Institute of Health and Welfare (2012). "Dementia in Australia". Cat. no. AGE 70. Canberra: AIHW.

Ayalon L, Bachner YG, Dwolatzky T, and Heinik J (2012). "Preferences for end-of-life treatment: Concordance between older adults with dementia or mild cognitive impairment and their spouses". Int Psychogeriatr ***24:**1798–804.*

Bains J, Birks J and Dening T (2002). In Dening T, ed. "Antidepressants For Treating Depression in Dementia". The Cochrane Database of Systematic Reviews *(4):CD003944.* doi:*10.1002/14651858.CD003944.*

Barclay, TR; Brasure, M; Nelson, VA and Kane, RL (2018). "Pharmacologic interventions to prevent cognitive decline, mild cognitive impairment, and clinical Alzheimer-type dementia: A systematic review", Annals of Internal Medicine ***168**(1):39–51.* doi:10.7326/M17-1529.

Bergh S, Selbaek G, and Engedal K (2012). "Discontinuation of antidepressants in people with dementia and neuropsychiatric symptoms (DESEP study):

double blind, randomized, parallel group, placebo controlled trial". Br Med J ***344****:12.*

Boustani M, Peterson B, Hanson L, Harris R, and Lohr KN (2003). "Screening for dementia in primary care: a summary of the evidence for the U.S. Preventive Services Task Force", Annals of Internal Medicine ***138****(11):927–37.* doi:10.7326/0003-4819-138-11-200306030-00015.

British Dental Association (2017). *"Can poor oral health lead to dementia?",* British Dental Journal ***223****(11):840. d* oi:10.1038/sj.bdj.2017.1064.

Budson AE and O'Connor MK (2017). "Seven steps to managing your memory: What's normal, what's not, and what to do about It", New York: Oxford University Press.

Budson AE and Solomon PR (2021). "Memory loss, Alzheimer's disease, and dementia: A practical guide for clinicians", 3rd Edition, Philadelphia: Elsevier, Inc.

*Bunn F, Burn AM, Goodman C, Rait G, Norton S, Robinson L et al. (2014). "Comorbidity and dementia: A scoping review of the literature". BMC Med ****192.****

*Burns A and Iliffe S (2009). "Dementia". British Medical J ****338****: b75. doi:10.1136/bmj.b75.*

Burns A, Cohen-Mansfield J, Cooper C, Fox N, Gitlin LN, Howard R, Kales HC, Larson EB, Ritchie K, Rockwood K, Sampson EL, Samus Q, Schneider LS, Selbæk G, Teri L and Mukadam N (2017). "Dementia prevention, intervention, and care", Lancet ***390*** *(10113): 2673– 2734.* doi:10.1016/ S0140-6736(17)31363-6.

Butler M, McCreedy E, Nelson VA, Desai P, Ratner E, Fink HA, Hemmy LS, McCarten JR, Barclay TR, Brasure M, Davila H, and Kane RL (2018). "Does Cognitive Training Prevent Cognitive Decline?: A Systematic Review". Annals of Internal Medicine ***168****(1):63–8.* doi:10.7326/M17- 1531. *(U.S.) Centers for Disease Control and Prevention (CDC&P) (2022). "Dementia risk reduction". https://www.cdc.gov/aging/publications/ features/dementia-risk-reduction-june-2022/index.html.*

Cerejeira J, Lagarto L, and Mukaetova-Ladinska EB (2012). "Behavioral and psychological symptoms of dementia", Frontiers in Neurology. ***3****: 73.* doi:10.3389/fneur.2012.00073.

Chang-Quan H, Hui W, Chao-Min W, Zheng-Rong W, Jun-Wen G, Yong-Hong L et al. (2011). "The association of antihypertensive medication use with risk of cognitive decline and dementia: A meta-analysis of longitudinal studies". Int J Clin Pract **65:**1295–305.

Clionsky E and Clionsky M (2023). "Dementia prevention: Using your head to save your brain", Johns Hopkins Press, Baltimore, 276 pages.

Creavin ST, Wisniewski S, Noel-Storr AH, Trevelyan CM, Hampton T, Rayment D et al. (2016). "Mini-Mental State Examination (MMSE) for the detection of dementia in clinically unevaluated people aged 65 and over in community and primary care populations". The Cochrane Database of Systematic Reviews(1):CD011145. doi:10.1002/14651858.CD011145. pub2.

Cullen B, O'Neill B, Evans JJ, Coen RF, and Lawlor BA (2007). "A review of screening tests for cognitive impairment", Journal of Neurology, Neurosurgery, and Psychiatry **78**(8):790– 9. doi:10.1136/jnnp.2006.095414.
(U.S.) Department of Health and Human Services (DHHS) (2022). "Can I prevent dementia? https://www.alzheimers.gov/life-with-dementia/can-i-prevent-dementia.

Dougall NJ, Bruggink S, and Ebmeier KP (2004). "Systematic review of the diagnostic accuracy of 99mTc-HMPAO-SPECT in dementia", The American Journal of Geriatric Psychiatry **12**(6):554-70. doi:10.1176/appi. ajgp.12.6.554.

European Association for Palliative Care. "White Paper defining optimal palliative care in older people with dementia; A Delphi study".

Fink, HA, Jutkowitz E, McCarten JR, Hemmy LS, Butler M, Davila H Ratner E, Calvert C, Lampit A, Hallock H, and Valenzuela M (2014). "Computerized cognitive training in cognitively healthy older adults: A systematic review and meta-analysis of effect modifiers". PLoS Medicine **11**(11):e1001756. doi:10.1371/journal.pmed.1001756.

Fink HA, Jutkowitz E, McCarten JR, Hemmy LS, Butler M, Davila H, Ratner E, Calvert C, Barclay TR, Brasure M, Nelson VA, and Kane RL (2018). "Pharmacologic interventions to prevent cognitive decline, mild cognitive impairment, and clinical Alzheimer-type Dementia: A systematic review", Annals of Internal Medicine **168**(1):39–51. doi:10.7326/M17-1529.

(U.S.) Food and Drug Administration (2014). "Information for Healthcare Professionals: Conventional Antipsychotics". fda.gov. 2008-06-16.

Fymat AL (2018a). "Dementia treatment: Where do we stand?", *Journal of Current Opinions in Neurological Science* **3**(1):1-3. 599.603.

Fymat AL (2019a). "On dementia and other cognitive disorders", *Journal of Clinical Research in Neurology* **2**(1):1-14.

Fymat AL (2019b). "Dementia: A review", *Journal of Clinical Psychiatry and Neuroscience* **1**(3):27- 34.

Fymat AL (2019c). "Dementia with Lewy bodies: A review", *Journal of Current Opinions in Neurological Science* **4**(1);15-32.

Fymat AL (2019d). "Our two interacting brains: Etiologic modulations of neurodegenerative and gastroenteric diseases", *Journal of Current Opinions in Neurological Science* **4**(2):50-4.

Fymat AL (2019e). "What do we know about Lewy body dementias?" *Journal of Psychiatry and Psychotherapy* (Editorial) **2**(1)-013:1-4. doi:10.31579/ JPP.2019/018.

Fymat AL (2020a). "Dementia: Should we reorient our approach to treatment?" *EC Journal of Psychology & Psychiatry* **9**(12):1-3.

Fymat AL (2020b). "Dementia: What is its causal etiology?" *International Journal of Neuropsychology and Behavioral Sciences* **1**(1):19-22.

Fymat AL (2020c). "Dementia: Fending Off The Menacing Disease... And What You Can Do About It", Tellwell Talent Publishers, pp 488. ISBN: 978-0-2288-4146-3 (Hardcover); 978-0-2288- 4145-6 (Paperback).

Fymat AL (2021). "On potentially reversible forms of dementia", *Journal of Current Opinions in Neurological Science* **6**(1):101-8.

Fymat AL (2022). "Dementia: Eliminating its potentially reversible forms", *Proc. European Union Academy of Sciences*. Pages 270-7.

*Gleason OC (2003). "Delirium", American Family Physician. **67**(5): 1027–34.*

*Glind van de EMM, van Enst WA, van Munster BC, Olde RMG, Scheltens P, Scholten RJ et al. (2013). "Pharmacological treatment of dementia: A scoping review of systematic reviews". Dement Geriatr Cogn Disord **36**:211–8.*

Hall CB, Lipton RB, Sliwinski M, Katz MJ, Derby CA, and Verghese J (2009). "Cognitive activities delay onset of memory decline in persons who develop dementia". Neurology 73(5):356– 61. doi:10.1212/ wnl.0b013e3181b04ae3.

Harris D. (2009). "Withholding and withdrawing life sustaining treatment in advanced dementia: How and when to make these difficult decisions". *Geriatr Aging* **12:**403–7.

Herr K, Karp JF, and Weiner DK (2007). "Pain in persons with dementia: complex, common, and challenging", The Journal of Pain *8(5):373–8.* doi:*10.1016/j.jpain.2007.03.003.*

Hoffmann F, van den Bussche H, Wiese B, Schön G, Koller D, Eisele M et al. (2011). "Impact of geriatric comorbidity and polypharmacy on cholinesterase inhibitors prescribing in dementia". BMC Psychiatry *11.*

Iadecola C (2013). "The pathobiology of vascular dementia", Neuron. *80 (4): 844-66.* doi:*10.1016/j.neuron.2013.10.008.*

Jick H, Zornberg GL, Jick SS, Seshadri S, and Drachman DA (2000). "Statins and the risk of dementia". Lancet *356:1627–31.*

Jorm AF (2004). "The Informant Questionnaire on cognitive decline in the elderly (IQCODE): a review", International Psychogeriatrics *16(3):275-93.* doi:*10.1017/S1041610204000390.*

Karlawish JH and Clark CM (2003). "Diagnostic evaluation of elderly patients with mild memory problems", Annals of Internal Medicine *138(5):411–9.* doi:*10.7326/0003-4819-138-5- 200303040-00011.*

Kunik ME, Snow AL, Molinari VA, Menke TJ, Souchek J, Sullivan G et al. (2003). "Health care utilization in dementia patients with psychiatric comorbidity". Gerontologist *43:86–91.*

Lüders S and Schrader J (2015). "Dementia and hypertension". Dtsch Med Wochenschr *140:1599–603.*

Langa KM and Levine DA (2014). "The diagnosis and management of mild cognitive impairment: a clinical review", JAMA *312(23):2551-61.* doi:*10.1001/jama.2014.13806.*

Laver K, Cumming RG, Dyer SM, Agar MR, Anstey KJ, Beattie E et al. (2016). "Clinical practice guidelines for dementia in Australia". Med J Aust *204.*

Lee AY (2011). "Vascular dementia". Chonnam Medical Journal. *47 (2): 66-71.* doi:*10.4068/cmj.2011.47.2.66.*

Liao JN, Chao TF, Liu CJ, Wang KL, Chen SJ, Tuan TC et al. (2015). "Risk and prediction of dementia in patients with atrial fibrillation - A nationwide population-based cohort study". Int J Cardiol *199:25–30.*

Lin JS, O'Connor E, Rossom RC, Perdue LA, and Eckstrom E (2013). "Screening for cognitive impairment in older adults: A systematic review for the U.S. Preventive Services Task Force". Annals of Internal Medicine **159**(9):601–12. doi:10.7326/0003-4819-159-9-201311050- 00730.

Livingston G, Sommerlad A, Orgeta V, Costafreda SG, Huntley J, Ames D, Ballard C, Banerjee S,

Kavirajan H, and Schneider LS (2007). "Efficacy and adverse effects of cholinesterase inhibitors and memantine in vascular dementia: a meta-analysis of randomised controlled trials", The Lancet. Neurology. **6** (9): 782–92. doi:10.1016/s1474-4422(07)70195-3.

Livingston G et al. (2020). "Dementia prevention, intervention, and care". The Lancet. doi.org/10.1016/S0140-6736(20)30367-6.

Lleó A, Greenberg SM, and Growdon JH (2006). "Current pharmacotherapy for Alzheimer's disease". Annual Review of Medicine. **57** (1): 513-33. doi:10.1146/annurev.med.57.121304.131442.

Lolk A and Gulmann NC (2006). "Psychopharmacological treatment of behavioral and psychological symptoms in dementia". Ugeskrift for Laeger (in Danish) **168**(40):3429–32.

Loy CT, Schofield PR, Turner AM, and Kwok JB (2014). "Genetics of dementia", Lancet **383** (9919): 828–40. doi:10.1016/s0140-6736(13)60630-3.

Lyketsos CG, Steinberg M, Tschanz JT, Norton MC, Steffens DC, Breitner JC et al. (2000). "Mental and behavioral disturbances in dementia: Findings from the Cache County Study on memory in aging". Am J Psychiatry **157:**708–14.

Malouf R and Grimley EJ (2008). "Folic acid with or without vitamin B12 for the prevention and treatment of healthy elderly and demented people". The Cochrane Database of Systematic Reviews (4): CD004514. doi:10.1002/14651858.CD004514.pub2.

McCleery J, Cohen DA, and Sharpley AL (2016). "Pharmacotherapies for sleep disturbances in dementia". The Cochrane Database of Systematic Reviews. **11** (11):CD009178. doi:10.1002/14651858.CD009178.pub3.

McGuinness B, Craig D, Bullock R, Malouf R, and Passmore P (2014). "Statins for the treatment of dementia". The Cochrane Database of Systematic Reviews. **7** (7):CD007514. doi:10.1002/14651858.CD007514.pub3.

MD Guidelines (2009). "Dementia definition", Reed Group.

Melis RJ, Marengoni A, Rizzuto D, Teerenstra S, Kivipelto M, Angleman SB *et al.* (2013). "The influence of multimorbidity on clinical progression of dementia in a population-based cohort". PLoS One **8:**e84014.

Nasreddine ZS, Phillips NA, Bédirian V, Charbonneau S, Whitehead V, Collin I, Cummings JL, and Chertkow H (2005). "The Montreal Cognitive Assessment, MoCA: a brief screening tool for mild cognitive impairment", Journal of the American Geriatrics Society ***53****(4):695– 9. doi:10.1111/j.1532-5415.2005.53221.x.*
(U.S.) National Institute on Aging (NIA), U.S. Department of Health and Human Services (2021). "What is dementia?" https://www.nia.nih.gov/health/what-is-dementia.

(U.S.) National Institute on Aging (2022). "Reducing your risk of dementia". https://order.nia.nih.gov/sites/default/files/2022-05/dementia-risk-tip-sheet.pdf.

(U.K.) National Institute for Clinical Excellence (NICE) (2014). *"Dementia overview",* pathways.nice.org.uk.

(U.S.) National Library of Medicine (NLM) (2015). "Dementia", MedlinePlus (14 May).

Ott A, Stolk RP, Van Harskamp F, Pols HA, Hofman A, Breteler MM et al. (1999). "Diabetes mellitus and the risk of dementia: The Rotterdam Study". Neurology ***53****:1937–42.*
Page A, Potter K, Clifford R, McLachlan A, and Etherton-Beer C (2015). "Prescribing for Australians living with dementia: study protocol using the Delphi technique". BMJ Open ***5****:e008048.*
Page AT, Potter K, Clifford R, McLachlan AJ, and Etherton-Beer C (2016). "Medication appropriateness tool for co-morbid health conditions in dementia: consensus recommendations from a multi- disciplinary expert panel", Internal Medicine Journal. ***46****(10): 1189-97. doi:10.1111/imj.13215.*
Page AT, Clifford RM, Potter K, Seubert L, McLachlan AJ, Hill X, King S, Clark V, Ryan C, Parekh N, and Etherton-Beer CD (2017). "Exploring the enablers and barriers to implementing the Medication Appropriateness

Tool for Co-morbid Health conditions during Dementia (MATCH- D) criteria in Australia: A qualitative study". BMJ Open *7*(8):e017906. doi: 10.1136/bmjopen- 2017-017906.

Parsons C, Hughes CM, Passmore AP, and Lapane KL (2010). "Withholding, discontinuing and withdrawing medications in dementia patients at the end of life: A neglected problem in the disadvantaged dying?" Drugs Aging *27:*435–9.

Reeve E, Simon Bell J, and Hilmer SN (2016). "Barriers to optimizing prescribing and deprescribing in older adults with dementia: A narrative review". Curr Clin Pharmacol *10:*168–77.

Rolinski M, Fox C, Maidment I, and McShane R (2012). "Cholinesterase inhibitors for dementia with Lewy bodies, Parkinson's disease dementia and cognitive impairment in Parkinson's disease", The Cochrane Database of Systematic Reviews. *3* (3): CD006504. doi:10.1002/14651858. CD006504.pub2.

Rosenbloom MH, Smith S, Akdal G, and Geschwind MD (2009). "Immunologically mediated dementias". Current Neurology and Neuroscience Reports (Review) *9*(5):359– 67. doi:10.1007/s11910-009-0053-2.

Sadock BJ and Sadock VA (2008). "Delirium, Dementia, and Amnestic and Other Cognitive Disorders and Mental Disorders Due to a General Medical Condition", Kaplan & Sadock's Concise Textbook of Clinical Psychiatry (3rd ed.). Philadelphia: Wolters Kluwer/Lippincott Williams & Wilkins. p. 52. ISBN 978-0-7817-8746-8.

Şahin CE (2014). "Management of Behavioral and Psychological Symptoms of Dementia". Noro psikiyatri arsivi. *51*(4):303–12. doi:10.5152/ npa.2014.7405.

Schneider LS, Dagerman KS, and Insel P (2005). "Risk of death with atypical antipsychotic drug treatment for dementia: Meta-analysis of randomized placebo-controlled trials". JAMA *294:*1934–43.

Schofield P (2005). "Dementia associated with toxic causes and autoimmune disease". International Psychogeriatrics (Review). 17 Suppl 1:S129–47. doi:10.1017/s1041610205001997.

Schubert CC, Boustani M, Callahan CM, Perkins AJ, Carney CP, Fox C *et al.* (2006). "Comorbidity profile of dementia patients in primary care: Are they sicker?" *J Am Geriatr Soc* **54:**104–9.

Seitz DP, Gill SS, Herrmann N, Brisbin S, Rapoport MJ, Rines J et al. (2013). "Pharmacological treatments for neuropsychiatric symptoms of dementia in long-term care: A systematic review". Int Psychogeriatr *25*:185–203.

Shega J, Emanuel L, Vargish L, Levine SK, Bursch H, Sampson EL, Ritchie CW, Lai R, Raven PW, and Blanchard MR (2005). "A systematic review of the scientific evidence for the efficacy of a palliative care approach in advanced dementia", International Psychogeriatrics *17*(1): 31–40.

Shub D and Kunik ME (2009). "Psychiatric Comorbidity in Persons With Dementia: Assessment and Treatment Strategies". Psychiatric Times *26*(4).

Smith T, Maidment I, Hebding J, Madzima T, Cheater F, Cross J et al. (2014). "Systematic review investigating the reporting of co-morbidities and medication in randomized controlled trials of people with dementia". Ageing *43*:868–72.

Snowdon DA (2003). "Healthy aging and dementia: Findings from the Nun Study". Annals of Internal Medicine *139*(5 Part_2):450–4. doi:10.7326/0003-4819-139-5_Part_2-200309021- 00014.

Stein PS, Desrosiers M, Donegan SJ, Yepes JF, and Kryscio RJ (2007). "Tooth loss, dementia, and neuropathology in the Nun Study". The Journal of the American Dental Association *138*(10):1314–22. doi:10.14219/jada. archive.2007.0046.

Taghizadeh-Larsson A, and Osterholm JH (2014)." How are decisions on care services for people with dementia made and experienced? A systematic review and qualitative synthesis of recent empirical findings". Int Psychogeriatr *26*:1849–62.

Teng EL and Chui HC (1987). "The Modified Mini-Mental State (3MS) examination". The Journal of Clinical Psychiatry *48*(8):314–8.

Umphred D (2012). Neurological rehabilitation (6th ed.). St. Louis, Mo.: Elsevier Mosby. p.838. ISBN 978-0-323-07586-2.

Weitzel T, Robinson S, Barnes MR, Berry TA, Holmes JM, Mercer S et al. (2011). "The special needs of the hospitalized patient with dementia", Medsurg Nursing *20*(1):13–8, quiz 19.

Welsh TJ, Gladman JR, and Gordon AL (2014). "The treatment of hypertension in people with dementia: A systematic review of observational studies". BMC Geriatr *14.*

Wolfson C, Wolfson DB, Asgharian M, M'Lan CE, Østbye T, Rockwood K et al. (2001). "A reevaluation of the duration of survival after the onset of dementia". N Engl J Med **344:***1111–6*

Woods B, O'Philbin L, Farrell EM, Spector AE, and and Orrell M (2018). *"Reminiscence therapy for dementia"*. Cochrane Database Syst Rev. ***3:*** *CD001120.pub3. doi:10.1002/14651858.*

World Health Organization (2012). "Dementia Fact Sheet N0. 362" *(April 2012).*

World Health Organization (2021). "Global status report on the public health response to dementia" ISBN 978-92-4-003324-5.

> **Epilepsy:**

Fymat AL (2017a). "Epilepsy: A review", *J of Current Opinions on Neurological Science* **1**(5):240-54.

Fymat AL (2017b). "Neurological disorders and the blood brain barrier: 1. Epilepsy", *J of Current Opinions on Neurological Science* 1(6):277-93.

Fymat AL (2022). "Epilepsy: The Electrical Storm In The Brain", Tellwell Talent Publishers, pp 412. ISBN-978-0-2288-8203-9 (Hardcover); 978-0-2288-8203-9; 978-0-2288-8202-2 (Paperback). https://portal.tellwell.ca/Tellwell/design/187051.

Fymat AL (2023). "Epilepsy: Surgical and non-surgical management and treatment", *Current Opinions in Neurological Science* **8(**1):1-26.

> **Huntington's disease:**

Barnat M, Capizzi M, Aparicio E, Boluda S, Wennagel D, Kacher R, Kassem R, Lenoir S, Agasse F, Braz BY, and Liu J-P (2020). "Huntington's disease alters human neurodevelopment". Science ***369****(6505):787–93.* doi:10.1126/science.aax3338. ISSN 0036-8075.

Labbadia J and Morimoto RI (2013). "Huntington's disease: Underlying molecular mechanisms and emerging concepts". Trends in Biochemical Sciences ***38****(8):378–85.*
doi:10.1016/j.tibs.2013.05.003.

Purves DE, Sánchez AM, Mejía-Toiber J, and Massieu L (2008). "Excitotoxic neuronal death and the pathogenesis of Huntington's disease". Archives of Medical Research *39(3):265–76. doi:10.1016/j.arcmed.2007.11.011.*

➢ Lyme disease:

Fymat AL (2020). "Lyme Disease: The Dreadful Invader, Evader, and Imitator… And What You Can Do About It", Tellwell Talent Publishers, pp 278. ISBN: 978-0-2288-3198-3 (Hardcover); 978- 0-2288-3199-0 (Paperback).

Fymat AL (2023a). "Lyme disease neurological implications: I. Symptomatology and etiology". *Neurology and Psychology Research Journal* **5**(2):1-24.

Fymat AL (2023b). "Lyme disease neurological implications: II. Diagnostic methodology". *Neurology and Psychology Research Journal* **5**(2):1-26.

Fymat AL (2023c). "Lyme disease neurological implications: III. Neuroborreliosis and other diseases transmitted by the Lyme tick vector". *Neurology and Psychology Research Journal* **5**(2):1-26.

Fymat AL (2023d). "Lyme disease neurological implications: IV. Symptoms management, treatment, and human vaccine development". *Neurology and Psychology Research Journal* **5**(2):1-32.

➢ Multiple sclerosis:

Fymat AL (2023a). "Multiple Sclerosis: The Progressive Demyelinating Autoimmune Disease", Tellwell Talent Publishers pp 504. ISBN: 978-0-2288-9292-2 (Hardcover); 978-0-2288-3 (Paperback). https://portal.tellwell.ca/Tellwell/Design/212669.

Fymat AL (2023b). "Multiple sclerosis: I. Symptomatology and etiology", *Journal of Neurology and Psychology Research* **4**(2):1-46. https://researchnovelty.com/articles.php?journal_id=5.

Fymat AL (2023c). "Multiple sclerosis: II. Diagnosis and symptoms management", *Journal of Neurology and Psychology Research* **4**(2):1-21. https://researchnovelty.com/articles.php? journal_id=5.

Fymat AL (2023d). "Multiple sclerosis: III. Treatment and prognosis", *Journal of Neurology and Psychology Research* 4(2):1-46. https://researchnovelty.com/articles.php?journal_id=5.

Irvine KA and Blakemore WF (2008). "Remyelination protects axons from demyelination-associated axon degeneration". Brain ***131***(6):1464–77. doi:10.1093/brain/awn080.

Kaufman DM and Milstein MJ (2013). Kaufman DM and Milstein MJ (eds.), "Chapter 15 - Multiple Sclerosis", *Kaufman's Clinical neurology for psychiatrists (Seventh Edition), Philadelphia: W.B. Saunders, pp. 329–49,* ISBN 978-0-7234-3748-2.

(U.S.) National Institute of Neurological Disorders and Stroke (2020). "Multiple sclerosis: Hope through research".

Stys PK and Tsutsui S (2019). "Recent advances in understanding multiple sclerosis". F1000Research ***8:2100.*** doi:10.12688/f1000research.20906.1.

➤ *Multiple system atrophy:*

Fymat AL (2023a). "Multiple System aArophy: The Chronic, Progressive, Neurodegenerative Synucleopathic Disease", Tellwell Talent Publishers, pp. 302. ISBN: 978-0-2288-9493-8 (Hardcover); 978-0-2288-9492-1 (Paperback). https://portal.tellwell.ca/Tellwell/Design/256783.

Fymat AL (2023b). "Multiple system atrophy: Symptoms management and treatment", *Journal of Neurology and Psychology Research* 4(1):1-37.

➤ **Parkinson's disease:**

Crossman AR (2000). "Functional anatomy of movement disorders". Journal of Anatomy *196(Pt 4) (4):519–25.* doi:10.1046/j.1469-7580.2000.19640519.x.

Elbaz A, Carcaillon L, Kab S, and Moisan F (2016). "Epidemiology of Parkinson's disease". Revue Neurologique ***172(1):14–26. doi:10.1016/j. neurol.2015.09.012.***

Fymat AL (2017a). "Parkinson's disease and other movement disorders: A review", *Journal of Current Opinions in Neurological Science* **2**(1):316-43.

Fymat AL (2017b). "Neurological disorders and the blood-brain barrier: 2. Parkinson's disease and other movement disorders", *Journal of Current Opinions in Neurological Science* **2**(1)362-83.

Fymat AL (2018). "Blood-brain barrier permeability and neurological diseases", *Journal of Current Opinions in Neurological Science* (Editorial) **2**(2):411-14.

Fymat AL (2019). "Viruses in the brain…? Any connections to Parkinson's and other neurodegenerative diseases?" *Proceedings of the European Union Academy of Sciences,* 2019 Newsletter, pages 249-52.

Fymat AL (2020a). "Recent research developments in Parkinson's disease", *Current Opinions in Neurological Science* **5**(1):12-30.

Fymat AL (2020b). "Parkinson's: What is known about the disease and what can be done about it?" *Journal of Clinical Research in Neurology* 3(2):1-12.

Fymat, AL (2020c). "Parkin… ss..oo..nn: Elucidating The Disease… And What You Can Do About It", Tellwell Talent Publishers, pp 258, 6 April 2020. ISBN: 978-0-2288-2874-7 (Hardcover); 978- 0-2228-2875-4 (Paperback).

Hill-Burns EM, Debelius JW, Morton JT, Wissemann WT, Lewis MR, Wallen ZD, Peddada SD, Factor SA, Molho E, ZabetianCP, and Knight R (2017). "Parkinson's disease and Parkinson's disease medications have distinct signatures of the gut microbiome: PD, Medications, and Gut Microbiome". Movement Disorders ***32**(5):739–49.* doi:10.1002/mds.26942.

> ### Tourette's syndrome:

Fymat AL (2023a). "Tourette: The Self-Under-Siege Neurodevelopmental And Neuropsychiatric Motor Syndrome", Tellwell Talent Publishers pp. 466. ISBN: 978-1-7794-1027-6 (Hardcover); 978-1-7794-1026-6 (Paperback). https://portal.tellwell.ca/Tellwell/Design/256783.

Fymat AL (2023b). "Tourette's syndrome: I. Symptomatology and etiology", *Journal of Neurology and Psychology Research* **5**(1):1-34. https:// researchnovelty.com/articles.php?journal_id=5.

Fymat AL (2023c). "Tourette's syndrome: II. Diagnosis and symptoms management", *Journal of Neurology and Psychology Research* **5**(1):1-27. https://researchnovelty.com/articles.php? journal_id=5.

Fymat AL (2023d). "Tourette's syndrome: III. Treatment and prognosis", *Journal of Neurology and Psychology Research* **5**(1):1-39. https:// researchnovelty.com/articles.php?journal_id=5.

Fymat AL (2023e). "Tourette's syndrome: IV. Research and latest updates", *Journal of Neurology and Psychology Research* **5**(1):1-12. https:// researchnovelty.com/articles.php?journal_id=5.

> ➤ **Why the infant brain remembers:**

Akers KG *et al.* (2014). "Hippocampal neurogenesis regulates forgetting during adulthood and infancy". *Science* 344:598– 602.

Alberini CM and Travaglia A (2017). "Infantile amnesia: A critical period of learning to learn and remember". *J Neurosci.* **37:**5783– 95.

Squire LR and Dede AJO (2015). "Conscious and unconscious memory systems". *Cold Spring Harb Perspect Biol* **7**, a021667.

Vhringer IA *et al.* (2017). "The development of implicit memory from infancy to childhood: On average performance levels and interindividual differences". *Child Dev.* **89:**370-82.

> ➤ **Memory and time**:

Bejan A (2019). "Why The Days Seem Shorter As We Get Older". Cambridge University Press.

Lazarus AA (1978). "In the Mind's Eye". New York: Rawson.

> ➤ **Memory and the aging brain:**

Abrams L and Farrell MT (2012). "Language processing in normal aging". *Running Head: Language in Aging.*

Arnáiz E and Almkvist O (2003). "Neuropsychological features of mild cognitive impairment and preclinical Alzheimer's disease". *Acta Neurologica Scandinavica* Supplementum **179:**34–41. doi:10.1034/j.1600-0404.107. s179.7.x.

Baddeley AD, Anderson MC, and Eysenck MW (2015). "Memory". East Sussex: Psychology Press.

Bender AR, Naveh-Benjamin M, and Raz N 2010). "Associative deficit in recognition memory in a lifespan sample of healthy adults". *Psychology and Aging* **25**(4):940–8. doi:10.1037/a0020595.

Budson AE and Price BH (2005). "Memory dysfunction". The New England Journal of Medicine **352** (7):692–9. doi:10.1056/NEJMra041071.

Budson AE and Price BH (2005). "Memory dysfunction in clinical practice". *Discovery Medicine* **5** (26):135–41.

Cabeza R (2002). "Hemispheric asymmetry reduction in older adults: the HAROLD model". *Psychology and Aging* **17**(1):85–100. doi:10.1037/0882-7974.17.1.85.

Craik FI, Luo L, and Sakuta Y (2010). "Effects of aging and divided attention on memory for items and their contexts". *Psychology and Aging* **25**(4):968–79. doi:10.1037/a0020276.

Family Caregiver Alliance (2020). "Caring for adults with cognitive and memory impairment". www.caregiver.org.

Fleischman DA, Wilson RS, Gabrieli JD, Bienias JL, and Bennett DA (2004). "A longitudinal study of implicit and explicit memory in old persons". *Psychology and Aging* **19**(4):617–25. doi:10.1037/0882-7974.19.4.617.

Hedden T and Gabrieli JD (2004). "Insights into the aging mind: a view from cognitive neuroscience". *Nature Reviews, Neuroscience* **5**(2):87–96. doi:10.1038/nrn1323.

Glisky EL (2007). "Changes in Cognitive Function in Human Aging", in Riddle DR (ed.) "Brain aging: Models, methods, and mechanisms", *Frontiers in Neuroscience,* CRC Press/Taylor & Francis, ISBN 9780849338182

Hanna-Pladdy B and MacKay A (2011). "The relation between instrumental musical activity and cognitive aging". *Neuropsychology* **25**(3):378–86. doi:10.1037/a0021895.

Harvard Medical School (2011). "Improving memory and treating memory loss".

Henry JD, MacLeod MS, Phillips LH, and Crawford JR (2004). "A meta-analytic review of prospective memory and aging". *Psychology and Aging* **19**(1):27–39. doi:10.1037/0882-7974.19.1.27.

Howard MW, Youker TE, and Venkatadass VS (2008). "The persistence of memory: Contiguity effects across hundreds of seconds". *Psychonomic Bulletin & Review* **15**(1):58–63. doi:10.3758/PBR.15.1.58.

Isaacowitz DM, Wadlinger HA, Goren D, and Wilson HR (2006). "Selective preference in visual f fixation away from negative images in old age? An eye-tracking study". *Psychology and Aging* **21**(1): 40–8. doi:10.1037/0882-7974.21.1.40.

Jak AJ, Bangen KJ, Wierenga CE, Delano-Wood L, Corey-Bloom J, and Bondi MW (2009). "Contributions of neuropsychology and neuroimaging to understanding clinical subtypes of mild cognitive impairment".

International Review of Neurobiology **84:**81–103. doi:10.1016/S0074-7742(09)00405-X. ISBN 9780123748331.

Johnson MK, Hashtroudi S, and Lindsay DS (1993). "Source monitoring". *Psychological Bulletin* **114** (1):3–28. doi:10.1037/0033-2909.114.1.3.

Johnson MK, Reeder JA, Raye CL, and Mitchell KJ (2002). "Second thoughts versus second looks: An age-related deficit in reflectively refreshing just-activated information". *Psychological Science* **13**(1): 64–7. doi:10.1111/1467-9280.00411.

Kahana M (2002). "Age dissociates recency and lag recency effects in free recall". *Journal of Experimental Psychology. American Psychological Association* **28**(3):530–40. doi:10.1037/0278-7393.28.3.530.

Kuhlmann B (2011). "Older adults' use of metacognitive knowledge in source monitoring: Spared monitoring but impaired control". *Psychology and Aging. American Psychological Association.* **26**(1): 143–9. doi:10.1037/a0021055.

Levitt T, Fugelsang J, and Crossley M (2006). "Processing speed, attentional capacity, and age-related memory change". *Experimental Aging Research* **32**(3):263–95. doi:10.1080/03610730600699118.

Li KZ, Blair M, and Chow VS (2010). "Sequential performance in young and older adults: Evidence of chunking and inhibition". *Neuropsychology, Development, and Cognition. Section B, Aging, Neuropsychology and Cognition* **17**(3):270–95. doi:10.1080/13825580903165428.

Light LL (2000). "Memory changes in adulthood". In *Psychology and the aging revolution: How we adapt to longer life.*(pp. 73–97). Washington, DC: American Psychological Association.

LiveScience (2011). "Memory study explains 'senior moments', working memory & aging, and | multitasking abilities".

Lu T, Pan Y, Kao SY, Li C, Kohane I, Chan J, and Yankner BA (2004). "Gene regulation and DNA damage in the aging human brain". *Nature* **429**(6994):883-91. doi: 10.1038/nature02661.

Mather M and Carstensen LL (2005). "Aging and motivated cognition: The positivity effect in attention and memory" *Trends in Cognitive Sciences* **9**(10):496–502. doi:10.1016/j.tics.2005.08.005.

Maylor EA (1995). "Prospective memory in normal ageing and dementia". MRC CBU, Cambridge"

Mayo Clinic (2011). "Memory loss: 7 tips to improve your memory".

Mitchell KJ, Johnson MK, Raye CL, Mather M, and D'Esposito M (2000). "Aging and reflective processes of working memory: binding and test load deficits". *Psychology and Aging* **15**(3):527–41. doi:10.1037/0882-7974.15.3.527.

Morrone I, Declercq C, Novella JL, and Besche C (2010). "Aging and inhibition processes: The case of metaphor treatment". *Psychology and Aging* **25**(3):697–701. doi:10.1037/a0019578.

Mufson EJ, Binder L, Counts SE, DeKosky ST, de Toledo-Morrell L, Ginsberg SD *et al.* (2012). "Mild cognitive impairment: pathology and mechanisms". *Acta Neuropathologica* **123**(1):13– 30. doi:10.1007/s00401-011-0884-1.

Nairne JS (2000). "Forgetting". In *Encyclopedia of Psychology* **3:**386–9). Washington, DC; New York, NY: American Psychological Association. (U.S.) National Institute on Aging (2012). "Forgetfulness: Knowing when to ask for help". Nia.nih.gov.

(U.S.) National Institutes of Health. "Memory related resources".

Naveh-Benjamin M (2000). "Adult age differences in memory performance: Tests of an associative deficit hypothesis". *Journal of Experimental Psychology: Learning, Memory, and Cognition.* **26**(5): 1170–87. doi:10.1037/0278-7393.26.5.1170.

Neuroscience News (2020_. "Early-life education improves memory in old age, especially for women".

Light LL (1991). "Memory and aging: Four hypotheses in search of data". *Annual Review of Psychology* **42:**333–76. doi:10.1146/annurev. ps.42.020191.002001.

Nilsson LG (2003). "Memory function in normal aging". *Acta Neurologica Scandinavica. Supplementum* **179:**7–13. doi:10.1034/j.1600-0404.107. s179.5.x.

Portet F, Ousset PJ, Visser PJ, Frisoni GB, Nobili F, Scheltens P *et al.* (2006). "Mild cognitive impairment (MCI) in medical practice: A critical review of the concept and new diagnostic procedure:. Report of the MCI Working Group of the European Consortium on Alzheimer's Disease". *Journal of Neurology, Neurosurgery, and Psychiatry* **77**(6):714–8. doi:10.1136/ jnnp.2005.085332.

Provyn J (2011). "Effects of age on contextually mediated associations in paired associate learning". *Psychology and Aging. American Psychological Association.*

Rasmussen M and Laumann K (2013). "The academic and psychological benefits of exercise in healthy children and adolescents". *European Journal of Psychology of Education* **28**(3):945-62. http://www.jstor.org/stable/23581530

Ritchel M (2011). "Multitasking takes toll on memory, study finds". *New York Times.*

Abrams L and Farrell MT. "Language compensation and production in normal aging". *Handbook of Psychology and Aging* **6**:1–16.

Shanbhag NM, Evans MD, Mao W, Nana AL, Seeley WW, Adame A, Rissman RA, Masliah E, and Mucke L (2019). "Early neuronal accumulation of DNA double strand breaks in Alzheimer's disease". *Acta Neuropathol Commun.* **7**(1):77. doi: 10.1186/s40478-019-0723-5.

Suprenant A, Bireta T, and Farley L (2014). "A brief history of memory and aging." In Nairne JS (ed.). *The Foundations of Remembering.* pp. 108–20. ISBN 978-1-138-00621-8.

Swaab D. (2014). "We are our brains : A neurobiography of the brain", From the *Womb to Alzheimer's* (Vol. First edition). New York: Spiegel & Grau.

University of California in San Francisco (UCSF), Memory and Aging Center (2012). "Practical tips for daily life". Memory.ucsf.edu.

Verhaeghen P (2003). "Aging and vocabulary scores: A meta-analysis". *Psychology and Aging* **18**(2): 332–9. doi:10.1037/0882-7974.18.2.332.

Verhaeghen P and Cerella J (2002). "Aging, executive control, and attention: A review of meta- analyses". *Neuroscience and Biobehavioral Reviews* **26**(7):849–57. doi:10.1016/s0149- 7634(02)00071-4.

Vierck E. "Memory and aging" American Psychological Association (APA), Office on Aging and Committee on Aging.

Vilenchik MM and Knudson AG (2003). "Endogenous DNA double-strand breaks: Production, fidelity of repair, and induction of cancer". *Proc U.S. Natl Acad Sci* **100**(22):12871-6.

doi:10.1073/pnas.2135498100.

West RL (1996). "An application of prefrontal cortex function theory to cognitive aging". *Psychological Bulletin* **120**(2):272–92. doi:10.1037/0033-2909.120.2.272.

➢ **Autobiographical memory:**

Cahill L and McGaugh JL (1995). "A novel demonstration of enhanced memory associated with emotional arousal". *Consciousness and Cognition* **4:**410–21.

LePort AK, Mattfeld AT, Dickinson-Anson H, Fallon JH, Stark CEL, Kruggel F, Cahill L, and McGaugh JL (2012). "Behavioral and neuroanatomical investigation of Highly Superior Autobiographical Memory (HSAM)". *Neurobiology of Learning & Memory* **98:**78-92.

Parker ES, Cahill L, and McGaugh JL (2006). "A case of unusual autobiographical remembering". *Neurocase* **12**(1):35–49.

➢ **Musical memory:**

Davidow JY, Foerde K, Galván A, and Shohamy D (2016). "An upside to reward sensitivity: The hippocampus supports enhanced reinforcement learning in adolescence". *Neuron.* **92**(1):93-9.

Fuhrmann D, Knoll LJ, and Blakemore SJ (2015). "Adolescence as a sensitive period of brain development". *Trends in Cognitive Sciences* **19**(10):558-66.

Jakubowski K, Eerola T, Tillmann B, Perrin F, and Heine L (2020). "A cross-sectional study of reminiscence bumps for music-related memories in adulthood". *Music & Science* **3:** 2059204320965058.

➢ **Memory loss:**

(U.S.) National Institute on Aging (2022). "Understanding memory loss: What to do when you have trouble remembering".
https://www.nia.nih.gov/site- search/dW5kZXJzdGFuZGluZyBtZW1 vcnkgbG9zcw%3D%3D s.

➢ **Memory improvement:**

Manning JR and Kahana MJ (2012). "Interpreting semantic clustering effects in free recall". *Memory* **20**(5):511-7. doi:10.1080/09658211.2012.6830 10.

> **Cognitive testing:**

Alzheimer's Association (2022). ""Mild Cognitive Impairment (MCI)". https://www.alz.org/alzheimers- dementia/ what-is-dementia/ related_conditions/mild-cognitive-impairment
(U.S.) Centers for Disease Control and Prevention, U.S. Department of Health and Human Services (2011). "Cognitive Impairment: A call for action". https://www.cdc.gov/aging/pdf/ cognitive_ impairment/ cogimp_poilicy_final.

(U.S.) Centers for Disease Control and Prevention, U.S. Department of Health and Human Services (2020). "Healthy Brain Initiative". https:// www.cdc.gov/aging/healthybrain/index.htm

Cleveland Clinic, Cleveland (OH): Health Library: Diagnostics & Testing (2022). "Mild cognitive impairment". https://my.clevelandclinic.org/ health/articles/22306-cognitive-test

Cleveland Clinic, Cleveland (OH): Health Library: Diagnostics & Testing (2022). "Cognitive Test". https://my.clevelandclinic.org/health/ diseases/17990-mild-cognitive-impairment

Dhakal A and Bobrin BD (2020). "Cognitive Deficits". StatPearls Publishing. https://www.ncbi.nlm.nih.gov/books/NBK559052/

Mayo Clinic. Mayo Foundation for Medical Education and Research (1998-2022). Mild cognitive impairment (MCI): Diagnosis and treatment". https:// www.mayoclinic.org/diseases- conditions/mild-cognitive-impairment/ diagnosis-treatment/drc-20354583

Mayo Clinic. Mayo Foundation for Medical Education and Research (1998-2022). Mild cognitive impairment (MCI): Symptoms and causes". https:// www.mayoclinic.org/diseases- conditions/mild-cognitive-impairment/ symptoms-causes/syc-20354578

Merck Manual Consumer Version, Merck & Co. Inc. (2022). "Neurological examination". https://www.merckmanuals.com/home/brain,-spinal-cord,-and-nerve-disorders/diagnosis-of- brain,-spinal-cord,-and-nerve-disorders/neurologic-examination

Merck Manual Professional Version, Merck & Co. Inc. (2022). "How to assess mental status". https://www.merckmanuals.com/professional/neurologic-disorders/neurologic- examination/how-to-assess-mental-status

Michigan Medicine: University of Michigan, Ann Arbor (MI): Regents of the University of Michigan; (1995-2022}. "Mild Cognitive Impairment. https://www.uofmhealth.org/conditions- treatments/brain-neurological-conditions/mild-cognitive-impairment

(U.S.) National Institute on Aging (NIA), U.S. Department of Health and Human Services (2022). "Assessing cognitive impairment in older patients". https://www.nia.nih.gov/health/assessing- cognitive-impairment-older-patients

(U.S.) National Institute on Aging (NIA), U.S. Department of Health and Human Services (2021). "What Is mild cognitive impairment?". https://www.nia.nih.gov/health/what-mild-cognitive-impairment

Norris DR, Clark MS, and Shipley S (2016). "The mental status examination". *Am Fam Physician* https://www.aafp.org/afp/2016/1015/p635.html.

(U.S.) Preventive Services Task Force (2022). "Screening for cognitive impairment in older adults". https://www.uspreventiveservicestaskforce.org/Home/GetFile/1/482/dementes/pdf.

Xueyan L, Jie D, Shasha Z, Wangen L, and Haimei L (2018). "Comparison of the value of Mini-Cog and MMSE screening in the rapid identification of Chinese outpatients with mild cognitive impairment" https://journals.lww.com/mdjournal/Fulltext/2018/06010/Comparison_of_the_value_of_ Mini_Cog_and_MMSE.74.aspx

> **Cognitive recovery after a stroke:**

Maeshima S and Osawa A (2021). "Memory impairment due to stroke." *Exon Publications* 111–9.

O'Sullivan MJ *et al.* (2023). "Cognitive recovery after stroke: Memory." *Stroke* **54**(1):44–54.

Schouten EA *et al.* (2009). "Long-term deficits in episodic memory after ischemic stroke: Evaluation and prediction of verbal and visual memory performance based on lesion characteristics." *Journal of Stroke and Cerebrovascular Diseases* 18(2):128–38.

On treatment

> ### Diet and nutrition role in aging:

Di Giosia P, Stamerra CA, Giorgini P, Jamialahamdi T, Butler AE, and Sahebkar A (2022). "The role of nutrition in inflammaging". *Ageing Research Reviews* **77**:101596. doi:10.1016/j.arr.2022.101596.

Dyall SC (2015). "Long-chain omega-3 fatty acids and the brain: A review of the independent and shared effects of EPA, DPA and DHA". *Frontiers in Aging Neuroscience* **7**:52. doi:10.3389/fnagi.2015.00052.

Gardener SL, Rainey-Smith SR, Weinborn M, Bondonno CP, and Martins RN (2021). "Intake of products containing anthocyanins, flavanols, flavanones, and cognitive function: A narrative review". *Frontiers in Aging Neuroscience* **13**:640381. doi:10.3389/fnagi.2021.640381.

Heckner MK, Cieslik EC, Eickhoff SB, Camilleri JA, Hoffstaedter F, and Holland TM, Agarwal P, Wang Y, Dhana K, Leurgans SE, Shea K, Booth SL, Rajan K, Schneider JA, and Barnes LL (2022). "Association of dietary intake of flavonols with changes in global cognition and several cognitive abilities". *Neurology* **100**(7): e694–e702. doi:10.1212/WNL.0000000000201541.

Hutchinson AN, Tingö L, and Brummer RJ (2020). "The potential effects of probiotics and ω-3 fatty acids on chronic low-grade inflammation". *Nutrients* **12**(8):2402.doi:10.3390/nu12082402.

Kent K, Charlton KE, Netzel M, and Fanning K (2017). "Food-based anthocyanin intake and cognitive outcomes in human intervention trials: A systematic review". *Journal of Human Nutrition and Dietetics* **30**(3):260–74. doi:10.1111/jhn.12431.

Lee J, Venna VR, Durgan DJ, Shi H, Hudobenko J, Putluri N, Petrosino J, McCullough LD, and Bryan RM (2020). "Young versus aged microbiota transplants to germ-free mice: Increased short- chain fatty acids and improved cognitive performance". *Gut Microbes* **12**(1):1814107. doi:10.1080/19490976.2020.1814107.

Moore K, Hughes CF, Ward M, Hoey Leane, and McNulty Helene (2018). "Diet, nutrition and the aging brain: Current evidence and new directions".

Proceedings of the Nutrition Society **77**(2):152–63. doi:10.1017/S0029665117004177.

> ➢ **Creatine and creatine supplementation as a treatment:**

Antonio J (2021). "Common questions and misconceptions about creatine supplementation: What does the scientific evidence really show?". Journal of the International Society of Sports Nutrition **18** *(1):13. doi:10.1186/ s12970-021-00412-w.*

Antonio J, Candow DG, Forbes SC, Gualano B, Jagim AR, Kreider RB, Rawson ES, Smith-Ryan AE, Vandusseldorp TA, Willoughby DS, and Ziegenfuss TN (2021). "Common questions and misconceptions about creatine supplementation: What does the scientific evidence really show?". Journal of the International Society of Sports Nutrition **18**(13):13. doi:10.1186/ s12970- 021-00412-w.*

Avgerinos KI, Spyrou N, Bougioukas KI, and Kapogiannis D (2018). "Effects of creatine supplementation on cognitive function of healthy individuals: A systematic review of randomized controlled trials". Experimental Gerontology **108**:166–73. doi:10.1016/j.exger.2018.04.013.*

Balsom PD, Söderlund K, and Ekblom B (1994). "Creatine in humans with special reference to creatine supplementation". Sports Medicine **18**(4):268–80. doi:10.2165/00007256-199418040-00005.*

Barcelos RP, Stefanello ST, Mauriz JL, Gonzalez-Gallego J, and Soares FA (2016). "Creatine and the liver: Metabolism and possible interactions". Mini Reviews in Medicinal Chemistry **16** *(1): 12– 8.* doi:10.2174/1389557 515666150722102613. *(The process of creatine synthesis occurs in two steps, catalyzed by L-arginine:glycine amidinotransferase (AGAT) and guanidinoacetate N- methyltransferase (GAMT), which take place mainly in kidney and liver, respectively. This molecule plays an important energy/pH buffer function in tissues, and to guarantee the maintenance of its total body pool, the lost creatine must be replaced from diet or* de novo *synthesis.)*

Bender A, Auer DP, Merl T, Reilmann R, Saemann P, Yassouridis A, et al. (2005). "Creatine supplementation lowers brain glutamate levels in Huntington's disease". Journal of Neurology **252**(1): 36–41. doi:10.1007/ s00415-005-0595-4.*

Bender A and Klopstock T (August 2016). "Creatine for neuroprotection in neurodegenerative disease: end of story?". Amino Acids *48*(8):1929–40. doi:10.1007/s00726-015-2165-0.

Benton D and Donohoe R (2011). "The influence of creatine supplementation on the cognitive functioning of vegetarians and omnivores". The British Journal of Nutrition *105*(7):1100–5. doi:10.1017/S0007114510004733.

Braissant O, Henry H, Béard E, and Uldry J (2011). "Creatine deficiency syndromes and the importance of creatine synthesis in the brain". Amino Acids *40*(5):1315–24. doi:10.1007/s00726-011-0852-z.

Brosnan JT, da Silva RP, Brosnan ME (2011). "The metabolic burden of creatine synthesis". Amino Acids *40*(5):1325–31. doi:10.1007/s00726-011-0853-y.

Brosnan ME and Brosnan JT (2016). "The role of dietary creatine". Amino Acids *48*(8):1785–91. doi:10.1007/s00726-016-2188-1. *(*The daily requirement of a 70-kg male for creatine is about 2 g; up to half of this may be obtained from a typical omnivorous diet, with the remainder being synthesized in the body... More than 90% of the body's creatine and phosphocreatine is present in muscle (Brosnan and Brosnan, 2007), with some of the remainder being found in the brain (Braissant *et al.* 2011).... Creatine synthesized in liver must be secreted into the bloodstream by an unknown mechanism (Da Silva *et al.* 2014a)

Cannan RK and Shore A (1928). "The creatine-creatinine equilibrium. The apparent dissociation constants of creatine and creatinine". The Biochemical Journal *22*(4):920–9. doi:10.1042/bj0220920.

Chilibeck PD, Kaviani M, Candow DG, and Zello GA (2017). "Effect of creatine supplementation during resistance training on lean tissue mass and muscular strength in older adults: A meta- analysis". Open Access J Sports Med *8*:213-26. doi: 10.2147/OAJSM.S123529.

Cooper R, Naclerio F, Allgrove J, and Jimenez A (2012). "Creatine supplementation with specific view to exercise/sports performance: an update". Journal of the International Society of Sports Nutrition *9* (1):33. doi:10.1186/1550-2783-9-33. *(*Creatine is produced endogenously at an amount of about 1 g/d. Synthesis predominately occurs in the liver, kidneys, and to a lesser extent in the pancreas. The remainder of the creatine available to the body is obtained through the diet at about 1 g/d for an omnivorous diet. 95% of the bodies creatine stores are found in the skeletal muscle and the remaining 5% is distributed in the brain, liver, kidney, and testes.)

Dechent P, Pouwels PJ, Wilken B, Hanefeld F, and Frahm J (1999). "Increase of total creatine in human brain after oral supplementation of creatine-monohydrate". *Am J Physiol.* **277**(3):R698- 704. doi: 10.1152/ajpregu.1999.277.3.

Dolan E, Gualano B, and Rawson ES (2019). "Beyond muscle: the effects of creatine supplementation on brain creatine, cognitive processing, and traumatic brain injury". European Journal of Sport Science ***19**(1):1–14. doi:10.1080/17461391.2018.1500644. ISSN 1746-1391. PMID 30086660.*

Folin O and Denis W (1912)"Protein metabolism from the standpoint of blood and tissue analysis".. Journal of Biological Chemistry ***12**(1):141–61.* doi:10.1016/S0021-9258(18)88723-3.

Forbes SC, Cordingley DM, Cornish SM, Gualano B, Roschel H, Ostojic SM, Rawson ES, Roy BD, Prokopidis K, Giannos P, and Candow DG (2022). "Effects of creatine supplementation on brain function and health". *Nutrients* **14**(5):921. doi: 10.3390/nu14050921.

Graham AS and Hatton RC (1999). "Creatine: a review of efficacy and safety". Journal of the American Pharmaceutical Association ***39**(6):803–10, quiz 875–7. doi:10.1016/s1086- 5802(15)30371-5.*

Green AL, Hultman E, Macdonald IA, Sewell DA, and Greenhaff PL (1996). "Carbohydrate ingestion augments skeletal muscle creatine accumulation during creatine supplementation in humans". The American Journal of Physiology ***271**(5 Pt 1):E821-6.* doi:10.1152/ajpendo.1996.271.5.E821.

Hanna-El-Daher L and Braissant O (2016). "Creatine synthesis and exchanges between brain cells: What can be learned from human creatine deficiencies and various experimental models?". Amino Acids ***48**(8):1877–95.* doi:10.1007/s00726-016-2189-0.

Hersch SM, Schifitto G, Oakes D, Bredlau AL, Meyers CM, Nahin R, and Rosas HD (2017). "The CREST-E study of creatine for Huntington disease: A randomized controlled trial". Neurology ***89**(6): 594–601. doi:10.1212/WNL.0000000000004209.*

Jäger R, Harris RC, Purpura M, and Francaux M (2007). "Comparison of new forms of creatine in raising plasma creatine levels". Journal of the International Society of Sports Nutrition ***4**:17.* doi:10.1186/1550-2783-4-17.

Kious BM, Kondo DG, and Renshaw PF (2019). "Creatine for the treatment of depression". Biomolecules **9**(9):406. doi: 10.3390/biom9090406.

Kreider RB, Kalman DS, Antonio J, Ziegenfuss TN, Wildman R, Collins R et al. (2017). "International Society of Sports Nutrition position stand: safety and efficacy of creatine supplementation in exercise, sport, and medicine". Journal of the International Society of Sports Nutrition ***14****:18. doi:10.1186/s12970-017-0173-z.*

Passwater RA (2005). Creatine. *McGraw Hill Professional. p. 9. I* SBN 978-0-87983-868-3.

Pastula DM, Moore DH, and Bedlack RS (2012). "Creatine for amyotrophic lateral sclerosis/motor neuron disease". The Cochrane Database of Systematic Reviews ***12****:CD005225. doi:10.1002/14651858.CD005225. pub3.*

Persky AM and Brazeau GA (2001). "Clinical pharmacology of the dietary supplement creatine monohydrate". Pharmacological Reviews ***53****(2):161–76.*

Prokopidis K, Giannos P, Triantafyllidis K, Konstantinos K, Kechagias KS, Forbes SC, Candow DG (2023). "Effects of creatine supplementation on memory in healthy individuals: A systematic review and meta-analysis of randomized controlled trials". *Nutrition Reviews **81**(4):416–27.* doi:10.1093/nutrit/nuac064.

Prokopidis K, Giannos P, Triantafyllidis K, Konstantinos K, Kechagias KS, Forbes SC, a d Candow DG (2023)."Author's reply: Letter to the Editor: Double counting due to inadequate statistics leads to false-positive findings in "Effects of creatine supplementation on memory in healthy individuals: A systematic review and meta-analysis of randomized controlled trials". Nutrition Reviews doi:10.1093/nutrit/nuac111.

Rawson ES and Venezia AC(2011). "Use of creatine in the elderly and evidence for effects on cognitive function in young and old". Amino Acids ***40****(5):1349–62. doi:10.1007/s00726-011- 0855-9. ISSN 0939-4451.*

Solis MY, Artioli GG, Otaduy MCG, Leite C da C, Arruda W, Veiga RR et al. (2017). "Effect of age, diet, and tissue type on PCr response to creatine supplementation". Journal of Applied Physiology *(Bethesda, Md : 1985) 2017;123:407–14.* https://doi.org/10.1152/JAPPLPHYSIOL.00248.2017/

Stoppani J (2004). "Creatine new and improved: Recent high-tech advances have made creatine even more powerful. Here's how you can take full advantage of this super supplement". Muscle & Fitness.

Stout JR, Antonio J, Kalman E, eds. (2008). "Essentials of Creatine in Sports and Health". Humana. ISBN 978-1-59745-573-2.

Verbessem P, Lemiere J, Eijnde BO, Swinnen S, Vanhees L, Van Leemputte M et al. (2003). "Creatine supplementation in Huntington's disease: A placebo-controlled pilot trial". Neurology **61**(7): 925–30. doi:10.1212/01. wnl.0000090629.40891.4b.

Volek JS, Ballard KD, and Forsythe CE (2008). "Overview of Creatine Metabolism". In Stout JR, Antonio J, Kalman E (eds.). Essentials of Creatine in Sports and Health. Humana. pp. 1–23. ISBN 978-1-59745-573-2.

Wallimann T (2007). "Introduction – Creatine: Cheap ergogenic supplement with great potential for health and disease". In Salomons GS, Wyss M (eds.). Creatine and Creatine Kinase in Health and Disease. Springer. pp. 1 –16. I SBN 978-1-4020-6486-9.

Xiao Y, Luo M, Luo H, and Wang J (2014). "Creatine for Parkinson's disease". The Cochrane Database of Systematic Reviews **2014** (6):CD009646. doi:10.1002/14651858.cd009646.pub2.

Yazigi SM, de Salles Painelli V, Artioli GG, Roschel H, Otaduy MC, and Gualano B. (2022). "Brain creatine depletion in vegetarians? A cross-sectional 1H-magnetic resonance spectroscopy (1H- MRS) study". The British Journal of Nutrition 2014;111:1272–4. https://doi.org/10.1017/S0007114513003802

> **Medication Appropriateness Tool for Comorbid Health conditions during Dementia (MATCH-D):**

Alexopoulos GS, Streim J, Carpenter D, and Docherty JP (2004). "Using antipsychotic agents in older patients". Expert Consensus Panel for Using Antipsychotic Drugs in Older Patients. *J Clin Psychiatry.* 2004;65 Suppl 2:5-99; discussion 100-102; quiz 103-4.

American Geriatrics Society (2015). "Beers Criteria Update Expert Panel" (updated beers criteria for potentially inappropriate medication use in older adults). *J Am Geriatr Soc* **63**:2227–46.

Barry PJ, Gallagher P, Ryan C, and O'Mahony D (2007). "START (screening tool to alert doctors to the right treatment): An evidence-based screening tool to detect prescribing omissions in elderly patients". *Age Ageing* **36:**632–8.

Beers MH (1997). "Explicit criteria for determining potentially inappropriate medication use by the elderly an update". *Arch Intern Med* **157:**1531–6.

Bell JS, LeCouteur DG, McLachlan AJ, Chen TF, Moles RJ, Basger BJ *et al.* (2012). "Improving medicine selection for older people: Do we need an Australian classification for inappropriate medicines use?" *Aust Fam Physician* **41:**49.

Drewes YM, den Elzen WPJ, Mooijaart SP, de Craen AJ, Assendelft WJ, and Gussekloo J (2011). "The effect of cognitive impairment on the predictive value of multimorbidity for the increase in disability in the oldest old: the Leiden 85-plus study". *Age Ageing* **40:** 352–7.

Farrall AJ and Wardlaw JM (2009). "Blood-brain barrier: Ageing and microvascular disease- systematic review and meta-analysis". *Neurobiol Aging* **30:**337–52.

Formiga F, Fort I, Robles MJ, Riu S, Sabartes O, Barranco E *et al.* (2009). "Comorbidity and clinical features in elderly patients with dementia: Differences according to dementia severity". *J Nutr Health Aging* **13:**423–7.

Gallagher P and O'Mahony D (2008). "STOPP (Screening Tool of Older Persons' potentially inappropriate prescriptions): application to acutely ill elderly patients and comparison with Beers' criteria". *Age Ageing* **37:**673–9.

Giron MST, Wang HX, Bernsten C, Thorslund M, Winblad B, and Fastbom J (2001). "The appropriateness of drug use in an older nondemented and demented population". *J Am Geriatr Soc* **49:** 277–83.

Hilmer SN, McLachlan AJ, and LeCouteur DG (2007). "Clinical pharmacology in the geriatric patient". *Fundam Clin Pharmacol* **21:**217–30.

Hilmer SN (2008). "ADME-tox issues for the elderly". *Expert Opin Drug Metab Toxicol* **4:**1321–31.

Holmes HM, Hayley DC, Alexander GC, and Sachs GA (2006). "Reconsidering medication appropriateness for patients late in life". *Arch Intern Med* **166:**605–9.

Holmes HM, Min LC, Yee M, Varadhan R, Basran J, Dale W *et al.* (2013). "Rationalizing prescribing for older patients with multimorbidity: considering time to benefit". *Drugs Aging* **30:**655–6.

Holt S, Schmiedl S, and Thürmann PA (2010). "Potentially inappropriate medications in the elderly: the PRISCUS list". *Dtsch Ärztebl Int* **107:**543–11.

Laroche ML, Charmes JP, Merle L. Potentially inappropriate medications in the elderly: A French consensus panel list". *Eur J Clin Pharmacol* **63:**725–31.

Lindblad CI, Hanlon JT, Gross CR, Sloane RJ, Pieper CF, Hajjar ER *et al.(2006).* "Clinically important drug-disease interactions and their prevalence in older adults". *Clin Ther* **28:**1133– 43.

Marriott J and Stehlik P (2012). "A critical analysis of the methods used to develop explicit clinical criteria for use in older people". *Age Ageing* **41:**441–50.

McLean AJ and LeCouteur DG (200). "Aging biology and geriatric clinical pharmacology". *Pharmacol Rev* **56:**163–84.

O'Mahoney D, O'Sullivan D, Byrne S, O'Connor MN, Ryan C, and Gallagher P (2015). "STOPP/ START criteria for potentially inappropriate prescribing in older people: Version 2". *Age Ageing* **44:**213–18.

Page AT, Etherton-Beer CD, Clifford RM, Burrows S, Eames M, and Potter K (2015). "Deprescribing in frail older people: Do doctors and pharmacists agree?" *Res Social Adm Pharm* **12:**438–49.

Roberts H, Greenwood N, and Lang (2019). "Speech and language therapy best practice for patients in prolonged disorders of consciousness: A modified Delphi study". *Commun Disord.* **54**(5):841- 54. doi: 10.1111/1460-6984.12489.

Saxby N, Ford K, Beggs S, Battersby M, and Lawn S (2020). "Developmentally appropriate supported self-management for children and young people with chronic conditions: A consensus". Patient Educ Couns. **103**(3):571-81. doi: 10.1016/j.pec.2019.09.029.

Scott IA, Hilmer SN, Reeve E, Potter K, LeCouteur D, Rigby D *et al.* (2015). "Reducing inappropriate polypharmacy: The process of deprescribing". JAMA Intern Med **175:**827–34.

Somers M, Rose E, Simmonds D, Whitelaw C, Calver J, and Beer C (2010). "Quality use of medicines in residential aged care". *Aust Fam Physician* **39:**413–16.

Tinetti ME, McAvay GJ, Fried TR, Allore HG, Salmon JC, Foody JM *et al.* (2008). "Health outcome priorities among competing cardiovascular, fall injury, and medication-related symptom outcomes". *J Am Geriatr Soc* **56:**1409–6.

Van Spall HGC, Toren A, Kiss A, and Fowler RA (2007). "Eligibility criteria of randomized controlled trials published in high-impact general medical journals: A systematic sampling review". *JAMA* **297:**1233–40.

> **Treatment: Other**

Fymat AL (2019). "Electromagnetic therapy for neurological and neurodegenerative diseases: I. Peripheral brain stimulations". *Open Access Journal of Neurology and Neurosurgery* **12**(2):30- 47. doi:10.19080/OAJNN.2019.12.555833.

Fymat AL (2020a). "Electromagnetic therapy for neurological and neurodegenerative diseases: II. Deep brain stimulation". *Open Access Journal of Neurology and Neurosurgery* **13**(1):1-17. doi: 19080/OAJNN.2020.13.555855.

Fymat AL (2020b). "Nanobiotechnology-based drugs for the treatment of neurological disorders", *Journal of Pharmaceutical Bioprocessing* **8**(3):1-3.

On prevention and risk factors

Larson EB (2022). "Risk factors for cognitive decline and dementia". https://www.uptodate.com/contents/search.

(U.S.) Department of Health and Human Services (DHHS) (2022). "Physical activity guidelines for Americans". https://health.gov/paguidelines/second-edition.

(U.S.) National Institute of Neurological Disorders and Stroke (2022). "Sleep apnea". https://www.ninds.nih.gov/health-information/disorders/sleep-apnea.

Watson NF *et al.* (2015). "Recommended amount of sleep for a healthy adult: A joint consensus statement of the American Academy of Sleep Medicine and Sleep Research Society". *Journal of Clinical Sleep Medicine.* doi.org/10.5664/jcsm.4758.

Memory and artificial intelligence

Jain V (2023). "How AI could lead to a better unerstanding of the brain", Nature 1(623):247-50.

va n de Ven GM and Tolias AS (2020). "The brain's memory abilities inspire AI experts in making neural networks less 'forgetful'", Science News, September 17, 2020.

van de Ven GM, Siegelmann HT, and Tolias AS (202o). "Brain-inspired replay for continual learning with artificial neural networks". *Nature Communications* 11**(1) doi: 10.1038/s41467- 029-17866-2.**

The European Human Brain Project

"An algorithm for large-scale brain simulations – News" (2020). www.humanbrainproject.eu.

Epstein R (2016). Weintraub P (ed.). "Your brain does not process information and it is not computer". Aeon Essays.

Frégnac Y and Laurent G (2014). "Neuroscience: Where is the brain in the Human Brain Project?". *Nature* **513**(7516):27–9. doi:10.1038/513027a.

Kreyer AC and Wang LX (2022). "Collaborating neuroscience online: The case of the Human Brain Project forum". PLOS ONE. **17**(12): e0278402. doi:10.1371/journal.pone.0278402.

Naddaf M (2023). "Europe spent €600 million to recreate the human brain in a computer. How did it go?". *Nature* 620(7975):718–20. doi:10.1038/d41586-023-02600-x.

"Overview - Human Brain Project" (2013). www.humanbrainproject.eu.

Theil S (2015). "Trouble in Mind". Scientific American **313**(4):36–42. doi:10.1038/scientificamerican1015-36.

Additional references

Fymat AL (2017a). "Nanoneurology: Drug Delivery Across the Brain Protective Barriers", *Journal of Nanomedicine Research* **5**(1):1-4, 00105. doi: 10:15406/jnmr/2017.05.00105.

Fymat AL (2017b). "Therapeutics delivery behind, through and beyond the blood-brain barrier", *Open Access Journal of Surgery* **5**(1):1-9; 555654. doi: 10.19080/OAJS.2017.05.555654.

Fymat AL (2018a). "Roles of nanomedicine in clinical neuroscience", *Global Journal of Nanomedicine* **4**(1):13-5. doi:10.19080/GJN.2018.04.555629.

Fymat AL (2018b). "Neutrophils-mediated treatment of neurodegenerative and other inflammatory diseases", *Journal of Clinical Research in Neurology* **1**(1):1-5.

Fymat AL (2018c). "Blood brain barrier permeability and neurological diseases", *J of Current Opinions on Neurological Science* **2**(2);411-4.

Fymat AL (2018d). "Regulating the brain's autoimmune system: The end of all neurological disorders?", *J of Current Opinions on Neurological Science* **2**(3):475-9.

Fymat AL (2018d). "Harnessing the immune system to treat cancers and neurodegenerative diseases", *J of Clinical Research in Neurology* **1**(1):1-14.

Fymat AL (2020). "Neuroradiology and its role in neurodegenerative diseases", *Journal of Radiology and Imaging Science* **1**(1):1-14. (Journal closed and transferred to: *Journal of Neuroradiology and Nanomedicine)* **5**(1):1-14.

Illustrations

Figures

Tables

Sidebars

Glossary

A

Acetylcholine: A chemical messenger that plays a vital role in memory and learning.

Advanced therapy medicinal products: Medicines for human use that are based on genes, tissues or cells.

Adrenoleukodystrophy (ALD) or **diffuse myelinoclastic sclerosis (DMS):** A disease linked to the X- chromosome. It is a result of fatty acid buildup caused by failure of peroxisomal fatty acid beta oxidation which results in the accumulation of very long chain fatty acids in tissues throughout the body.

Agnosia: Lack of perception.

Agrypnia: A complete lack of sleep.

Akathisia: A movement disorder characterized by a subjective feeling of inner restlessness accompanied by mental distress and an inability to sit still. A state of agitation, distress, and restlessness that is an occasional side-effect of antipsychotic and antidepressant drugs.

Alexander's disease (AD): A very rare autosomal dominant leukodystrophy, which is a neurological condition caused by anomalies in the myelin protecting nerve fibers in the brain. The most common type is the infantile form. Adult-onset forms of AD are less common than the juvenile ones. The symptoms sometimes mimic those of Parkinson's disease or multiple sclerosis, or may present primarily as a psychiatric disorder. AD is a progressive and often fatal disease.

Alzheimer's disease (AD): A neurodegenerative disease that causes a large number of nerve cells in the brain to die. These changes make it hard for a person to remember things, have clear thinking, and make good judgments. It usually starts slowly and progressively worsens. It is the cause of 60%–70% of cases of dementia. The most common early symptom is progressive memory loss and difficulty in remembering recent events. As the disease advances, symptoms can include problems with language, disorientation (including easily getting lost), mood swings, loss of motivation, self-neglect, and behavioral issues. Gradually, bodily functions are lost, ultimately leading to death. The cause of AD is poorly understood. The strongest genetic risk factor is from an allele of APOE. Other risk factors include a history of head injury, clinical depression, and high blood pressure. Initial symptoms are often mistaken for normal brain aging. Good nutrition, physical activity, and engaging socially are known to be of benefit generally in aging, and may help in reducing the risk of cognitive decline. No treatments can stop or reverse its progression, though some may temporarily improve symptoms.

Amaurosis *fugax*: A painless temporary loss of vision in one or both eyes that appears as a "black curtain coming down vertically into the field of vision", monocular blindness, dimming, fogging, or blurring. Duration depends on the cause of the vision loss.

Amnesia: A neurological disorder whose key defining characteristic is a temporary but almost total disruption of short-term memory with a range of problems accessing older memories. A person in a state of transient global amnesia (TGA) exhibits no other signs of impaired cognitive functioning but recalls only the last few moments of consciousness.

Anterograde: A disruption of **short-term memory.**

> **Childhood (or infantile):** The relative lack of memories from early childhood.

> **Transient global:** A neurological disorder whose key defining characteristic is a temporary but almost total disruption of **short-term memory** with a range of problems accessing **older memories.**

Amyloid-related imaging abnormality (ARIA): A temporary swelling in areas of the brain that usually resolves over time.

Amyotrophy: Muscle wasting.

Amyotrophic lateral sclerosis (ALS) also known as Lou Gehrig's disease**:** A rare neurodegenerative disease that results in the progressive loss of motor neurons that control voluntary muscles. It is the most common form of the motor neuron diseases. About 15% develop frontotemporal dementia.

Anastomotic: Conjoined.

Anomia: Speech and language difficulties. Difficulty finding the correct word(s).

Anosognosia: Lost insight of the disease process and its limitations.

Anticholinergics (anticholinergic agents): Substances (for example, *Atropine*) that block the action of the neurotransmitter called acetylcholine (ACh) at synapses in the central and peripheral nervous system. These agents inhibit the parasympathetic nervous system by selectively blocking the binding of ACh to its receptor in nerve cells. The nerve fibers of the parasympathetic system are responsible for the involuntary movement of smooth muscles present in the gastrointestinal tract, urinary tract, lungs, sweat glands, and many other parts of the body. In broad terms, anticholinergics are divided into two categories in accordance with their specific targets in the central and peripheral nervous system and at the neuromuscular junction: Antimuscarinic agents, and antinicotinic agents (ganglionic blockers, neuromuscular blockers). The term "anticholinergic" is typically used to refer to antimuscarinics which competitively inhibit the binding of ACh to muscarinic acetylcholine receptors. Such agents do not antagonize the binding at nicotinic acetylcholine receptors at the neuromuscular junction, although the term is sometimes used to refer to agents which do so.

Anthocyanins: **Polyphenols, a family of plant-based compounds that are increasingly associated with health benefits. They can also provide a brain boost, lower** blood pressure, **and contribute to better cardiovascular health.**

Aortic dissection: A tear in the aorta.

Aphasia: The inability to comprehend or formulate language because of damage to specific brain regions. It can be due to stroke, head trauma, epilepsy, brain tumors, brain damage and brain infections, or neurodegenerative diseases (such as dementias). In the case of progressive aphasia, the four aspects of communication (spoken language production and comprehension, and written language production and comprehension) must have significantly declined over a short period of time. Impairments in any of these aspects can impact on functional communication. Intelligence, however, is unaffected. Aphasia also affects visual language such as sign language. In contrast, the use of formulaic expressions in everyday communication is often preserved. One prevalent deficit in the aphasias is a difficulty in finding the correct word (anomia). Aphasia is related to the individual's language cognition.

Apraxia: Difficult execution of movements; difficulties in writing, drawing, dressing, coordination, and planning.

Associative effect: The access to the memory performance of an elder person, which is attributed to their difficulty in creating and retaining cohesive episodes.

Asterixis: "Flapping tremor" of the hand when the wrist is extended.

Ataxia telangectasia (AT) or **ataxia–telangiectasia syndrome (ATS)** or **Louis–Barre syndrome (LBS):** A rare, neurodegenerative, autosomal recessive disease causing severe disability. Ataxia refers to poor coordination and telangiectasia to small dilated blood vessels, both of which are hallmarks of the disease. It impairs certain areas of the brain including the cerebellum, causing difficulty with movement and coordination. It also weakens the immune system, causing a predisposition to infection. Further, it prevents repair of broken DNA, increasing the risk of cancer.

Atheroma: Arterial wall swelling.

Athetosis: A symptom characterized by slow, involuntary, convoluted, writhing movements of the fingers, hands, toes, and feet and in some cases, arms, legs, neck and tongue. It is often accompanied by the symptoms of cerebral palsy, as it is often a result of this physical disability.

Atrophy: Muscle wasting.

Attention: The cognitive ability that allows a person to deal with the inherent processing limitations of the human brain by selecting information for further processing.

Attentional resources limitation effect: The lesser capability of dividing attention between two tasks so that tasks with higher attentional demands are more difficult to complete due to a reduction in mental energy.

Autophagy: A form of intracellular phagocytosis in which a cell actively consumes damaged organelles or misfolded proteins by encapsulating them into an autophagosome, which fuses with a lysosome to destroy the contents of the autophagosome.

Autosomal dominant: The pattern of inheritance characteristic of some genetic disorders. Autosomal means that the gene in question is located on one of the numbered, or non-sex, chromosomes. Dominant means that a single copy of the mutated gene (from one parent) is enough to cause the disorder.

B

Balo concentric sclerosis (BCS) also formerly known as **leuko-encephalitis periaxialis concentrica:** A disease in which the white matter of the brain appears damaged in concentric layers, leaving the axis cylinder intact. It is a demyelinating disease similar to standard MS, but with the particularity that the demyelinated tissues form concentric layers.

Basal ganglia disease: A group of physical problems caused by the failure of the basal ganglia (nuclei) to properly suppress unwanted movements or to properly prime upper motor neuron circuits to initiate motor function. Hypokinetic disorders that can lead to the inability to suppress unwanted movements.

Behavioral flexibility: That flxibility to efficiently and appropriately adapt to different situations and changing environmental demands (including the speed of adaptation) and to the capacity to develop solutions to novel problems or novel solutions to old problems.

Biological aging: A complex process that involves molecular damage, metabolic imbalance, immune system changes, and increased susceptibility to environmental stressors and disease.

Blepharospasm: Any abnormal contraction of the orbicularis oculi muscle.

Brain herniation: A potentially deadly side effect of very high pressure within the skull that occurs when a part of the brain is squeezed across structures within the skull. The brain can shift across such structures as the falx cerebri, the tentorium cerebelli, and even through the foramen magnum (the hole in the base of the skull through which the spinal cord connects with the brain). Herniation can be caused by a number of factors that cause a mass effect and increase intracranial pressure (ICP), including traumatic brain injury (IBI), intracranial hemorrhage, or brain tumor.

Brain plasticity: The brain's ability to change structure and function.

Brain scan: A type of test a doctor may use to look for changes in the brain. While a person lies down, an instrument takes pictures to show normal and problem areas of the brain.

Breakthrough Device Designation: An FDA designation given to medical devices with preliminary evidence of clinical effectiveness compared to other available treatments.

C

CAMFAK or **CAMAK syndrome (ca**taracts, **m**icrocephaly, **fa**ilure to thrive, and **k**yphoscoliosis.) A rare inherited neurological disease, characterized by peripheral and central demyelination of nerves, similar to that seen in Cockayne's syndrome. The disease may occur with or without failure to thrive and arthrogryposis. Severe intellectual deficit and death within the first decade are typical.

Canavan's disease (CD) or **Canavan–Van Bogaert–Bertrand (CBD) disease:** A rare and fatal autosomal recessive degenerative disease that causes progressive damage to nerve cells and loss of white matter in the brain. It is one of the most common degenerative cerebral diseases of infancy. Symptoms of the most common (and most serious) form of CD typically appear in early infancy usually between the first three to six months of age. CD then progresses rapidly from that stage, with typical cases involving intellectual disability, loss of previously acquired motor skills, feeding difficulties, abnormal muscle tone (i.e., initial floppiness - hypotonia - that may eventually translate into spasticity), poor head control, and megalocephaly (abnormally enlarged head). Paralysis, blindness, or seizures may also occur.

Cataplexy: A sudden and transient episode of muscle weakness accompanied by full conscious awareness. It is, typically triggered by emotions such as laughing, crying, or terror. It is caused by an autoimmune destruction of hypothalamic neurons.

Catatonic: Being unable to move or respond to the outside world.

Cholinesterase: An enzyme that breaks down acetylcholine.

Chorea (or **choreia**, occasionally): An abnormal involuntary movement disorder, one of a group of neurological disorders called dyskinesias.

Hemichorea: Chorea of one side of the body, such as chorea of one arm but not both (analogous to hemiballismus).

Sydenham: Named after the English physician Thomas Sydenham (10 September 1624 – 29 December 1689). He was the discoverer of the disease, Sydenham's chorea (also known as St Vitus' Dance and rheumatic chorea), a disorder characterized by rapid, uncoordinated jerking movements primarily affecting the face, hands and feet. It is an autoimmune disease that results from childhood infection with Group A beta-hemolytic Streptococcus. It is reported to occur in 20–30% of people with acute rheumatic fever and is one of the major criteria for it, although it sometimes occurs in isolation. The disease occurs typically a few weeks, but up to 6 months, after the acute infection, which may have been a simple sore throat (pharyngitis). It is more common in females than males, and most cases affect children between 5 and 15 years of age. Adult onset of Sydenham's chorea is comparatively rare, and the majority of the adult cases are recurrences following childhood Sydenham's chorea.

Choreoathetosis: The occurrence of involuntary movements in a combination of chorea (irregular migrating contractions) and athetosis (twisting and writhing).

Choroid plexus papilloma (CPP): A rare benign neuroepithelial intraventricular lesion found in the choroid plexus. It leads to increased cerebrospinal fluid production, thus causing increased intracranial pressure and hydrocephalus.

Chunking: The combination of to-be-remembered pieces of information, such as numbers or letters, into a smaller number of units (or "chunks"), making them easier to remember.

Clinical trials: Prospective biomedical or biobehavioral research studies on human participants designed to answer specific questions about biomedical or biobehavioral interventions, including new treatments (such as novel vaccines, drugs, dietary choices, dietary supplements, and medical devices) and known interventions that warrant further study and comparison.

Cockayne's syndrome (CS) or **Neill-Dingwall syndrome (NDS):** A rare and fatal autosomal recessive neurodegenerative disorder characterized by growth failure, impaired development of the nervous system, abnormal sensitivity to sunlight (photosensitivity), eye disorders and premature aging. Problems with any or all of the internal organs are possible. It is associated with a group of disorders called leukodystrophies, which are conditions characterized by degradation of neurological white matter.

Cognitive reserve: The ability of an individual to demonstrate no cognitive signs of aging despite an aging brain.

Confabulations: Invented memories.

Conflating: Combining two or more sets of information, texts, ideas, etc. into one.

Congenital distal spinal muscular atrophy (DSMA): A hereditary condition characterized by muscle wasting (atrophy), particularly of distal muscles in legs and hands, and by early-onset contractures (permanent shortening of a muscle or joint) of the hip, knee, and ankle.

Contiguity effect: Stimuli that occur close together in the associated time.

Contracture: A permanent shortening of a muscle or joint.

Corticotrophin-releasing factor (CRF): A hormone associated with the production of stress and found in high levels in people experiencing various forms of anxiety. It exerts a protective effect on the brain, including the memory changes brought on by Alzheimer's.

Cramming: Studying in one long, continuous period.

Cytoplasmic cell death (also called **Type III**): Another way programmed cell death can also occur via non-apoptotic processes.

D

Declining memory effect: The memory decline during the aging process and the lesser capacity to hold information.

Deep brain stimulation (DBS): A surgical treatment which aims to reduce tics and seizures that could not be controlled with medication, and where surgery to treat their cause is not possible.

Degenerative condition: A condition that continues to get worse.

Dementia: The general name for a decline in cognitive functioning, meaning changes to a person's thinking, remembering, reasoning, and behavior that make daily life and activities difficult to manage.

It impacts a person's ability to do everyday activities. This typically involves memory impairment; disruption in thought patterns, thinking, and behavior; emotional problems; difficulties with language; and decreased motivation. The symptoms may be described as occurring in a continuum over several stages. A diagnosis of dementia requires the observation of a change from a person's usual mental functioning and a greater cognitive decline than what is caused by normal aging. Several diseases and injuries to the brain such as a stroke can give rise to dementia. However, the most common cause is Alzheimer's disease. Dementia is also described as a spectrum of disorders with causative subtypes based on a known disorder, such as Parkinson's disease for Parkinson's disease dementia (PDD), Huntington's disease for Huntington's disease dementia (HDD), vascular disease for vascular disease dementia (VDD), HIV infection causing HIV dementia (HIVD); frontotemporal lobar degeneration for frontotemporal dementia (FTLD); or Lewy body disease for dementia with Lewy bodies (DLB), and prion diseases. Subtypes of neurodegenerative dementias may also be based on the underlying pathology of misfolded proteins such as synucleinopathies, and tauopathies. More than one type of dementia existing together is known as mixed dementia (MD).

Diffuse myelinoclastic sclerosis or **Schilder's disease:** A very infrequent neurodegenerative disease that presents clinically as pseudotumoral demyelinating lesions, making its diagnosis difficult. It is considered one of the borderline forms of multiple sclerosis.

Distal hereditary motor neuropathies (dHMN): A genetically and clinically heterogeneous group of motor neuron diseases that result from genetic mutations in various genes and are characterized by degeneration and loss of motor neuron cells in the anterior horn of the spinal cord and subsequent muscle atrophy.

Dopamine: A neurotransmitter that plays a role in pleasure and learning. It might be involved in the activation of boundary and event cells. Dopamine and the brain's normal internal rhythm that affects learning and memory (the theta rhythm) could be the essential beat at which the boundary and event cells need to fire.

Dravet's syndrome (DS) or **severe myoclonic epilepsy of infancy (SMEI):** An autosomal dominant genetic disorder which causes a catastrophic form of epilepsy. It is characterized by prolonged febrile and non-febrile seizures within the first year of a child's life. It progresses to other seizure types like myoclonic and partial seizures, psychomotor delay, and ataxia. It is characterized by cognitive impairment, behavioral disorders, and motor deficits. It is also associated with sleep disorders including somnolence and insomnia.

Dysarthria: A speech sound disorder resulting from neurological injury of the motor component of the motor–speech system. A condition in which problems occur with the muscles that help produce speech, often making it very difficult to pronounce words. It is unrelated to problems with understanding language (that is, dysphasia or aphasia), although a person can have both. It leads to impairments in intelligibility, audibility, naturalness, and efficiency of vocal communication. Dysarthria that has progressed to a total loss of speech is referred to as anarthria.

Dyskinesia: Abnormal and involuntary muscle movements, including movements similar to tics or chorea and diminished voluntary movements.

Dysphagia: Difficulty swallowing.

Dystonia: A neurological hyperkinetic movement disorder in which sustained or repetitive muscle contractions result in twisting and repetitive movements or abnormal fixed postures. The movements may resemble a tremor. Dystonia is often intensified or exacerbated by physical activity, and symptoms may progress into adjacent muscles.

E

Elaborative rehearsal: One of the most effective known encoding technique.

Emgram cells: Neurons activated during acquisition of a memory and reactivated during memory recall in the part of the hippocampus called the dentate gyrus.

Encephalitis: Inflammation of the brain. The severity can be variable with symptoms including reduction or alteration in consciousness, headache, fever, confusion, a stiff neck, and vomiting. Complications may include seizures, hallucinations, trouble speaking, memory problems, and problems with hearing.

Encephalopathy: Any disorder or disease of the brain, especially chronic degenerative conditions. It does not refer to a single disease, but rather to a syndrome of overall brain dysfunction. The hallmark is an altered mental state or delirium. Characteristic of the altered mental state is impairment of the cognition, attention, orientation, sleep–wake cycle and consciousness.

- **Wernicke encephalopathy:** It can co-occur with Korsakoff alcoholic syndrome, characterized by amnestic-confabulatory syndrome: retrograde amnesia, anterograde amnesia, confabulations (invented memories), poor recall and disorientation.
- **Anti-NMDA receptor encephalitis:** The most common autoimmune encephalitis. It can cause paranoid and grandiose delusions, agitation, hallucinations (visual and auditory), bizarre behavior, fear, short-term memory loss, and confusion.
- **HIV encephalopathy:** It can lead to dementia.
- **Hashimoto's encephalopathy:** A neurological condition characterized by encephalopathy, thyroid autoimmunity, and good clinical response to corticosteroids. It is associated with Hashimoto's thyroiditis.

Engram: The transient or enduring change in our brain that results from encoding an experience.

Epigenetic clock: An epigenetic biomarker of tissue age.

Epilepsy: A group of non-communicable neurological disorders characterized by recurrent epileptic seizures, which are a clinical manifestation of an abnormal, excessive, purposeless, and synchronized electrical discharge in the brain cells called neurons.

Epileptic seizure: The clinical manifestation of an abnormal, excessive, purposeless, and synchronized electrical discharge in the brain cells called neurons.

Excitotoxic cell death: The cell death caused by glutamate receptors that can cause neurodegenerative conditions that affect memory.

Exophthalmos: Bulging eyes.

Exposure therapy: A technique often used to reduce or eliminate learned fear by repeatedly exposing people to a fear-provoking stimulus in the absence of a negative or aversive outcome.

F

Flashback: The reaction felt by an individual when the memory of a trauma is cued by an experience in the present as though the traumatic experience is happening again.

Flavanols: Compounds found in high levels in unprocessed cocoa that might benefit cognition.

Foix-Alajouanine syndrome (FAS) or **subacute ascending necrotizing myelitis (SANM):** A disease caused by dural arteriovenous malformation of the spinal cord that present in the lower thoracic or lumbar spinal cord, numbness; loss of sensation and sphincter dysfunction, and disseminated nerve cell death in the spinal cord.

Foville's syndrome (FS): It is caused by the blockage of the perforating branches of the basilar artery in the region of the brainstem known as the pons. It is most frequently due to lesions such as vascular disease and tumors involving the dorsal pons.

Free radicals: Unstable atoms produced naturally in the body as a byproduct of normal functions within the body. They cause damage to cell membranes and DNA. Over time, this can lead to inflammation, premature skin aging, and a host of age-associated diseases.

Friedreich's ataxia (FA): An autosomal-recessive genetic disease that causes difficulty walking, a loss of coordination in the arms and legs, and impaired speech that worsens over time.

Frontotemporal dementia: A medical condition caused by damage to the nerve cells in the brain. The signs can occur in both younger and older adults. These signs may include unusual behaviors, emotional problems, trouble communicating, difficulty with work, or difficulty with walking.

G

Gaucher's disease (GD): A genetic disorder in which the enzyme glucocerebroside accumulates in cells and certain organs. It is characterized by bruising, fatigue, anemia, low blood platelet count, and enlargement of the liver and spleen.

Glutamate: The most common neurotransmitter in the brain. It can excite nerve cells to their death through a process known as excitotoxicity.

Glutamate regulators: They control the amount of glutamate in the central nervous system to an optimal level.

Glymphatic system: The lymphatic drainage system of the brain.

Healthy aging index (HAI) - A score that assesses neurocognitive function among other correlates of health through the years.

Hemiballismus (or **hemiballism**): A basal ganglia syndrome resulting from damage to the sub- thalamic nucleus in the basal ganglia. It is a rare hyperkinetic movement disorder that is characterized by violent involuntary limb movements on one side of the body and can cause significant disability. It affects both sides of the body and is much rarer.

Hereditary spastic paraplegia (HSP) or hereditary spastic paraparesis (HSP), or familial spastic paraplegia (FSP), or French settlement disease (FSD), or Strumpell disease (SD), or Strumpell-Lorrain disease.(SLD): A group of inherited diseases whose main feature is a progressive gait disorder. The disease presents with progressive stiffness (spasticity) and contraction in the lower limbs. It is different from cerebral palsy.

Herpetology: The branch of zoology concerned with the study of amphibians including frogs, toads, salamanders, newts, and caecilians (gymnophiona) and reptiles (including snakes, lizards, amphisbaenids, turtles, terrapins, tortoises, crocodilians, and tuataras). Birds, which are cladistically included within Reptilia, are traditionally excluded here.

Hippocampal theta rhythm: A specific type of electrical activity that can be observed in the hippocampus and other brain structures in numerous species of mammals.

Humanitarian device exemption (HDE): An FDA provision for rare diseases or conditions experienced by relatively few patients among whom it has been difficult to gather evidence to demonstrate effectiveness.

Huntington's disease (HD) (also known as **Huntington's chorea**): A mostly inherited incurable neurodegenerative disease. Earliest symptoms are often subtle problems with mood or mental/ psychiatric abilities. A general lack of coordination and an unsteady gait often follow. It is also a basal ganglia disease causing a hyperkinetic movement disorder known as chorea. As the disease advances, uncoordinated, involuntary body movements of chorea become more apparent. Physical abilities gradually worsen until coordinated movement becomes difficult and the person is unable to talk. Mental abilities generally decline into dementia, depression, apathy and impulsivity at times.

Hydrocephalus or **Normal pressure hydrocephalus (NPH):** A condition in which an accumulation of cerebrospinal fluid (CSF) occurs within the brain. This typically causes increased pressure inside the skull. Older people may have headaches, double vision, poor balance, urinary incontinence, personality changes, or mental impairment. The four types of hydrocephalus are communicating, non-communicating, *ex vacuo*, and normal pressure.

Hypercapnia: A concentration of carbon dioxide higher than normal level.

Hyperfocus: Unusual prolonged and intense level of attention for interesting or rewarding tasks.

Hyperthymesia, also known as **hyperthymestic syndrome** or **highly superior autobiographical memory (HSAM):** A condition that leads people to be able to remember an abnormally large number of their life experiences in vivid detail.

Hypokinesia: The reduced range of movements.

Hyponatremia: Low sodium.

Hypoventilation (or **respiratory depression) syndrome (RDS):** A condition occurring when ventilation is inadequate to perform needed respiratory gas exchange, causing an increased concentration of carbon dioxide (hypercapnia) and respiratory acidosis.

Hypoxemia: A drop in the percentage of oxygen in the circulation to a lower than normal level.

I

Iatrogenic: Treatment-induced.

Ichthyology: The branch of zoology devoted to the study of fish, including bony fish (Osteichthyes), cartilaginous fish (Chondrichthyes), and jawless fish (Agnatha). According to FishBase, 33,400 species of fish had been described as of October 2016, with approximately 250 new species described each year.

Inhibition effect: Taking longer time in recalling or recognizing an item, and making more frequent errors.

Inhibitory control effect: The inability to prevent the suppression of irrelevant information in working memory and, correspondingly, the limited capacity for relevant information.

J

Jactitation: Restlessness while in bed,

K

Kernicterus: The rapidly increasing unconjugated bilirubin that crosses the blood-brain-barrier in infants.

Krabbe's disease (KD) or **globoid cell leukodystrophy (GCL)** or **galactosylceramide lipidosis (GSL):** A rare and often fatal lysosomal storage disease that results in progressive damage to the nervous system. It involves dysfunctional metabolism of sphingolipids and is inherited in an autosomal recessive pattern. The buildup of unmetabolized lipids adversely affects the growth of the nerve's protective myelin sheath.

L

Lennox-Gastaut syndrome (LGS): A complex, rare, and severe childhood-onset epilepsy characterized by multiple and concurrent seizure types including tonic seizure, cognitive dysfunction, and abnormal aspect on electroencephalogram (EEG). Typically, it presents in children aged 3–5 years and most of the time persists into adulthood. It has been associated with perinatal injuries, congenital infections, brain malformations, brain tumors, genetic disorders such as tuberous sclerosis and several gene mutations. Sometimes, LGS is observed after infantile epileptic spasm syndrome (formerly called West's syndrome).

Lethologica: The tip-of-the-tongue phenomenon when trying to remember a person, an action, an event, etc.

Lyme disease (or Lyme *borreliosis*): A tick-borne zoonotic disease that affects humans and animals. It is a bacterial, vector-borne infection due to *borrelia* (a helicoid spirochete) that is transmitted by bites from the *Ixodes* tick. *Borrelia* includes a dozen species (36 as of the end of 2018, but others may still be discovered).

M

Marburg multiple sclerosis (MMS) or **acute fulminant multiple sclerosis:** One of the MS borderline diseases. Other diseases in this group are neuromyelitis optica (NMO), Balo concentric sclerosis (BCS), Schilder's disease (SD), and for some as tumefactive multiple sclerosis (TMS).

Meige's syndrome (MS) or Brueghel's syndrome (BS) or oral facial dystonia OFD): A type of dystonia. A combination of two forms of dystonia, blepharospasm and oromandibular dystonia (OMD). The combination of upper and lower dystonia is called cranial-cervical dystonia.

Melatonin: A hormone naturally produced by the pineal gland in the brain's center in response to darkness. It helps regulate the circadian clock and sleep. Synthetic forms can be taken as a supplement to help induce sleep.

Memory: Various forms include: Autobiographical; declarative (see explicit); emotional: episodic: explicit; implicit; intrusive; k*inesthetic (see implicit); l*ong term (or semantic); motor; non- declarative (see implicit); objective; procedural (see implicit); photographic; prospective; semantic (see long-term memory); sensory (v*erbal; visual-spatial or iconic; auditory or echoic; olfactory; and haptic); s*hort-term (also known as active);spatial: and working).

Memory athlete: **S**omeone who participates in memory competitions, which can involve a variety of tests of memory ability. Competitors train their ability to recall information with the aid of mental techniques called mnemonics. Memory sport includes international competitions (the World Memory Championships launched in 1991) as well as national and lower-level contests.

Memory "boundaries": The idea that memories can have hard and soft starting and ending points.

Memory champion: A person who can accomplish impressive feats of memory not because of a radical difference in cognitive functioning relative to other people, but through training and the use of techniques for enhancing memory.

Metabolic syndrome (MS): The combination of high blood pressure, high blood sugar, elevated triglyceride levels, and abdominal obesity.

Migraine: A genetically influenced complex neurological disorder characterized by episodes of moderate-to-severe headache, most often unilateral, and generally associated with nausea and light and sound sensitivity. Other characterizing symptoms may include vomiting, cognitive dysfunction, allodynia, and dizziness. Although primarily considered to be a headache disorder, migraine is better thought of as a spectrum disease rather than a distinct clinical entity. It is associated with psychiatric disorders (major depression, bipolar disorder, anxiety disorders, and obsessive–compulsive disorder).

Mnemonic: Tricks and techniques for remembering information that is difficult to recall. An example is the mnemonic "Richard Of York Gave Battle In Vain" to remember the first letters of the colors of the rainbow in order of their wave lengths: Red, Orange, Yellow, Green, Blue, Indigo, and Violet.)

Mnemonic devices: Mental techniques. Ways of enhancing memory that can involve elaboration— connecting what one is trying to remember to other information in memory—organizing to-be- remembered details more efficiently in memory, and making use of mental visualization.

Morvan's syndrome (MS) or **fibrillary chorea** (in French: *la chorée fibrillaire*)**:** A rare, life- threatening autoimmune disease describing patients with multiple, irregular contractions of the long muscles, cramping, weakness, pruritus, hyperhidrosis, insomnia, and delirium. This rare disorder is characterized by severe insomnia or complete lack of sleep (agrypnia) for weeks or months in a row, and associated with autonomic alterations consisting of profuse perspiration with characteristic skin miliaria (also known as sweat rash), tachycardia, increased body temperature, and hypertension.

Multiple system atrophy (MSA) or **striatonigral degeneration (SND):** A rare neurodegenerative disorder characterized by autonomic dysfunction, tremors, slow movement, muscle rigidity, and postural instability (collectively known as parkinsonism) and ataxia. This is caused by progressive degeneration of neurons in several parts of the brain including the basal ganglia, inferior olivary nucleus, and cerebellum. MSA often presents with some of the same symptoms as Parkinson's disease. It is distinct from multisystem proteinopathy, multiple organ dysfunction syndrome.

Myoclonus: A brief, involuntary, irregular (lacking rhythm) twitching of a muscle, a joint, or a group of muscles, different from clonus, which is rhythmic or regular. It describes a medical sign and, generally, is not a diagnosis of a disease. Myoclonic twitches, jerks, or seizures are usually caused by sudden muscle contractions (positive myoclonus) or brief lapses of contraction (negative myoclonus).

Myelitis: Inflammation of the spinal cord which can disrupt the normal responses from the brain to the rest of the body, and from the rest of the body to the brain. It can cause the myelin and axon to be damaged resulting in symptoms such as paralysis and sensory loss. It is classified in several categories depending on the area or the cause of the lesion; however, any inflammatory attack on the spinal cord is often referred to as transverse myelitis.

N

Narcolepsy: A chronic neurological syndrome of hypothalamic disorder that involves a decreased ability to regulate sleep–wake cycles. Symptoms often include periods of excessive daytime sleepiness and brief involuntary sleep episodes, vivid hallucinations or an inability to move (sleep paralysis) while falling asleep or waking up. Narcolepsy paired with cataplexy is an autoimmune disorder. There are two main characteristics of narcolepsy: excessive daytime sleepiness and abnormal REM sleep.

Necrosis: Death of tissue.

Neuroleptic malignant syndrome (NMS): A rare but life-threatening reaction that can occur in response to neuroleptic or antipsychotic medication.

Neuromyelitis optica (NMO) and NMO spectrum disorders (NOSD): Autoimmune diseases characterized by acute inflammation of the optic nerve: optic neuritis (ON) and spinal cord (myelitis). Episodes of ON and myelitis can be simultaneous or successive. A relapsing disease course is common, especially in untreated patients.The etiology remains unknown (idiopathic NMO).

Neurotrophic: Act to destroy nerve tissue and create inflammation.

N-methyl-D-aspartic acid (NMDA): A receptor antagonist that stops calcium from invading the neurons and causing nerve injury.

Nosography: A description or classification of diseases.

Nosology: The branch of medical science that deals with the classification of diseases.

Nostalgia: A longing for the past, an experience often described as bittersweet.

Nystagmus: Rapid, involuntary eye movements.

O

Obsessions: Persistent unwanted thoughts, mental images, or urges that generate feelings of anxiety, disgust, or discomfort.

Obsessive compulsory/behavioral disorder (OC/BD): A mental and behavioral disorder in which an individual has intrusive thoughts (an obsession) and feels the need to perform certain routines (compulsions) repeatedly to relieve the distress caused by the obsession, to the extent where it impairs general function.

Off-label medicines: Not FDA-approved medicines intended for the diagnosis, prevention or treatment of rare diseases. They are called "orphan" because under normal market conditions (i.e. in the absence of an orphan regulation), the pharmaceutical industry has little interest in developing and marketing products intended for only a small number of patients, when the high cost of bringing a medicinal product to market may not be recovered by the expected sales of the product.

Ornithology: The scientific study of birds.

Osteoarthritis (OA): A type of degenerative joint disease that results from breakdown of joint cartilage and underlying bone.The most common symptoms are joint pain and stiffness. Other symptoms may include joint swelling, decreased range of motion, and, when the back is affected, weakness or numbness of the arms and legs. It is believed to be caused by mechanical stress on the joint and low grade inflammatory processes.

Optogenetic: Light-based.

Oxydative stress: The physiological stress on the body that is caused by the cumulative damage done by free radicals inadequately neutralized by antioxidants and that is held to be associated with aging.

Palsy: A medical term referring to various types of paralysis or paresis, often accompanied by weakness and the loss of feeling and uncontrolled body movements such as shaking. Specific kinds of palsy include: Bell's palsy, bulbar palsy, cerebral palsy, conjugate gaze palsy, Erb's palsy (or brachial palsy), Fazio-Lande infantile palsy, spinal muscular atrophy, progressive supranuclear palsy, squatter's palsy, and **third nerve palsy.**

Pantothenate kinase-associated neurodegeneration (PKAN) **(**formerly called Hallervorden–Spatz syndrome, HSS), is a genetic degenerative disease of the brain that can lead to parkinsonism, dystonia, dementia, and ultimately death. Neurodegeneration in PKAN is accompanied by an excess of iron that progressively builds up in the brain. PKAN is caused by loss of function of the enzyme PANK2, due to bi-allelic genetic mutations. It follows autosomal recessive inheritance. This enzyme is the first step in the pathway converting vitamin B5 into coenzyme A. There are currently no treatments that modify disease progress, though there are a number of medications and therapies that can help improve symptoms and there is active research into treatments.

Paraphasia: **Speech difficulties due to an inability to recall vocabulary, incorrect word substitutions.**

Paresis: **Paralytic dementia.**

Parkinson's disease (PD): **A chronic degenerative disorder of the central nervous system (CNS) that mainly affects the motor system. The symptoms usually emerge slowly and, as the disease worsens, non-motor symptoms become more common. Early symptoms are tremor, rigidity, slowness of movement, and difficulty with walking. Problems may also arise with cognition, behavior, sleep, and sensory systems. Parkinson's disease dementia becomes common in advanced stages of the disease. The motor symptoms of the disease result from the death of nerve cells in the substantia nigra, a region of the midbrain that supplies dopamine to the basal ganglia. The cause of this cell death is poorly understood, but involves the aggregation of the protein alpha-synuclein into Lewy bodies within the**

neurons. Collectively, the main motor symptoms are known as parkinsonism or a parkinsonian syndrome. The cause of PD is unknown, but a combination of genetic and environmental factors are believed to play a role.

Parkinsonism: **A clinical syndrome characterized by tremor, bradykinesia (slowed movements), rigidity, and postural instability. It usually leads to dementia with Lewy bodies (DLB), Parkinson's disease dementia (PDD), and many other conditions.**

Pharmacovigilance: The science and activities related to the detection and reporting of side effects of a medicine, together with measures to minimize these risks.

Phosphorylation: The addition of a chemical group to a protein, which affects its activity levels in biochemical reactions.

Posterior cortical atrophy (PCA) or **Benson's syndrome (BS):** A rare form of dementia considered a visual variant or an atypical variant of Alzheimer's disease (AD). It causes atrophy of the posterior part of the cerebral cortex, resulting in the progressive disruption of complex visual processing. In rare cases, PCA can be caused by dementia with Lewy bodies (DLB) and Creutzfeldt–Jakob disease (CJD).

Primary lateral sclerosis (PLS): A very rare neuromuscular disease characterized by progressive muscle weakness in the voluntary muscles. It only affects upper motor neurons.

Primary progressive aphasia (**PPA**): A type of neurological syndrome in which language capabilities slowly and progressively become impaired. The symptoms that accompany PPA depend on what parts of the left hemisphere are significantly damaged. It results from continuous deterioration in brain tissue, which leads to early symptoms being far less detrimental than later symptoms. Eventually, almost every patient becomes mute and completely loses the ability to understand both written and spoken language. Many, if not most of those with PPA experience impairment of memory, short-term memory formation and loss of executive functions.

Priming: Refers to activating behavior through the power of unconscious suggestion.

Prion: An abnormal protein. Infectious prions are misfolded proteins that can cause normally folded proteins to also become misfolded.

Processing speed effect: The processing information decrease with age, causing the inability to use working memory efficiently and rendering more difficult those cognitive tasks that rely on quick processing speed.

Progressive muscular atrophy (PMA) also called **Duchesne–Aran disease (DAD)** or **Duchesne– Aran muscular atrophy (DAMA):** A disorder characterized by the degeneration of lower motor neurons, resulting in generalized, progressive loss of muscle function.

Progressive supranuclear palsy (PSP): A late-onset neurodegenerative disease involving the gradual deterioration and death of specific volumes of the brain. The condition leads to symptoms including loss of balance, slowing of movement, difficulty moving the eyes, and cognitive impairment. PSP may be mistaken for other types of neurodegeneration such as PD, frontotemporal dementia (FTD), and Alzheimer's disease (AD). The cause of the condition is uncertain, but involves the accumulation of the tau-protein within the brain.

Proteopathies: Diseases associated with the aggregation of misfolded proteins.

Psychogenic: Having a psychological origin or cause rather than a physical one.

R

Registry: A collection of information about individuals, usually focused around a specific diagnosis or condition.

Reliability: The degree to which different diagnosticians agree on a diagnosis.

Repetitive transcranial magnetic stimulation (rTMS)**:** An emerging therapeutic modality for seizure suppression.

Repurposed medicine: A medicine already approved for human use in a certain indication and for which researchers or clinicians identify new disease(s) that the medicine could treat (i.e. a new indication).

Research domain criteria (RdoC): A research framework by the (U.S.) National Institute of Mental Health (NIMH) for new approaches to investigating mental disorders, integrating many levels of information (from genomics and circuits to behavior and self-reports) to explore basic dimensions of functioning that span the full range of human behavior from normal to abnormal.

Restless legs syndrome (RLS) or **Willis–Ekbom disease (WED):** Generally, a long-term disorder that causes a strong urge to move one's legs. This is often described as aching, tingling, or crawling in nature. Additionally, many have limb twitching during sleep, a condition known as periodic limb movement disorder.

Reye's syndrome: A rapidly worsening brain disease. Symptoms may include vomiting, personality changes, confusion, seizures, and loss of consciousness.

S

Sclerosis (or **sclerosus**): The Latin names of a few disorders. The hardening of tissue and other anatomical features.

Self-efficacy: The sense of control that people have over their own lives and destiny. A strong sense of self-efficacy has also been linked to lowered stress levels.

Semantic network model: One way of thinking about memory organization. This model suggests that certain triggers activate associated memories.

Senior moment: A memory deficit that appears to have a biological cause.

Sensory-gating: The physiologic process whereby redundant environmental stimuli are filtered out in the early stages of perception. Impairment of sensory gating gives rise to altered sensory perception.

Sequential performance: The execution of a series of steps needed to complete a routine.

Serial position effect: The role played in informaion recall by the order of information.

Skin miliaria: Sweat rash.

Sleep apnea (SA): A sleep disorder in which pauses in breathing or periods of shallow breathing during sleep occur more often than normal. It may be either obstructive sleep apnea or central sleep apnea, or a combination of both. It is associated with a wide array of effects, including increased risk of car accidents, hypertension, cardiovascular disease, myocardial infarction, stroke, atrial fibrillation, insulin resistance, higher incidence of cancer, and neurodegeneration. Alzheimer's disease (AD) and severe obstructive sleep apnea are connected because there is an increase in the protein beta-amyloid as well as white-matter damage.

Source information: One type of episodic memory that declines with old age.

Spasmodic torticollis (ST) or **cervical dystonia (CD):** An extremely painful, predominantly idiopathic, chronic neurological movement disorder causing the neck to involuntarily turn to the left, right, upwards, and/or downwards. Both agonist and antagonist muscles contract simultaneously.

Spasticity: Progressive stiffness.

Spinal cord compressiom (SCC): A form of myelopathy in which the spinal cord is compressed. Causes can be bone fragments from a vertebral fracture, a tumor, abscess, ruptured intervertebral disc or other lesion.

Spinal muscular atrophy (SMA): A genetically and clinically heterogeneous group of rare debilitating disorders characterized by the degeneration of lower motor neurons and subsequent atrophy of various muscle groups in the body.

Status dystonicus (SD): A serious and potentially life-threatening disorder which occurs in people who have primary or secondary dystonia. Symptoms consist of widespread severe muscle contractions.

Stiff-person syndrome (**SPS**) or **stiff-man syndrome (SMS):** A rare neurologic disorder of unclear cause characterized by progressive muscular rigidity and stiffness. Chronic pain, impaired mobility, and lumbar hyperlordosis are common symptoms.

Stroke: A medical condition in which poor blood flow to the brain causes cell death. There are two main types: ischemic (due to lack of blood flow) or hemorrhagic (due to bleeding). Both cause parts of the brain to stop functioning properly. Signs and symptoms may include an inability to move or feel on one side of the body, problems understanding or speaking, dizziness, or loss of vision to one side. If symptoms last less than one or two hours, the stroke is a 'transient ischemic attack' (TIA), also called a 'mini-stroke'. A hemorrhagic stroke may also be associated with a severe headache.The biggest risk factor for stroke is high blood pressure. Other risk factors include high blood cholesterol, tobacco smoking, obesity, diabetes mellitus, a previous TIA, end-stage kidney disease, and atrial fibrillation.

Subacute sclerosing panencephalitis (SSPE) also **known as Dawson disease (DD):** A rare form of progressive brain inflammation caused by a persistent infection with the measles virus. The condition primarily affects children, teens, and young adults. It is almost always fatal.

Surrogate endpoint: A marker (such as with a laboratory measurement, radiographic image, physical sign or other measure) that is thought to predict clinical benefit but is not itself a measure of clinical benefit. The use of a surrogate endpoints can considerably shorten the time required prior to receiving FDA approval.

Sustained attention: A measure of the ability to attend to, and respond to, stimuli for an extended period of time.

Synaptic plasticity: The ability of nerve cells to modify the strength of their connections.

Syringobulbia: A medical condition in which syrinxes, or fluid-filled cavities, affect the brainstem (usually the lower brainstem). The exact cause is often unknown, but may be linked to a widening of the central canal of the spinal cord. This may affect one or more cranial nerves, resulting in various kinds of facial palsies. Sensory and motor nerve pathways may be affected by interruption or compression of nerves.

Syringomyelia: Refers to a disorder in which a cyst or cavity (called syrinx) forms within the spinal cord. The cyst can expand and elongate over time, destroying the spinal cord. The damage may result in loss of feeling, paralysis, weakness, and stiffness in the back, shoulders, and extremities. It may also cause a loss of the ability to feel extremes of hot or cold, especially in the hands. It may also lead to a cape-like bilateral loss of pain and temperature sensation along the upper chest and arms.

Syrinx: Fluid-filled cavity.

T

Tauopathy: A neurodegenerative disease involving the aggregation of the tau-protein into neurofibrillary or gliofibrillary tangles in the human brain. Tangles are formed by hyperphosphorylation of the microtubule protein known as tau, causing the protein to dissociate from microtubules and form insoluble aggregates.

Taxonomy: (See also nosology.)

Theurgy: The operation or effect of a supernatural or divine agency in human affairs.

Tics: Problems in which a part of the body moves repeatedly, quickly, suddenly, and uncontrollably. Movements or sounds that take place "intermittently and unpredictably out of a background of normal motor activity", having the appearance of "normal behaviors gone wrong". They may also occur in "bouts of bouts", which may vary among people. They can occur in any body part, such as the face, shoulders, hands, or legs.

Tourette's syndrome: A common inherited, neurodevelopmental, neuropsychiatric, motor disorder that may cause sudden, unwanted, and uncontrolled rapid and repeated movements or vocal sounds called tics. It is not a degenerative condition.

Tourettism: Secondary causes of tic disorders.

Transglutaminases: Human enzymes ubiquitously present in the human body and in the brain in particular.

Transient global amnesia (TGA): A sudden, temporary loss of memory of unclear cause.

Tremor: An involuntary, somewhat rhythmic, muscle contraction and relaxation involving oscillations or twitching movements of one or more body parts.

V

Vagus nerve stimulation: to improve behavioral controlN A non-invasive electrical stimulation of the vagus nerve that affects cognitive functions, and inhibitory and tic control in patients with tic disorders.

Vascular myelopathy (VM): Refers to an abnormality of the spinal cord in regard to its blood supply.

W

Weber's syndrome (WS) or midbrain stroke syndrome (MSS) or superior alternating hemiplegia (SAH): A form of stroke that affects the medial portion of the midbrain. It involves oculomotor fascicles in the interpeduncular cisterns and cerebral peduncle so it characterizes the presence of an ipsilateral lower motor neuron type oculomotor nerve palsy and contralateral hemiparesis or hemiplegia.

West's syndrome (WS): Epileptic spasms is an uncommon-to-rare epileptic disorder in infants, children and adults. Other names for it are "generalized flexion epilepsy", "infantile epileptic encephalopathy", "infantile myoclonic encephalopathy", "jackknife convulsions", and "massive myoclonia".

White matter hyperintensities: A sign of cardiovascular-related brain damage linked to high blood pressure in older adults. Increased volume of white matter hyperintensities are linked to decreased memory performance in older adults, and are a predictor of Alzheimer's disease.

Wilson's disease (WD): A genetic disorder in which excess copper builds up in the body. Symptoms are typically related to the brain and liver. Liver-related symptoms include vomiting, weakness, fluid build-up in the abdomen, swelling of the legs, yellowish skin, and itchiness. Brain-related symptoms include tremors, muscle stiffness, trouble in speaking, personality changes, anxiety, and psychosis. WD is caused by a mutation in the Wilson disease protein (ATP7B) gene. This protein transports excess copper into bile, where it is excreted in waste products. The condition is autosomal recessive. For people to be affected, they must inherit a mutated copy of the gene from both parents. Diagnosis may be difficult and often involves a combination of blood tests, urine tests and a liver biopsy. Genetic testing may be used to screen family members of those affected. WD is typically treated with dietary changes and medication. Complications of WD can include liver failure, liver cancer, and kidney problems. A liver transplant may be helpful to those for whom other treatments are not effective or if liver failure occurs. WD occurs in about one in 30,000 people. Symptoms usually begin between the ages of 5 and 35 years. It was first described in 1854 by German pathologist Friedrich Theodor von Frerichs and is named after British neurologist Samuel Wilson.

Abbreviations & Acronyms

A

AA: Alzheimer's Association (formerly Alzheimer's Disease and Related Disorders Association, ADRDA)

AAMI: Age-Associated Memory Impairment (same as ARMI)

AAN: American Academy of Neurology

AAO: American Academy of Ophthalmology

AAP: American Psychiatric Association

Aβ: β-amyloid protein

ABA: Amoebic Brain Abscess

ACIAP: **A**tttention deficit; **C**ontiguity; **I**nhibitory control decline; **A**ttentional resources limitation; **P**rocessing

ACh: Acetylcholine

ACS: Alternating Current Stimulation

AD: Alcohol Dementia

AD: Alexander's disease

AD: Alpers' disease

AD: Alzheimer's Disease

ADD: AD Dementia

ADE: Acute Disseminated Encephalomyelitis

ADEAR: (U.S.) (NIH/NIA) Alzheimer's and related Dementias Education And Referral

ADH: Associative Deficit Hypothesis

ADHD: Attention Deficit Hyperactivity Disorder

ADL: Activities of Daily Living

ADL: AdenoLeukoDystrophy

AE: Adverse Events

AFMS: Acute Fulminant Multiple Sclerosis

AGE: Advanced Glycation End-products

AHA: American Heart Association

AI: Artificial Intelligence

ALD: AdrenoLeukoDystrophy

ALS: Amyotrophic Lateral Sclerosis (or Lou Gehrig's disease)

ALSD: ALS Dementia

AM: Active memory

AM: Auditory Memory (see also Echoic)

AM: Autobiographical Memory

AMTS: Abbreviated Mental Test Score

ANDA: Abbreviated NDA

ANS: Autonomous NS

APA: American Psychiatric Association

APP: Amyloid Precursor Protein

APS: (U.S.) American Philosophical Society

ADRDA: Alzheimer Disease and Related Disorders Association (now the Alzheimer's Association)

ARIA: Amyloid-Related Imaging Abnormalities

ARMI: Age-Related Memory Impairment (same as AAMI)

ASD: Autism Spectrum Disorder

ASIC: Application-Specific Integrated Circuits

AT: Ataxia Telangectasia

ATMP: Advanced Therapy Medicinal Products

ATP: Adenosine TriPhosphate
ATS: Ataxia Telangiectasia Syndrome
AUD: Alcohol Use Disorder

B

BBB: Blood-Brain Barrier
BCS: Balo Concentric Sclerosis
B(CSF)B: Blood–CerebroSpinal Fluid Barrier
BD: Behcet's disease
BD: Bipolar Disorder
BDD: (FDA's) Breakthrough Device Designation
BGD: Basal Ganglia Disease
BLA: Biologic License Application
BP: Bell's palsy
BRAIN: (U.S.-NIH) Brain Research through Advancing Innovative Neurotechnologies
BS: Benson's Syndrome
BS: Brueghel's syndrome
BSE: Bovine Spongiform Encephalopathy
BST: Brain Stimulation Therapies
BT: Behavioral Therapy

C

Caspases: Cysteine-Aspartic Acid Proteases
CAT: Computerized Axial Tomography
CBD: Cannabidiol
CBD: CorticoBasal Dementia
CBBD: Canavan–Van Bogaert–Bertrand Disease
CBER: (FDA) Center for Biologics Evaluation and Research
CBG: CorticoBasal Ganglia
CBT: Cognitive Behavioral Therapy
CCMD: Chinese Classification and Diagnostic Criteria of Mental Disorders
CD: Canavan's Disease
CD: Celiac Disease
CD: Cervical Dystonia
CD: Childen's Dementia

CD: Cortical Dementia
CDC&P: (U.S.) Center for Disease Control & Prevention
CDER: (FDA) Center for for Drug Evaluation and Research
cdSMA: congenital distal Spinal Muscular Atrophy
CE: Cerebral Edema
CES: Cranial Electrotherapy Stimulation
CID: Chronic Inflammatory Conditions
CJD: Creutzfeldt-Jacob Disease
CNS: Central NS
COPD: Chronic Obstructive Pulmonary Disease
CP: Cranial Pressure
CPP: Choroid Plexus Papilloma
CPR: CardioPulmonary Resuscitation
Cr: Creatine
CRF: Corticotrophin-Releasing Factor (a stress hormone)
CRO: Contract Research Organization
CS: Cockayne's syndrome
CSA: Central Sleep Apnea
CSF: CerebroSpinal Fluid
CSH: Chronic Subdural Hematoma
CST: Cavernous Sinus Thrombosis
CT: Clinical Trial
CT: Computerized Tomography
cTBS: continuous TBS
CTE: Chronic Traumatic Encephalopathy
CTP: Clinical Trial Protocol
CV: Cerebral Vasculitis
CVD: CerebroVascular Disease
CVDD: CVD Dementia
CX: Cerebrotendinous Xanthomatosis

D

DAMA: Duchesne –Aran Muscular Atrophy
DBS: Deep Brain Stimulation
DCS: Direct Current Stimulation
DD: Dawson's disease
DHHS: (U.S.) Department of Health and Human Services

dhMN: distal Hereditary Motor
   Neuropathies
DLB: Dementia with Lewy Bodies
DLPFC: DorsoLateral PreFrontal Cortex
DM: Declarative Memory
   DMD: Duchesne's Muscular Dystrophy
DMS: Diffuse Myelinoclastic Sclerosis
DPA: Dentatorubal Pallidoluysian Atrophy
DS: Dravet's Syndrome
DSB: (DNA's) Double-Strand Break
DSM: (APA) Diagnostic & Statistical Manual
   of Mental Disorders
DSM-5: *DSM-5th edition*
DSM-TR: DSM-Text Revision

E

EACT: Excitatory Amino Acid Transporter
EAS: Experimental & Applied Science
ECT: ElectroConvulsive Therapy
EEG: Electroencephalography
ELISA: Enzyme-Linked ImmunoSorbent
   Assay
EM: Echoic Memory
EM: Emotional Memory
EM: *Erythema Migrans*
EM: Explicit Memory
EOD: Early Onset Dementia
EP: Episodic Memory
ESD: Early Stage Dementia
ETS: ElectroTherapy Stimulation

F

FA: Friedreich's Ataxia
FAS: Foix-Alajouanine Syndrome
FAST: Functional Assessment Staging
   Scale
FC: Fibrillary Chorea
FCI: Fixed Cognitive Impairment
FDA: (U.S.) Food & Drug Administration
FFI: Fatal Familial Insomnia
fMRI: functional MRI
FS: Foville's Syndrome
FSD: French Settlement Disease

FSP: Familial Spastic Paraplegia
FTD: FrontoTemporal Disorder
FTDD: FTD Dementia
FTLD: FrontoTemporal Lobar Degeneration
FXS: Fragile-X Syndrome
FXTAS: Fragile X-associated Tremor/Ataxia
   Syndome

G

GA: Glutaric Aciduria
GABA: Gamma-AminoButyric Acid
GCL: Globoid Cell Leukodystrophy
GD: Gaucher's Disease
GDS: Geriatric Depression Scale
GEL: Genetics, Environment, Lifestyle
GPi: Globus Pallidus internum
GSL: GalactoSylceramide Lipidosis
GWAS: Genome-Wide Association Studies

H

HAD: HIV-Associated Dementia
HAI: Healthy Aging Index
HBP: (European) Human Brain Project
HC: Huntington's Chorea
HD: Huntington's Disease
HDD: HD Dementia
HDE: (FDA's) Humanitarian Device
   Exemption
HDG: HydroxyDeoxyGuanosine
HDL: High Density Lipoprotein
HE: Hashimoto's Encephalitis
HIV: Human Immunodeficiency Virus
HIVE: HIV Encephalitis
HIVAD: HIV-Associated Dementia
HM: Haptic Memory
HSAM: Highly Superior Autobiographical
   Memory
HSP: Hereditary Spastic Paraparesis
HSP: Hereditary Spastic Paraplegia
HSV: Herpes Simplex Virus
HTT: Huntingtin gene

I

ICC: Interstitial Cell of Cajal
ICD: (WHO) International Statistical Classification of Diseases and Related Health Problems
ICP: IntraCranial Pressure
iFLP: infantile Fazio-Lande Palsy
IM: Implicit Memory
IMD: Immunologically-Mediated Dementia
IND: Investigational New Drug
IPG: Implantable Pulse Generator
IRB: Institutional Review Board

K

KD: Krabbe's disease
KLD: Klein-Levin Disease
KM: Kinesthetic Memory
KP: Korsakoff's Psychosis

L

LBD: Lewy Body Dementia
LBD: Lewy Body Disease
LBDD: LBD Dementia
LBS: Louis–Barre syndrome
LD: Lyme Disease
LE: Limbic Encephalitis
LEC: Local Ethics Committee
LEPC: LeukoEncephalitis Periaxialis Concentrica
LGS: Lennox-Gastaut Syndrome
LMA: Lateral Motor Area
LMN: Lower Motor Neurons
LNB: Lyme *NeuroBorrelliosis*
LNS: Lesch-Nyhan syndrome
LOD: Late Onset Dementia
LS: Leigh's Syndrome
LSD: Late Stage Dementia
LTM: Long-Term Memory

M

MATCH-D: Medications Appropriateness Tool for Co-Morbid Health – Dementia
MBD: Marchiafava–Bignami Disease

MCI: Mild Cognitive Impairment
MCLD: MetaChromatic LeukoDystrophy
MCP: Myelinolysis Central Pontine
MCSS: Multiple CerebroSpinal Sclerosis
MD: Mixed Dementia
mDNA: mitochondrial DNA
MDS: Mild Dementia Stage
MDS: (U.S.) Movement Disorders Society
MDDS: Mitochondrial DNA Depletion Syndrome
MGD: Millard–Gubler Disease
MID: Multi-Infarct Dementia
MM: Motor Memory
MMS: Marburg Multiple Sclerosis
MMSE: Mini Mental State Exam
MND: Motor Neuron Diseases
MNS: Median Nerve Stimulation
MOI: Monoamine Oxidase Inhibitor
MRA_ Magnetic Resonance Angiography
MRI: Magnetic Resonance Imaging
MRS: Magnetic Resonance Spectroscopy
MS: Meige's syndrome
MS: Morvan's Syndrome
MS: Multiple Sclerosis
MSA: Multiple System Atrophy
MSD: Middle Stage Dememtia
MSS: Midbrain Stroke Syndrome
MST: Magnetic Seizure Therapy
MSUD: Maple Syrup Urine Disease
mTBI: mild TBI

N

NAC: Non-Abeta Component
NAS: (U.S.) National Academy of Sciences
NCCIH: (U.S.) National Center for Complementary and Integrative Health
NCL: Neuronal Ceroid Lipofuscinosis
NDA: New Drug Application
NDD: NeuroDegenerative Disease(s)
NDDD: NDD Dementia
NDM: Non-Declarative Memory
NDS: Neill-Dingwall Syndrome
NEI: (U.S.) National Eye Institute

NFT: NeuroFibrillary Tangles

NIA: (U.S.) National Institute on Aging

NIH: (U.S.) National Institutes of Health

NIMH: (U.S.) National Institute of Mental Health

NINDS: U.S.) National Institute for Neurological Disorders & Stroke

NLM: (U.S.) National Library of Medicine

NMDA: N-Methyl-D-aspartic Acid

NMO: NeuroMyelitis Optica

NMOSD: NMO Spectrum Disorders

NMS: Neuroleptic Malignant Syndrome

NORT: Novel Object Recognition Task

NOSD: NO Spectrum Disorder

NPD: Niemann-Pick Disease

NPH: Normal Pressure Hydrocephalus

NPI: NeuroPsychiatric Inventory

NS: Nervous System

NSAID: Non-Steroidal Anti-Inflammatory Drugs

O

OA: OsteoArthritis

OCD: Obsessive Compulsive Disorder

OFD: Oral Facial Dystonia

OM: Olfactory Memory

ON: Optic Neuritis

ORA: Orexin Receptor Antagonist

OS: Oxidative Stress

OSA: Obstructive Sleep Apnea

OTC: Over-The-Counter

P

PBP: Progressive Bulbar Palsy

PCA: Posterior Cortical Atrophy

PCD: Programmed Cell Death

PCr: PhosphoCreatine

PCR: Polymerase Chain Reaction

PD: Parkinson's Disease

PD: Primary Dementia

PD: Pugilistic Dementia

PDD: PD Dementia

PDM: Psychodynamic Diagnostic Manual

PDUFA: (U.S.) Prescription Drug User Fee Act

PET: Positron Emission Tomography

PHF: Paired Helical Filaments

PHSA: (U.S.) Public Health Service Act

Pib-PET: Pittsburgh PET

PID: Progressively Irreversible Dementias

PKAN: Pantothenate Kinase- Associated Neurodegeneration

PKU: PhenylKetonUria

PLS: Primary Lateral Sclerosis

PM: Procedural Memory

PM: Prospective Memory

PMA: Progressive muscular Atrophy

PMD: Pelizaeus-Merzbacher Disease

PMD: Psychodynamic Diagnostic Manual

PML: Progressive Multifocal Leukoencephalopathy

PNS: Peripheral NS

PPA: Primary Progressive Aphasia

PSP: Progressive Supranuclear Palsy

p-tau: phosphorylated-tau protein

PTSD: Post-Traumatic Stress Disorder

PUD: Peptic Ulcer Disease

PUMNS: Penn Upper Motor Neuron Score

Q

QOL: Quality Of Life

R

RCT: Randomized CT

RD: Reversible Dementias

RDoC: Research Domain Criteria (a project of NIMH)

RDS: Respiratory Depression Syndrome

RE: Reye's Encephalopathy

RER: Recency, Emotion, and Repetition

RLS: Restless Legs Syndrome

RNS: Random Noise Stimulation

ROH: Research Opportunities in Humans

RS: Reye's syndrome

RSD: Reversible Secondary Dementia

rTMS: repetitive Transcranial Magnetic Stimulation
RVR: Regional Volume Reduction

S

SA: Sleep Apnea
SAE: Serious AE
SAH: Superior Alternating Hemiplegia
SANM: Subacute Ascending Necrotizing Myelitis
SASE: Sub-Acute Sclerosing Encephalitis
SCA: SpinoCerebellar Ataxia
SCC: Spinal Cord Compression
SCI: Subjective Cognitive Impairment
SD: Schilder's Disease
SD: Senility Dementia
SD: Status Dystonicus
SD: Strumpell Disease
SD: Syphilitic Dementia
sEEG: stereo EEG
SES: SocioEconomic Status
SFS: San Filippo's Syndrome
SLD: Strumpell-Lorrain disease
SLE: Systemic Lupus Errhythematosus
SM: Semantic Memory
SM: Sensory Memories

SM: Spatial Memory
SM: Subjective Memory
SMA: Spinal Muscular Atrophy
SMA: Supplementary Motor Area
SMEI: Severe Myoclonic Epilepsy of Infancy
SMS: Stiff-Man Syndrome
SND: StriatoNigral Degeneration
SP: Sub-Project (of HBP)
SPS: Stiff Person Syndrome
SPECT: Single Photon Emission Computed Tomography
SREAT: Steroid-Responsive Encephalopathy Associated with Autoimmune Thyroiditis
SS: Sjogren's Syndrome
SSB: (DNA's) Single-Strand Break
SSD: Sick Sinus Syndrome
SSPE: Subacute sclerosing panencephalitis
ST: Spasmodic Torticollis
STAC: Scaffolding Theory of Aging and Cognition
STM: Short-Term Memory

T

tACS: transcranial ACS

TBI: Traumatic Brain Injury
TBS: Theta Burst Stimulation
tDCS: transcranial DCS
TER: Time, Emotion, and Repetition
tETS: transcranial ETS
TES: Transcranial Electrotherapy Stimulation
TGA: Transient Global Amnesia
TIA: Transient Ischemic Attack
TMS: Transcranial Magnetic Stimulation
TMS: Tumefactive Multiple Sclerosis
TNRD: TriNucleotide Repeat Disorders
TNS: Trigeminal Nerve Stimulation
tRNS: transcranial RNS
TS: Tourette's Syndrome

TSD: Tay-Sachs Disease
tUSS: Transcranial US
tVNS: transcutaneous VNS

U

UMN: Upper Motor Neurons
USS: Ultrasound Stimulation

V

vCJD: variant CJD
VD: Vascular Dementia
VD: Vascular Disease
VDD: VD Dementia
VE: Viral Encephalitis
VM: Vascular Myelopathy

VM: Verbal Memory

VM: Viral Meningitis

VNS: Vagus Nerve Stimulation

VM: Visual Memory

W

WD: Whipple's Disease

WD: Wilson's Disease

WE: Wernicke's Encephalitis

WE: Wernicke's Encephalopathy

WED: Willis–Ekbom Disease

WHO: World Health Organization

WM: Working Memory

WS: Weber's Syndrome

WS: West's Syndrome

Y

YOD: Young Onset Dementia

Drugs & Supplements

A

Aducanumab/Aduhelm®

B

Belsomra
Benzodiazepines/Diazepam)
Brexpiprazole/Rexulti®

C

Cannabinoids
Cholinesterase inhibitor
Cincalcet
Citalopram/Celexa®)
Creatine

D

Detrol LA
Donepezil/Aricept®
Doxepin/Silenor®
Dronabinol

E

Escitalopram/Lexapro®
Estazolam/Promos®
Eszopiclone/Lunesta®

F

Fampridine
Fluoxetine/Prozac®
Folate/Vitamin B-12
Fruitflow-II

G

Galantamine/Razadyne®
Ginkgo Biloba

L

Lecanemab/Leqembi®
Lunesta
Luteolin

M

Melatonin
Memantine/Namenda®
Memantine+ Donepezil/Namzaric®
Minocycline

N

N-Methyl-D-aspartic Acid (NMDA)
    glutamate
Non-benzodiazepine hypnotics

O

Orexin receptor antagonist (ORA)

P

Panax Ginseng
Paroxetine/Paxil®
Phosphatidylserine-Omega
Piracetam

R

Ramelteon/Rozerem®

Resveratrol
Rivastigmine/Exelon®
Rozerem

S

Salbutamol
Selective serotonin re-uptake inhibitors
    (SSRI)
Sertraline/Zoloft®
Sevoflurane
Statins
Suvorexant/Belsomra®

T

Tacrine
Temazepam/Restoril®
Trazodone/Desyrel®
Triazolam/Halcion®

V

Vilazodone

Z

Zaleplon/Sonata®
Zolpidem/Ambien®/Intermezzo®/
    Zolpimist®

Diseases/ Disorders/ Syndromes

A

Acidemia
    Organic
Adrenoleukodystrophy, X-linked
Agrypnia
AIDS
Akathisia
Alexander's disease
Allodynia
Alpers' disease (or mitochondrial DNA
    depletion syndrome)
Alzheimer's disease
Amaurosis *fugax*
Amnesia
Anterograde
    Transcranial global
Amoebic brain abscess caverni
Amyotrophic lateral sclerosis
Anomia
Anti-NMDA receptor encephalitis
Aphasia
Acute
    Primary progressive
Apnea
Apneustic respiration
Asthma

Ataxia
    Fragile X-associated syndrome
    Spinocerebellar types 2, 17 dominant
        inheritance
    Telangectasia (or Louis–Barre
        syndrome)
Athetosis
Atrial fibrillation
Atrophy
    Cerebral
    Congenital distal
    Dentatorubal pallidoluysian
    Posterior cortical
    Progressive muscular
    Spinal muscular
Axonal injury (diffuse)

B

Balo concentric sclerosis (or
    leukoencephalitis periaxialis
    concentrica)
Basal ganglia disease
Behcet's disease
Benson's syndrome
Blepharospasm
Blindness
Brain herniation

Brain tumor
Brueghel's syndrome

C

CAMFAK syndrome
Canavan's disease (or Canavan–Van
    Bogaert– Bertrand disease)
Cancer (brain)
Cardiac arrhythmias
Cardiovascular disease
Cataplexy
Cavernous sinus thrombosis
    Aseptic
    Septic
Celiac disease
Celiac sensitivity, non-gluten
Cerebral edema
Cerebrotendinous xanthomatosis
Cheyne-Stokes respiration
Cholera
Chorea
    Fibrillary (or Morvan's syndrome)
    Sydenham's
Choreoathetosis
Choroid plexus papilloma
Chronic inflammatory conditions
Chronic obstructive pulmonary disease
Chronic traumatic encephalopathy
Cockayne's syndrome (or Neill-Dingwall
    syndrome)
Cognitive impairment
    Fixed
    Mild (amnestic; non-amnestic)
    Subjective
Coma
Corpus callosum demyelination
Corticobasal degeneration
Cramping
Creutzfeld-Jakob disease

D

Dawson's disease
Dehydration

Delirium
Dementia
    Alcohol
    Alzheimer type
    Early onset
    Frontotemporal (or Pick's disease)
    HIV
    Juvenile
    Late onset
    Lewy bodies
    Mixed
    Multi-infarct
    Paralytic (aka general paresis;
        general paralysis of the insane)
    Parkinson type
    Pugilistica
    Senilitic
    Vascular
    with Lewy bodies
Dentatorubal pallidoluysian atrophy
Depression disorder
Devic's disease (or neuromyelitis optica)
Diabetes
Diffuse myelinoclastic sclerosis
Dizziness
Dravet's syndrome (or severe myoclonic
    epilepsy of infancy)
    Focal
    Generalized
Drowsiness
Duchesne–Aran disease (or muscular
    atrophy)
Dysarthria
Dyskinesia
Dysphagia
Dystonia
    Cervical
    Oral facial
    Oromandibular

E

Encephalitis
    Anti-NMDA receptor

Herpes viral
HIV
Japanese
Lethargica
Limbic
Viral
Wernicke's
Encephalopathy
    Chronic traumatic
    Degenerative
    Demyelinating
Episodic/paroxysmal
    Hashimoto's
    Subacute necrotizing
    Sub-acute sclerosing
Epidural abscess
Epilepsy
    Myoclonic
    Status epilepticus
    Extrapyramidal disorders

F

Fatal familial insomnia
Foville's syndrome
Foix-Alajouanine syndrome (or subacute
    ascending necrotizing myelitis)
Fragile X-associated tremor/ataxia
    syndome
French settlement disease
Friedreich's ataxia
Frontotemporal lobar degeneration
Functional neurological symptom disorder

G

Galactosylceramide lipidosis (or Krabbe's
    disease; or globoid cell leukodystrophy)
Gaucher's disease, type 3
Generalized anxiety disorder
Globoid cell leukodystrophy (or Krabbe's
    disease; or galactosylceramide
    lipidosis)
Glutaric aciduria type 1

H

Hallervorden–Spatz syndrome
Hallucinations
Hashimoto's encephalopathy
Headache
Hematoma
    Chronic dural
    Epidural
    Intracerebral
    Subdural
Hemiballismus
Hemorrhage
    Intracranial
    Subarachnoid
HIV encephalopathy
Huntington's chorea/disease
Hydrocephalus
    Acute
    Normal pressure
Hypercapnia
Hyperhidrosis
Hyper/hypotension
Hyponimia
Hypo/hypertension
Hypothyroidism
Hypotonia
Hypotonicity
Hypoventilation syndrome (or respiratory
    depression)
Hypoxic/ischemic injury

I

Illness anxiety disorder
Infantile epileptic spasm syndrome (or
    West's syndrome)
Influenza
Insomnia disorder (hyper-; hypo-)
    Fatal familial
Intracranial aneurysm
Intracranial idiopathic hyper/hypotension
Intracranial pressure
Insulin resistance

J

Jactitation

K

Klein-Levin disease
Korsakoff's psychosis
Krabbe's disease (or globoid cell
   leukodystrophy; or galactosylceramide
   lipidosis)

L

Leigh's disease/syndrome
Lennox-Gastaut syndrome
Lesch–Nyhan syndrome
Leukoencephalitis periaxialis concentrica
   (or Balo concentric sclerosis)
Leukodystrophy, metachromatic
Louis–Barre syndrome (or ataxia
   telangectasia)
Lyme neuroborreliosis
Lyme disease/syndrome

M

Malaria
Maple syrup urine disease
Marburg's multiple sclerosis (or acute
   fulminant multiple sclerosis)
Marchiafava–Bignami disease
Megalocephaly
Meige's syndrome
Meningitis
   Cryptococcal
Meningoencephalitis
Metachromatic leukodystrophy
Midbrain stroke syndrome (or Weber's
   syndrome; or superior alternating
   hemiplegia)
Migraine
Millard–Gubler disease
Mitochondrial DNA depletion syndrome (or
   Alpers' disease)
Motor neuropathy (distal hereditary)
Morvan's syndrome (or fibrillary chorea)

Movement disorders
Multiple cerebrospinal sclerosis
Multiple sclerosis
   Acute fulminant
   Disseminated
   Insular
   Local
   Marburg's
Multiple system atrophy
Muscular atrophy
Myelinolysis, central pontine
Myelitis (encephalo-, meningo-, polio-,
   transverse-)
Myelopathy (vascular)
Myocardial infarction
Myoclonus

N

Narcolepsy
Nausea
Necrosis
Neill-Dingwall syndrome (or Cockayne's
   syndrome)
Niemann-Pick disease type C
Neuroacanthocytosis
Neurocognitive disorders
Neurodegenerative diseases
Neuroleptic malignant syndrome
Neuronal ceroid lipofuscinosis
Neuromyelitis optica (or Devic's disease)
Neuromyelitis optica spectrum disorder
Neuronal ceroid lupofuscinosis
Neuropathy, distal hereditary motor
Neurosyphilis
Niemann-Pick disease
Non-gluten celiac sensitivity
Normal pressure hydrocephalus
Nystagmus

O

Organic acidemias
Osmotic demyelination syndrome
Osteoarthritis

P

Palsy:

    Bell's palsy

    Bulbar palsy.

    Cerebral palsy

    Conjugate gaze palsy

    Erb's palsy (or brachial palsy)

    Fazio-Lande infantile palsy

    Progressive bulbar

    Progressive supranuclear palsy

    Pseudobulbar palsy

    Spinal muscular atrophy (or wasting palsy).

    Squatter's palsy

    Third nerve palsy

Pantothenate kinase-associated neurodegeneration

Paraparesis

    Hereditary spastic

    Subacute sclerosing

Panencephalitis

Pantothenate kinase-associated neurodegeneration

Paralysis

Paraplegia

    Hereditary spastic

    Familial spastic

Parkinsonism

Parkinson's disease

Pelizaeus-Merzbacher disease/syndrome

Peptic ulcer disease

Phenylketonuria

Pick's disease (or frontotemporal dementia)

Post-hypercapnic apnea

Post-traumatic stress disorder

Prion and prion-like diseases

Progressive multifocal leukoencephalopathy

Progressive supranuclear palsy

Pruritus

Psychosis

R

Rabies

Eespiratory acidosis

Respiratory depression syndrome (or hypoventilation)

Restless legs syndrome

Reye's encephalopathy/syndrome

S

San Filippo syndrome, type B

Sarcoidosis

Schilder's disease

Seizures (epileptic)

Sclerosis (primary lateral)

Serotonin toxicity

Severe myoclonic epilepsy of infancy (or Dravet's syndrome)

Sick sinus syndrome

Sjogren's syndrome

Sleep apnea disorders

    Congenital central

    Hypoventilation syndrome

Sleep paralysis

Sleep-wake disorders (advanced phase)

Spasmodic torticollis

Spinal cord diseases (compression)

Spinal muscular atrophy (congenital distal)

Status dystonicus

Stiff-person/man syndrome

Striatonigral degeneration

Stroke

    Extradural hemorrhage

    Intracerebral

    Ischemic

    Lacunar

Subarachnoid

Subdural (or extradural hemorrhage)

    Transient ischemic attack

Strumpell disease

Strumpell-Lorrain disease

Subacute ascending necrotizing myelitis (or Foix- Alajouanine syndrome)

Subacute sclerosing panencephalitis

Superior alternating hemiplegia (or midbrain stroke syndrome; or Weber's syndrome)
Synucleinopathies
Syphilis
Syringobulbia
Syringomyelia
Systemic lupus errhythematosus

T

Tachycardia
Tauopathy
Tay-Sachs disease
Tourette's syndrome
Tourettism
Transient ischemic attack (or mini-stroke)
Trauma
Traumatic brain injury
Tremor
    Essential
    Intentional
Trinucleotide repeat disorders
Tripanosomasis
Tropical spastic paraparesis
    Acute
    Disseminated
Tumefactive multiple sclerosis
Tumors
    Lymphoma
    Glioma

U

Urea cycle disorders

V

Vascular disease
Vision problems
    Chemosis
    Exophthalmos
    Loss
Visual disturbances
Vitamin B12 deficiency
Vomiting

W

Weaknes
Weber's syndrome (or midbrain stroke syndrome; or superior alternating hemiplegia)
Wernicke's encephalopathy
West's syndrome (or formerly: infantile epileptic spasm syndrome)
Whipple disease
Willis–Ekbom disease
Wilson's disease

X

Xeroderma pigmentosum
X-linked adenoleukodystrophy

Subject Index

Author Index

Arrighi HM *R.18*
Arruda W *R.38*
Arsava EM **R.**2
Arsava EY **R.**2
Artioli GG *R.38*
Arumugam TV **R.**13
Arvanitakis WZ **R.**15
Asada T **R.**14
Asch DA *R.20*
Asgharian M *R.27*
Ashkan K **R.**7
Assendelft WJ *R.39*
Atlan G **R.**4
Audet JN **R.**11
Auer DP *R.36*
Augustine GJ **1.**8; **R.**7
Auwera van der S *R.19*
Avicenna **1.**5
Avgerinos KI *R.36*
Ayalon L *R.22*
Azevedo F **R.**2
Azoulay L **R.**1

B

Baddeley AD *R.30*
Bacekman L **R.**12
Bachner YG *R.22*
Bacon **14.**2
Bacyinski A **R.**2
Bains J *R.22*
Bak LK **R.**6
Baker LD **R.**11
Balfe M *R.20*
Ballard C *R.24*
Ballard KD *R.38*
Balo **6.**23; **G.**3
Balsom PD *R.36*
Banerjee S *R.24*
Bangen KJ *R.31*
Banich MT **R.**11
Barcelos RP *R.36*
Barclay TR *R.22, 23*
Barker P *R.9*

Barnat M *R.27*
Barnes C **R.**11
Barnes LL *R.10, 11, 35*
Barnes MR *R.27*
Baron IS *R.12*
Barranco E *R.39*
Barre **6.**37; **G.**3
Barres BA **R.**3
Barrett LF **R.**10
Barry PJ *R.39*
Bartzokis **10.**3
Barzilai N **R.**14
Basger BJ *R.39*
Basi GS *R.20*
Başkaya, MK **6.**34
Basran J *R.39*
Bastiaanssen TFS **R.**11
Battersby M *R.40*
Bauer, Scott **14.**28
Bauer T *R.20*
Baus, Bruce **3.**3
Beach TG *R.20*
Beal MF *R.17*
Bear MF **R.**2
Beach TG *R.20*
Béard E *R.36*
Beattie E *R.24*
Bédirian V *R.25*
Bedlack RS *R.37*
Beer C *R.40*
Beers MH *R.39*
Beggs S *R.40*
Behcet **8.**14; **14.**13, 26
Beinlich FRM **R.**6, 14
Bejan A *R.30*
Bekhtereva, Natalia **18.**2
Bell **6.**39; **14.**29, 32; **G.**14
Bell JS *R.39*
Bell SJ *R.26*
Belle van G *R.20*
Benabid, Alim Louis **18.**3
Bender A *R.36*
Bender AR *R.30*

Choi OW **R.**12

Chow VS **R.**31

Christensen DJ **R.**9

Chugani HT **R.**5

Chui HC **R.**27

Chung CG **R.**17

Churchland PS **R.**9

Cicero **14.**2

Cieslik EC **R.**35

Citri A **R.**4

Claesson MJ **R.**11

Clark BD **R.**3

Clark CM **R.**20, 24

Clark DD **R.**3

Clark MS **R.**34

Clark V **R.**25

Cleveland DW **R.**18

Clifford FR **R.**3

Clifford R **R.**25

Clifford RM **R.**25, 39

Clionsky E **R.**22

Clionsky M

Cobb M **R.**3

Cockayne **6.**23, 24; **9.**6; **G.**5

Côco LZ **R.**18

Coen RF **R.**23

Cohen DA **R.**25

Cohen-Mansfield J **R.**22

Coles LS **R.**12

Coles NS **R.**12

Collin I **R.**25

Collins R **R.**37

Colombo, Matteo Realdo (or Realdus Columbus) **1.**5, 7, 8

Colvin RA **R.**8

Compton RJ **R.**11

Condello S **R.**17

Connors MA **R.**2

Coon AL **R.**5

Cooper C **R.**22

Cooper R **R.**36

Cordingley DM **R.**37

Corey-Bloom J **R.**21, 31

Cornish SM **R.**37

Corrada M **R.**21

Cosgrove KP **R.**3

Costafreda SG **R.**24

Cotter PD **R.**11

Counts SE **R.**32

Cowan CSM **R.**11

Cowan WM **R.**3

Cowin SC **R.**3

Craen de AJ **R.**39

Craig D **R.**25

Craik F **R.**12

Craik FI **R.**30

Crawford J **R.**14

Crawford JR **R.**31

Creavin ST **R.**22

Creutzfeld **I.**12;**6.**5, 11-13, 18, 40; **8.**14, 20, 22; **9.**2, 4; **14.**6-8, 26; **23.**7; **24.**1-3, 5; **F.**1; **G.**15; **R.**21

Crichton-Browne, Sir James **1.**10

Crispie F **R.**11

Critchley HD **R.**4

Cross J **R.**26

Crossley M **R.**31

Crossman AR **R.**29

Crosson B **R.**12

Croteau DL **R.**18

Cryan JF **R.**11

Cullen B **R.**23

Cumming RG **R.**24

Cummings JL **R.**19, 25

Currò M **R.**17

Cushing, Harvey **1.**12, 14

D

Daffner KR **R.**20

Dagerman KS **R.**26

Dale W **R.**39

Damasio A **R.**3, 9

Dammer EB **R.**9

Dan Y **R.**4

Dandy, Walter Edward **1.**14

Daneman R **R.**3

Frank LL **R.**11

Freberg L **R.**9

Frégnac Y **R.**41

Frerichs, Friedrich Theodor von **G.**19

Fried TR *R.40*

Friedreich **6.**37-8; **G.**8

Friesen WV **R.**16

Frigeri T **R.**4

Frisoni GB R.20, 32

Frosch MP R.20

Fugelsang J R.31

Fuhrmann D R.33

Fulton, John Farquhar **1.**13

Fymat, Alain L **I.**1, 3; **7.**3; **8.**5, 18, 19;
    9.2, 7-10; **14.**4, 7, 10, 11, 14, 22-5, 30;
    17.3, 5; **20.**2; **R.**4, 12, 16, 17, 19, 23,
    27-9, 40, 41

G

Gabrieli J **R.**12

Gabrieli JD *R.30*

Gaillard F **R.**4

Gale SA R.20

Galen, of Pergamon (or Aelius Galenus, or
    Claudius) **1.**4, 5, 7; **14.**2

Gallagher P *R.39*

Galván A *R.33*

Galluzzi S R.20

Gamboa **6.**41

Garcia A **R.**12

Garcia MA **R.**12

Gardener SL *R.35*

Gastaut **6.**7, 26, 27, 40; **9.**3; **24.**1, 3; **G.**10

Gauba E **R.**13

Gaucher **6.**5, 13; **8.**2; **14.**3; **G.**8

Geddes J R.9

Gelder MG R.9

Gerasimov ES **R.**9

Geschwind MD R.17; R.26

Gianaros PJ **R.**4

Giannos P *R.37, 38*

Gibb R **R.**13

Gilbert DT **R.**10

Gill SS R.26

Ginsberg SD R.32

Giorgini P R.35

Giosia di P R.35

Giron MST R.39

Gitlin LN R.22

Gladman JR R.27

Gleason OC R.24

Glees P **R.**4

Glind van de EMM R.24

Glisky EL R.30

Goard M **R.**4

Goldberg EM **R.**3

Goldstein S **R.**4

Goila AK **R.**4

Golgi, Camillo **1.**11, 13; **2.**1, 4; **3.**12; **4.**2

Goll Y **R.**4

Golubeva AV **R.**11

Gomolka RS **R.**6, 14

Gonzalez-Gallego J R.36

Goodman C R.22

Gordon AL R.27

Goren D R.31

Gosche KM R.19

Gowers, Sir William **1.**10, 11

Grabe HJ R.19

Graff BJ R.19

Graham AS R.37

Gray, Henry **6.**3

Gray Marcus A **R.**4

Gray P **R.**9

Greeff R **R.**1

Green AL R.37

Green PS **R.**11

Greenberg SM R.25

Greenhaff PL R.37

Greenwood N R.40

Greiner LH R.21

Grierson AJ R.17

Grimley EJ R.25

Grodstein F **R.**10

Gross CG **R.**4

Gross CR *R.39*

Gross M **R.**16

Grossman LI **R.**5

*Growdon JH **R.**25*

Grut M **R.**12

Gruyter de W **R.**9

*Gualano B **R.**35, 37, 38*

Gual-Grau SS **R.**11

Gubler **6.**7

*Gulmann NC **R.**25*

Gusnard DA **R.**7

Gussekloo J **R.**39

Guttenplan S **R.**9

Guyton **R.**4

Guzzetta KE **R.**11

H

*Habes M **R.**19*

Häggmark A **R.**8

Haggstrom, Mikael **6.**22

Hahn O **R.**12

*Haimei L **R.**34*

*Hajjar ER **R.**39*

Hajjar IM **R.**9

Halitzki E **R.**11

*Hall CB **R.**24*

Hall J **R.**4

*Hall PH, **R.**18*

*Hatton RC **R.**37*

Hauglund NL **R.**6, 14

Haus, Bruce **3.**3

Hayley DC **R.**39

He JQ **R.**13

Heberden C **R.**12

*Hebding J **R.**26*

*Heckner MK **R.**35*

Hedden T **R.**12, 30

*Hegenscheid K **R.**19*

*Heine L **R.**33*

*Heinik J **R.**22*

Helenius H **R.**13

Hellier J **R.**4

Hallervorden **6.**15; **G.**14

*Hallock H **R.**23*

Hallström BM **R.**8

*Hampton T **R.**22*

Han SB **R.**10

*Hanefeld F **R.**37*

Haney MS **R.**12

Hanlon JT **R.**39

*Hanna-El-Daher L **R.**37*

Hanna-Pladdy B **R.**30

*Hansen LA **R.**21*

*Hanson L **R.**22*

Harasaka C **R.**13

Harerimana NV **R.**9

Hariri A **R.**2

Harris D **R.**24

*Harris R **R.**22*

*Harris RC **R.**37*

Harris SE **R.**12

*Harrison SL **R.**19*

*Harskamp van F **R.**25*

Hart WD **R.**9

Harter DH **R.**3

Harvey, William **1.**8, 9

Hashimoto **6.**8, 35; **8.**14; **14.**9, 13; **G.**7

Hashtroudi S **R.**31

Helmholtz von, Hermann Ludwig Ferdinand **1.**10, 11; **R.**6

Hemmy L **R.**16

*Hemmy LS **R.**22, 23*

Henkenius AL **R.**14

*Henry H **R.**36*

Henry JD **R.**31

Henseler, I **6.**18

*Herms J **R.**20*

Herophilus, of Chalcedon **1.**4

*Herr K **R.**24*

*Herrmann N **R.**26*

*Hersch SM **R.**37*

Hess, Walter Rudolph **1.**13

Jeppesen DK *R.17*

Jasinska AJ **R.**12

Jessel TM **R.**5, 7

Jiang CS **R.**12

Jick H R.24

Jie D R.34

Jimenez A R.36

Jin JS **R.**13, 14

Jiří V **R.**6

Johansen-Berg H **R.**7

Johnson E R.18

Johnson M R.20

Johnson MK R.31

Jones EG **R.**5

Jones R **R.**5

Jorm AF R.24

Joshi AU **R.**13

Julian T **R.**14

Jun-Wen G R.22

Jutkowitz E R.23

K

Kaasinen V **R.**13

Kab S R.29

Kacher R R.27

Kadakkuzha BM **R.**13

Kahana M R.31

Kahana MJ R.33

Kahl KG **R.**12

Kaiser LG **R.**13

Kalat J **R.**9

Kalman E R.38

Kane RL R.22

Kales HC R.22

Kalman DS R.37

Kampf C **R.**8

Kandel ER **R.**3, 5, 7

Kane RL **R.**10, *22, 23*

Kang JH **R.**9, 10

Kanwisher N **R.**4

Kao SY **R.**13, *31*

Kapogiannis D R.36

Karbowski K **R.**5

Karlawish JH R.20, 24

Karp JF R.24

Kassem R R.27

Katz LC **R.**7, 14

Katz MJ R.24

Kaufman DM R.28

Kaur A **R.**12

Kaviani M R.36

Kavirajan H R.24

Kawas C R.21

Kearney C **R.**10

Kebede AA **R.**3

Kechagias KS R.38

Keep R **R.**5

Keller A **R.**12

Keller JN **R.**13

Kemper SJ R.21

Kennard, Margaret Alice **1.**13

Kensinger EA **R.**13

Kent K R.35

Keohane K R.20

Kern F **R.**12

Kim MO R.17

Kim N **R.**9

Kimberley **R.**6

King S R.25

Kious BM R.37

*Kiss A R.4*0

Kivipelto M R.25

Klein **6.**7

Klocinski JL R.20

Kłopocka M **R.**2

Klopstock T R.36

Knight R R.29

Knoblich JA **R.**5

Knoll LJ R.33

Knudson AG R.32

Kober H **R.**10

Kochan NA **R.**13

Koffler MFGS **R.**12

Kohane I **R.**13, *31*

Kolb B **R.**10, 13

Koletsa T **R.**7

Koller D **R.**24

Kondo DG **R.**37

Konjevod M **R.**21

Konstantinos K **R.**38

Koob GF **R.**9

Korsakoff **6.**35; **8.**9, 15

Korte **6.**43

Koundal S **R.**11

Kozaki S **R.**14

Krabbe **6.**6, 25; **8.**14; **14.**14, 26; **G.**10

Kraepelin. Emil **7.**2

Krebs B **R.**20

Kreider RB **R.**35, 37

Kretzer RM **R.**5

Kretzschmar HA **R.**20

Kreyer AC **R.**41

Krivanek TJ **R.**20Kruggel F **R.**33

Kryscio RJ **R.**26

Kuffler, Stephen William **1.**14

Kuhlmann B **R.**31

Kukreti R **R.**18

Kukull WA **R.**20

Kunik ME **R.**24, 26

Kusk P **R.**6, 14

Kuzawa CW **R.**5

Kwak YD **R.**18

Kwok JB **R.**18, 25

L

Labbadia J **R.**27

Lagarto L **R.**22

Lai R **R.**26

LaMantia AS **R.**7

Lamb ME **R.**2

Lambert KG **R.**5

Lampit A **R.**23

Lancaster MA **R.**5

Lande **G.**14; **6.**37, 39

Lanfermann H **R.**12

Lang **R.**40

Langa KM **R.**24

Lange N **R.**5

Langner R **R.**12

Lapane KL **R.**26

Laroche ML **R.**39

Larsen WJ **R.**5

Larson EB **R.**20, 22, **4**0

Laterra J **R.**5

Latif-Hernandez A **R.**13

Launer LJ **R.**21

Laurent G **R.**41

Laver K **R.**24

Lawlor BA **R.**23

Lawn S **R.4**0

Laws SM **R.**18

Lazarus AA **R.**30

Leahy B **R.**14

LeCouteur D **R.4**0

LeCouteur DG **R.**39

Lee AY **R.**24

Lee CT **R.**5

Lee H **R.**11, 17

Lee IM **R.**10

Lee J **R.**35

Lee SB **R.**17

Leemputte van M **R.**38

Leeuwenhoek van, Antonie Philips **1.**8, 9

Lefebvre L **R.**11

Legate N **R.**16

Lehallier B **R.**12

Leigh **6.**6, 20

Leite C da C **R.**38

Lemiere J **R.**38

Lennox **6.**7, 26, 27, 30, 40; **9.**3; **24.**1, 3; **G.**10

Lenoir S **R.**27

Leonard WR **R.**5

LePort AK **R.**33

Lesch **6.**9

Leurgans SE **R.**10, 35

Levey AI **R.**9

Levin **6.**7

Levine DA **R.**24

Levine SK **R.**26

Levitt T **R.**31

Lewis ED **R.**3

Mandavilli BS **R.**13

Manning JR **R.***33*

Mao LL **R.**8

Mao W **R.***32*

Marburg **6.**23; **G.**10

Marchiafava **6.**7, 25; **F.**2

Marcusson J **R.**13

Mardinoglu A **R.**8

Marengoni A **R.***25*

Marin-Valencia I **R.**6

*Marizzoni M **R.***20*

Marjamaiki P **R.**14

Markesbery WR **R.**14, 16, 19, 21

Markram H **R.**3

Marriott J **R.***39*

Marshall LH **R.**6

Martin CA **R.**5

Martins RN **R.***35*

Marvin **6.**24

Maselli MA **R.**3

*Masliah E **R.***20, 32*

Massa, Niccolò **1.**5

*Massieu L **R.***27*

*Mather KA **R.***18, 31*

*Mather M **R.***31*

*Mattfeld AT **R.***33*

Mattson MP **R.**13*, 17*

Maudsley AA **R.**12

*Mauriz JL **R.***36*

Maylor EA **R.***31*

*Maynard S **R.***18*

*Mayou R **R.***9*

Mazure CM **R.**3

McAvay GJ **R.***40*

*McCarten JR **R.***22, 23*

*McCleery J **R.***25*

*McCormick WC **R.***20*

*McCreedy E **R.***22*

*McCullough LD **R.***35*

McDaniel M **R.**6

*McFeeley BM **R.***20*

*McGaugh JL **R.***33*

McGregor K **R.**12

*McGuinness B **R.***25*

McInerney F **R.***21*

Mckenzie-Rioch D **R.**9

*McLachlan A **R.***25, 39*

*McLachlan AJ **R.***39*

*McLean AJ **R.***39*

McLellan AT **R.**9

McNamara JO **R.**7

McNulty H **R.***35*

McReynolds MR **R.**13

*McShane R **R.***26*

McTiernan A **R.**11

Meguro K **R.**13

*Mehlen P **R.***16*

*Mehta DC **R.***20*

Meige **6.**5, 10; **G.**10

*Mejía-Toiber J **R.***27*

Melis RJ **R.***25*

*Mellick GD **R.***18*

Mendel E **R.**1

Mendell LM **R.**5

Mendes de Leon CF **R.**11

Méndez P **R.**4

*Menke TJ **R.***24*

*Mercer S **R.***27*

*Merl T **R.***36*

*Merle L **R.***39*

Merzbacher **8.**14; **14.**14, 26

*Merz J **R.***20*

Metere, Riccardo **1.**2

*Metter EJ **R.***21*

*Meyers CM **R.***37*

*Meyrelles SS **R.***18*

Mike **R.**7

Millard **6.**7

*Miller CC **R.***17*

*Milstein MJ **R.***28*

*Min LC **R.***39*

Minhas PS **R.**13

*Mimica N **R.***21*

*Mirra SS **R.***20*

Mitchell KJ **R.***31*

*Mitra J **R.***18*

Mitsios N **R.**8

Mittelstrass J **R.**9

*Mitteregger G **R.**20*

Miyakoshi LM **R.**6, 14

*M'Lan CE **R.**27*

Mobbs CV **R.**13, 14

Mochly-Rosen D **R.**13

*Moisan F **R.**29*

*Moles RJ **R.**39*

*Molho E **R.**29*

Molina D **R.**6

*Molinari VA **R.**24*

Møllgård K **R.**6, 14

Moloney GM **R.**11

Monfils, Lucien **6.**33

Moniz de, Abreu Freire Egas António
    Caetano **1.**13

Mooijaart SP *R.39*

Moon PK **R.**13

<u>Moore BA</u> *R.20*

*Moore DH **R.**37*

*Moore K **R.**35*

Moore SP **R.**6

*Montine TJ **R.**20*

Morgan J **R.**12

*Morgan JC **R.**18*

Mori Y **R.**6, 14

Moriarty GL **R.**10

Morillas E **R.**11

*Morimoto RI **R.**27*

Morningstar AR **R.**12

Morris CG **R.**8

*Morris J, **R.**19*

Morris MC **R.**11

Morris ME **R.**10

Morrison JH **R.**12

*Morrone I **R.**31*

*Mortimer JA **R.**19, 21*

*Morton JT **R.**29*

Morvan **6.**35-6; **G.**12

Mou Y **R.**14

Mrsulja BB **R.**6

*Mucke L **R.**32*

Mufson EJ *R.32*

*Mukadam N **R.**22*

Müller, Johannes Peter **1.**10, 11

Müller MS **R.**6

Munoz B **R.**11

*Munster van BC **R.**24*

*Mukaetova-Ladinska EB **R.**22*

Muzik O **R.**5

Myneni S **R.**12

N

*N*abais MF *R.18*

*Naclerio F **R.**36*

Naglieri J **R.**4

Någren K **R.**13

*Nahin R **R.**37*

Nairne JS **R.**32

*Nana AL **R.**32*

Nansen, Fridtjof **2.**4

*Nasreddine ZS **R.**25*

Nauta WJH **R.**9

Naveh-Benjamin M *R.30, 32*

Nedergaard M **R.**5, 6, 9, 14

*Nedic EG **R.**21*

Neill **G.**5; **6.**23

*Nelson PT **R.**20*

*Nelson VA **R.**22, 23*

Nestler EJ **R.**5

Neto MC **R.**11

Netter F **R.**6

*Netzel M **R.**35*

*Nicastri CM **R.**20*

Nicholson C **R.**6, 9

*Nikolac PM **R.**21*

*Nicolazzo JA **R.**20*

Niemann **8.**2, 14; **14.**3, 14, 26

Nieuwenhuys R **R.**6

Nihan **6.**9

Nilsson P **R.**8, 32

Nó, Rafael Lorente de **2.**4

*Nobili F **R.**32*

*Noel-Storr AH **R.**22*

*Norris DR **R.**34*

Riley KP **R.**14, 16

*Rines J **R.**26*

Rinne JO **R.**13, 14

Rioch, David McKenzie **1.**14

Rissman RA ***R.**32*

Ritchel M ***R.**32*

*Ritchie CW **R.**26*

*Ritchie K **R.**22*

Ritz NL **R.**11

*Riu S **R.**39*

Rizzuto D ***R.**25*

Roberge C **R.**12

Roberts H ***R.**40*

Robles MJ ***R.**39*

Robinson A ***R.**21*

*Robinson L **R.**22*

*Robinson S **R.**27*

Robinson TE **R.**13

*Rockwood K **R.**22, 27*

Rocque, BG **6.**34

Rodrigue KM **R.**14

*Rolinski M **R.**26*

*Rosas HD **R.**37*

*Roschel H **R.**37, 38*

*Rose E **R.**40*

*Rosenbloom MH **R.**26*

*Rossom RC **R.**24*

*Roy BD **R.**37*

Rozycka A **R.**7

Rubin A **R.**13

*Rubinsztein DC **R.**18*

Rudow G **R.**16

Rudy B **R.**3

*Ruitenberg A ***R.**21*

Ruscio J **R.**10

*Ryan C **R.**25, 39*

Ryan WS **R.**16

S

Sabartes O ***R.**39*

Sabati M **R.**12

Sabbatini RME **R.**7

Sachdev PS **R.**13, 14, *18*

Sachs **8.**2; **14.**3

Sachs GA ***R.**39*

Sacks FM **R.**11

Sadler T **R.**7

*Sadock BJ **R.**26*

*Sadock VA **R.**26*

*Saemann P **R.**36*

*Sahebkar A **R.**35*

*Şahin CE **R.**26*

*Sagud M **R.**21*

Sailasuta N **R.**1

*Sakuta Y **R.**30*

*Salles-Painelli de V **R.**38*

*Salmon JC ***R.**40*

Salob SP ***R.**20*

Salthouse T **R.**12

Sampaio-Baptista C **R.**7

*Sampson EL **R.**22, 26*

*Samus Q **R.**22*

Sancheti H **R.**15

*Sánchez AM **R.**27*

Sander D **R.**10

Sanders A **R.**14

Sanggaard S **R.**11

*Saso L **R.**18*

*Sauer A **R.**20*

Saver J **R.**7

Saxby N ***R.**40*

Scarmeas N **R.**14

Schacter DL **R.**10

Scheff SW **R.**13

*Scheibye-Knudsen M **R.**18*

*Scheltens P **R.**24, 32*

*Schenk D **R.**20*

*Schifitto G **R.**37*

*Schneider JA **R.**20, 35*

*Schneider LS **R.**24*

Schilder **6.**6, 21, 23; **G.**6

*Schmiedl S **R.**39*

Schmitt FA **R.**13

Schmitt, Francis O **1.**14

Schmitz B **R.**12

Schneider JA **R.**9, 10, 15

Sowell ER **10**.3, 4, 14

Spatz **6**.15; **G**.14

Spector, AE *R.27*

Spyrou N R.36

Squire LR **R**.8, *30*

Staley JK **R**.3

Stamerra CA *R.35*

Standring S **R**.8

Stark CEL *R.33*

Starr JM **R**.15

Stefanello ST R.36

Steffens DC R.25

Stehlik P R.39

Stein PS R.26

Steinberg M R.25

Stephenson J R.18

Steptoe A **R**.4

Stern Y **R**.14

Stevens B **R**.3

Stevnsner T R.17

Stewart WF R.21

Stijnen T R.21.

Stojanovic J **R**.9

Stokes **6**.35

Stolk RP R.25

Stoppani J R.38

Stout JR R.38

Streim J R.38

Strumpell **6**.39; **G**.8

Stys PK R.28

Suarez JI **R**.8

Such Y **R**.14

Sudo Y **R**.15

Suematsu M **R**.13

Sugiura Y **R**.13

Suhara T **R**.14, 15

Sullivan G R.24

Sun BL **R**.8

Sun JY **R**.8

Suprenant A *R.32*

Svob S R.21

Swaab D R.32

Swaminathan N **R**.8

Swammerdam, Jan (or Johannes) **1**.8, 9

Swanson LW **R**.8

Sweet JJ **R**.14

Swentosky A **R**.4

Swinnen S R.38

Sydenham, Thomas **G**.4

Sydor A **R**.5

T

Taghizadeh-Larsson A R.26

Tanada S **R**.15

Takano A **R**.15

Takano T **R**.9

Tamargo RJ **R**.5

Tang Y **R**.15

Tangney CC **R**.11

Tao L **R**.14

Tate WP R.21

Tay **8**.2; **14**.3

Taylor SF **R**.10

Teerenstra S R.25

Teng EL R.27

Teri L R.20, 22

Tessman PA **R**.8

Thal DR R.20

Thal LJ R.21

Thambisetty M **R**.9

Theil S **R**.41

Theoharides TC **R**.7

Thies B R.20

Thiyagarajan M **R**.9

Thompson LM R.18

Thompson PM **R**.14

Thornton DJ **R**.8

Thorslund M R.39

Thürmann PA R.39

Tillmann B *R.33*

Tinetti ME R.40

Tingö L R.35

Tiraboschi P R.21

Tolias AS 24.**40, 41**

Toga AW **R**.14

Toledo JB R.19

Wang C **R.**14

Wang E **R.**15

*Wang H **R.**18*

*Wang HX **R.**39*

*Wang J **R.**38*

*Wang KL **R.**24*

*Wang L **R.**20*

Wang LH **R.**8

Wang LX **R.**41

Wang Q **R.**13

*Wang R **R.**18*

Wang W **R.**2

Wang Y **R.**11, 15, *35*

Wangen L *R.34*

Wanlin Z **R.**13, 14

Ward M *R.35*

Warden A **R.**9

Wardlaw J **R.**11

Wardlaw JM *R.39*

*Watson NF **R.**40*

Weber **6.**7, 29, 30; **F.**2; **G.**18

Wegner DM **R.**10

Wei W **R.**13, 14

Weinberger D **R.**2

Weinborn M *R.35*

*Weiner DK **R.**24*

Weiner MW **R.**13

Weinstein N **R.**16

Weintraub P **R.**41

Weissman IL **R.**13

*Weitzel T **R.**27*

*Wekstein DR **R.**21*

Welcome SE **R.**14

*Welsh TJ **R.**27*

*Wenk GL **R.**21*

Wenzel D **R.**5

*Wennagel D **R.**27*

Wernicke, Carl (or Karl) **1.**11; **5.**2, 5, 9; **6.**8, 35, 40; **8.**9, 15; **9.**3; **24.**1

West RL *R.33*

West, William James **6.**7, 27; **G.**18

Weyandt LL **R.**4

Wezel, Andries van (or Vesalius, Andreas) **1.**5-7

Whalley LJ **R.**15

Whipple **8.**11, 14; **14.**9, 13

Whishaw IQ **R.**10, 13

White B **R.**9

*Whitehead V **R.**25*

*Whitelaw C **R.**40*

Wierenga CE **R.**12, *31*

*Wiese B **R.**24*

Wijdicks EFM **R.**9

Wildman DE **R.**5

*Wildman R **R.**37*

Wildt S **R.**16

*Wilken B **R.**37*

Willey, Glover Denis **16.**4

Williams SM **R.**7

Wilinson CW **R.**11

Willis, Thomas **I.**5; **1.**9; **3.**13; **4.**3, 6; **6.**15; **G.**16; **R.**6

*Willoughby DS **R.**35*

Wilson **8.**2; **14.**3; **G.**18

Wilson HR *R.31*

Wilson RS **R.**11, 15, *30*

Winblad B **R.**13, *39*

Winder NR **R.**15

Wingo AP **R.**9

Wingo TS **R.**9

*Wisniewski S **R.**22*

*Wissemann WT **R.**29*

*Wittfeld K **R.**19*

*Wolfson C **R.**27*

*Wolfson DB **R.**27*

Wong DF **R.**15

Woo JS **R.**12

*Woods B **R.**27*

Wouw van de M **R.**11

Wu WW **R.**5

Wyke M **R.**12

Wyss-Coray T **R.**13, 15

X

Xiao H **R.**14

Printed in the USA
CPSIA information can be obtained
at www.ICGtesting.com
LVHW060339030224
770541LV00026B/291

9 781779 415271